Intensive Care
A Concise Textbook

C. J. Hinds MB BS, MRCP, FFARCS
Consultant and Senior Lecturer
in Anaesthesia and Intensive Care
St Bartholomew's Hospital, London

Bruce
92

Baillière Tindall   London Philadelphia Toronto
Sydney Tokyo

Baillière Tindall 24–28 Oval Road
W.B. Saunders London NW1 7DX

West Washington Square
Philadelphia, PA 19105, USA

1 Goldthorne Avenue
Toronto, Ontario M8Z 5T9, Canada

ABP Australia Ltd, 44–50 Waterloo Road
North Ryde, NSW 2113, Australia

Harcourt Brace Jovanovich Japan Inc.
Ichibancho Central Building, 22–1 Ichibancho
Chiyoda-ku, Tokyo 102, Japan

© 1987 Baillière Tindall

First published 1987
Second printing 1988
Third printing 1992

Typeset by Scribe Design, Gillingham, Kent
Printed and bound in Great Britain at the University Press, Cambridge

British Library Cataloguing in Publication Data

Hinds, Charles J.
  Intensive care: a concise textbook.
  1. Critical care medicine
  I. Title
  616'.028   RC86.7

ISBN 0-7020-1150-9

Contents

Foreword

The practice of intensive care has expanded very rapidly during the past 20 years. New methods of investigation and treatment have led to a clearer understanding of acutely disordered physiology and to better methods of supporting vital functions, even when specific treatment for the disease initiating these abnormalities has either not changed or remains empirical.

The diversity of antecedent disorders, the number of systems deranged in the acutely sick, and the multiplicity of therapeutic regimens can easily fragment management. Skill in the practice of intensive care comes from assembling all the organ-specific information and recommendations into a logical and comprehensive policy, tailored to individual requirements and giving the right order of priority to different needs which, at times, are conflicting.

Dr Hinds has used this skill to produce a textbook covering the main issues of intensive care and, by writing as sole author, has achieved uniformity of style and standard while avoiding the overlap, repetition and potential for conflicting advice which beset the editor of multi-author works. He writes in impeccably clear and simple prose so that even difficult concepts are easy to understand. The term 'concise textbook' has been interpreted to include sufficient theory to satisfy those seeking a rational basis for management, and enough practical advice for decisions to be reached and safe policies to be implemented. The result is an excellent introductory text for both junior medical staff and intensive care nurses.

M.A. Branthwaite
MD FRCP FFARCS
Consultant Physician and Anaesthetist
Brompton Hospital, London SW3

Preface

Over the past two decades there has been considerable progress in the management of patients with acute life-threatening illnesses and this has contributed to the emergence of intensive care medicine as a discipline in its own right. It is now widely acknowledged that there is a need for appropriate specialist training in this subject and many recommend that those pursuing careers in anaesthesia, medicine or surgery, but who do not intend to specialize in intensive care, should also be familiar with the principles of managing critically ill patients. Accordingly, aspects of intensive care medicine are already included in the FFARCS examination, and it is now suggested that physicians in training should also gain experience in this field.

This book was conceived primarily as an introduction to intensive care medicine for doctors in training, although it is hoped that some of the contents will also be of interest to nurses specializing in intensive care. It is intended to be sufficiently comprehensive to provide a sound working knowledge of the discipline and yet concise enough to be read in its entirety. The contents are aimed particularly at those with little previous experience of intensive care who are embarking on clinical posts involving the management of critically ill patients, and those undertaking postgraduate examinations such as the FFARCS. With this in mind, I have attempted to summarize the important theoretical aspects of intensive care practice and discuss some of the current controversies, as well as making practical recommendations for treatment.

In preparing this book I have been most fortunate in receiving the invaluable assistance of many friends and colleagues at St Bartholomew's Hospital. In particular, I would like to thank Dr AD Blainey (Department of Chest Medicine), Dr DS Dymond (Department of Cardiology), Dr MJG Farthing (Department of Gastroenterology), Dr RN Greenwood (Department of Nephrology), Dr AP Hopkins (Department of Neurological Sciences), Dr Pamela F Prior (Department of Neurological Sciences) and Dr EJ Shaw (Department of Medical Microbiology) for their advice on specialist aspects of the text and illustrations. I am also deeply indebted to the Department of Medical Illustration at St Bartholomew's Hospital and Miss Teresa Lanigan for their expertise in preparing the figures and photographs. Finally, I am extremely grateful to my secretary, Mrs Annie Wright, for typing the manuscript.

Charles J. Hinds

To my wife and our respective parents,
whose unfailing support made this possible.

1
Introduction

Intensive care is a new branch of medicine which has progressed and expanded rapidly since its inception about 25 years ago. Intensive care medicine (or 'critical care medicine') is concerned predominantly with the management of patients with acute life-threatening conditions ('the critically ill') within the specialized environment of an intensive care unit, but also encompasses the resuscitation and transport of those who become acutely ill, or are injured, both elsewhere in the hospital and in the community.

The creation of intensive care units, and the subsequent development of intensive care medicine, owes much to the introduction of intermittent positive pressure ventilation (IPPV) for the treatment of patients with respiratory failure. The therapeutic potential of this technique was first recognized during the 1950s when it was used to support patients with respiratory failure due to neuromuscular disorders, such as poliomyelitis, or acute exacerbations of chronic obstructive airway disease (COAD), as well as occasionally those with postoperative respiratory insufficiency. The more widespread adoption of therapeutic IPPV (as opposed to its established role in anaesthesia) during the early 1960s prompted many institutions to create 'respiratory care units' to facilitate the management of patients requiring mechanical ventilation. At the same time, it was appreciated that patients who had undergone cardiac surgery (which was then associated with an appreciable mortality) could benefit from intensive postoperative care and that the complications of myocardial infarction could be detected and treated more effectively within designated 'coronary care' units. It also became apparent that other critically ill patients could be better managed within purpose-built units, fully equipped with monitoring and technical facilities, in which they could receive intensive nursing care and the constant attention of appropriately trained medical staff.

Subsequently, the scope of intensive care medicine has inevitably expanded to include the management of patients with a wide variety of underlying medical and surgical disorders. Moreover, patients with acute cardiorespiratory disturbances frequently develop failure of other organs or systems and, once the initial objective of sustaining life has been achieved, the primary disease must be diagnosed and appropriately treated. Thus, although intensive care medicine remains a discipline primarily concerned with the management of acute, major disturbances of cardiovascular and respiratory function, a co-ordinated, multidisciplinary approach is essential for optimal patient care.

RESULTS, COSTS AND PATIENT SELECTION

For many critically ill patients, intensive care is undoubtedly life-saving and resumption of a normal lifestyle is to be expected. In certain cases, e.g.

1

patients requiring mechanical ventilation for Guillain–Barré syndrome and those recovering from cardiac surgery, mortality rates should be very low and the majority will make a complete recovery. Furthermore, it is likely, though difficult to prove, that the elective admission of selected high-risk cases into the intensive care unit, particularly in the immediate postoperative period, can minimize morbidity and mortality, as well as reducing the demands on medical and nursing personnel on the general wards. Provided these patients are carefully selected, this may represent a particularly cost-effective use of intensive care facilities.

In the most seriously ill patients, however, immediate mortality rates are high; a significant number succumb soon after discharge from the intensive care unit and the quality of life for some of those who do survive may be poor. Thus, Cullen (1977) found that only 46% of a group of unstable patients who required intensive medical and nursing interventions were alive at one month and within 12 months the overall mortality had risen to 73%. Of those still alive at one year, 18% were still hospitalized and only 12% of the entire group were functioning as they had prior to their acute illness. Moreover, intensive care is expensive, particularly for those with the worst prognosis. Bellamy and Oye (1984) have reported that the total charges for patients with adult respiratory distress syndrome admitted to a medical intensive care unit ranged from US$9263 to as much as US$187 893 with a median cost of US$52 894; median daily charges were US$2430. In this, and other studies (Cullen, 1977; Turnbull et al, 1979), the non-survivors cost considerably more than the survivors, probably mainly because of the large quantities of blood and blood products usually required by the most seriously ill patients (Cullen, 1977). At present, as much as 20% of all costs in some hospitals in the USA are attributable to intensive care (Thibault et al, 1980) and it is likely that as new therapeutic techniques and agents become available these costs will continue to escalate. Unfortunately, similar data relating to intensive care practice in the UK are not currently available.

Inappropriate use of intensive care facilities has other implications (Jennett, 1984). The patient may experience unnecessary suffering and loss of dignity, while relatives may also have to endure considerable emotional pressures. In some cases, treatment may simply prolong the process of dying, or sustain life of dubious quality, and in others the risks of interventions may outweigh the potential benefits. Finally, skilled medical and nursing staff may be diverted from caring for patients elsewhere in the hospital and the ability of staff on general wards to manage seriously ill patients is diminished. As a consequence, in some hospitals in the USA even the presence of an intravenous infusion warrants admission to an intensive care unit (Downs, 1984). Jennett (1984) has summarized the circumstances in which intensive care may be harmful as: unnecessary, because routine care would have achieved the same result; unsuccessful, because the patient is too ill to recover; unsafe, because the risks of complications exceed the benefits; unkind, because the subsequent quality of life is unacceptable; or unwise, because of diversion of limited resources. Of these the last two are the most contentious.

Rational selection of those patients most likely to benefit from intensive care is therefore clearly desirable, both for a humane approach to the management of the critically ill and to ensure optimal use of relatively scarce resources. This involves not only identifying patients who will inevitably die, but also those who will make a good recovery even without intensive care. (In one medical intensive care unit in the USA approximately three-quarters of the patients were admitted solely for non-invasive monitoring; of these, only 10% subsequently required major interventions (Thibault et al, 1980).) However, except in the case of patients with disseminated, incurable malignancy or terminal chronic respiratory failure, the long-term prognosis is usually uncertain and it is therefore not possible to refuse admission when there is a prospect of recovery from the acute illness, however remote this may be. Although some have found a correlation between age and long-term survival (Cullen, 1977), the quality of life for the elderly who do survive is equivalent to that of younger patients (Cullen, 1977). Moreover, in a recent study, age did not influence either the cost or the outcome of patients admitted to a medical intensive care unit (Fedullo and Swinburne, 1983).

It is therefore rarely possible, or acceptable, to discriminate between critically ill patients before admission, and the decision as to whether to continue aggressive treatment in a patient who fails to respond to intensive care then assumes greater importance. For example, it has been shown that the ultimate outlook for patients who continue to require a high level of therapeutic intervention day after day is uniformly dismal (Cullen, 1977). Although such decisions can be extraordinarily difficult, the need for a humanitarian approach is now widely accepted and the legality of limiting therapy when the quality of life is threatened, or such treatment is considered futile, is being increasingly discussed. Nevertheless, clinicians in general remain understandably reluctant to adopt specific guidelines. Currently, decisions to limit therapy, or not to resuscitate in the event of cardiorespiratory arrest, are made jointly by the medical staff of the unit, the primary physician and the nurses, normally in consultation with the patient's family. It is usually not possible to involve the patient, although some may have communicated to a relative that in certain circumstances they would not wish to have their life prolonged, and in North America it is now possible to enact a 'living will' or 'right to die' document. Such key decisions must be taken by senior staff who are continuously involved in patient care and are regularly present on the unit.

Scoring systems

Various scoring systems have been described which can be used to assess the severity of an acute illness. These have included an assessment of the severity of the acute disturbance of physiological function (acute physiology and chronic health evaluation, APACHE) (Knaus et al, 1985), and a measure of the therapeutic effect expended on a patient (therapeutic intervention scoring system, TISS) (Keene and Cullen, 1983). These 'predictive indices' cannot predict with certainty the outcome in an individual patient; indeed they were not designed to do so, and physicians are therefore reluctant to accept the estimated probabilities of death as the basis for limiting or discontinuing treatment. Nevertheless, provided the scoring system used is appropriate to the type of patient being studied, they can accurately quantify the severity of illness, and predict the overall mortality, for a group of patients. They therefore allow meaningful comparisons between the results in different centres and may enable the efficacy of new forms of treatment to be assessed without recourse to controlled trials.

PLANNING AND DESIGN OF INTENSIVE CARE UNITS (Intensive Care Society—*Standards for Intensive Care Units*)

The type and size of unit suitable for a particular hospital depends on several factors, including the number of acute beds and the type of cases being treated. The Department of Health and Social Security recommends that approximately 1–2% of the acute beds of a general hospital should be allocated to intensive care, and suggests that this should be increased when there are special units within the hospital for cardiac and major vascular surgery, and neurosurgery (Department of Health and Social Security, 1970). The size of unit provided should also be governed by the fact that the minimum number of beds that is viable is four, while more than ten beds become difficult to manage (Ledingham, 1977).

Thus, as the number of cases for which intensive care is considered appropriate increases, it may be necessary to establish separate units, specializing in the management of particular problems. It is now common to have independent coronary care units, and, particularly in North America,

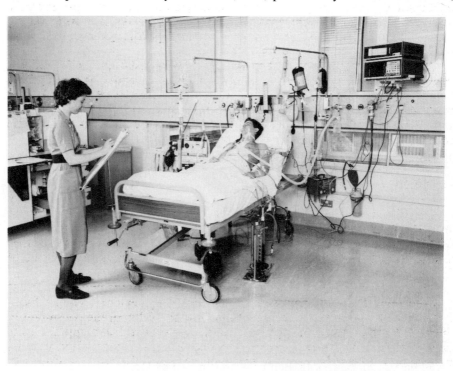

Fig. 1.1 Access to intensive care patients must be unrestricted. This is achieved by allowing adequate floor space for each bed area and by mounting equipment behind the bed.

larger institutions frequently possess separate neurosurgical, cardiac, general surgical, respiratory, and medical intensive care units. If this is the case, units should be in close proximity in order to make optimum use of pooled medical, nursing and technical staff, as well as equipment.

Intensive care units must be spacious in order to allow easy access to the patient despite the surrounding plethora of equipment; $20\,m^2$ per bed is recommended (Fig. 1.1) (Intensive Care Society—Standards for Intensive Care Units).

Each bed will be equipped with monitors, suction apparatus, humidifiers, ventilators, piped oxygen, air and a vacuum supply. A plentiful supply of mains sockets is essential, as are power points for mobile x-ray equipment. Facilities for haemodialysis may be provided at selected bed areas.

In order not to restrict access to the patient, this apparatus is often mounted on a rail system behind the bed. Less frequently, services are ceiling-mounted or delivered via a free standing bollard (Kerr et al, 1985).

There should preferably be a large, open-plan area containing several beds with some adjacent single- or double-bedded cubicles, the exact proportion being determined by the types of patient being treated. Single cubicles may be used to minimize the risks of cross-infection by isolating patients with impaired immune responses or those harbouring dangerous micro-organisms, and for mentally alert patients. Open plan areas make the most efficient use of nursing staff. As well as plenty of storage space, it is important to have adequate office accommodation, a staff rest room, a waiting area and overnight accommodation for relatives and an interview room. Other facilities may include a library and tutorial room as well as an on-site 'stat' laboratory.

Because the large amount of equipment in an intensive care unit produces considerable heat, air conditioning is required in order to maintain a reasonable working environment, although its value in preventing cross-infection is less well established. Finally, it is important for the psychological well-being of both patients and staff that all bed areas are well illuminated with natural daylight (Wilson, 1972) (see p. 103).

STAFFING (Ledingham, 1977)

It is essential that a suitably qualified doctor is immediately available throughout the day and night to deal with emergencies occurring on the unit. Often, this doctor will be an anaesthetist, but this is not essential provided that he is capable of emergency intubation and has a thorough knowledge of the techniques of ventilatory support and their complications.

The question as to who should be in overall charge of the unit is at present a vexed one. There is, however, a measure of agreement amongst those closely involved in intensive care that the 'base specialty' of the consultant in charge is largely irrelevant, provided that he is motivated and appropriately trained. It is to be hoped that over the next few years, recognized training programmes in intensive care will be established, available to any doctor with a postgraduate qualification, and that this will put an end to the destructive arguments between anaesthetists, physicians and surgeons as to who should control intensive care units.

The proportion of the consultant's time allocated to intensive care will depend largely on the size and type of hospital in which he works. In a large teaching hospital, most, or even all, of his sessions may be devoted to intensive care in order that teaching and research commitments can be fulfilled, while in some district general hospitals it may be appropriate to appoint a consultant 'with an interest in intensive care' who will also have an appreciable number of sessions in his base specialty. The on-call commitment will necessarily be shared between a number of suitably trained consultants. In many hospitals the intensive care unit is run by a group of several consultant anaesthetists, while in others the team consists of both anaesthetists and physicians.

An adequate complement of suitably trained nurses is crucial to the success of an intensive care unit. Ideally, on any one shift there should be one nurse for each patient and a sister in charge. Allowing for holidays, off-duty and sickness, this requires a total complement of five to six nurses, including one sister, per bed as well as a nursing officer who assumes overall responsibility. In practice, because of economic constraints and a shortage of suitably qualified personnel, this ideal is rarely achieved. Further problems are posed by the inevitable fluctuations both in patient numbers and in the degree of nursing care which each requires. Although the optimum bed occupancy is said to be approximately 80% (Ledingham, 1977), in many units this figure is closer to 60%. Furthermore, some units deal almost exclusively with seriously ill, ventilated patients, while others will admit a larger proportion of relatively stable cases mainly for observation. Thus, units which are adequately staffed when full of highly dependent patients will have an excess of nurses at other times. All too often these nurses are then seconded to other areas of the hospital, with disastrous effects on morale. The alternative is a relatively understaffed unit, unable to cope during periods of peak demand. In an attempt to solve this problem, and to achieve a balance between these two extremes, more exact methods of assessing the overall nursing requirements of a particular unit are being developed (Intensive Care Society—Standards for Intensive Care Units). A receptionist who can answer the telephone, attend to relatives and perform clerical duties is a valuable addition to the team and can relieve the nurses' work load.

Physiotherapists who are experienced in dealing with critically ill, ventilated patients perform a vital role in successful intensive care (see subsequent chapters) and must be integrated into the 'team'.

Adequate technical support for repair and maintenance of equipment is also essential. It is particularly important that on-site laboratory equipment, such as automated blood gas analysers, are subjected to a strict quality control programme performed by experienced laboratory staff (see Chapter 3).

Expert imaging (chest x-ray, ultrasound, computerized axial tomographic (CAT) scanning, etc) is an important aspect of intensive care and requires the services of expert radiographers, as well as close liaison with radiologists.

The psychological pressures on those who work in intensive care units are considerable, and this applies particularly to the nursing staff (Baxter, 1974; Tomlin, 1977). In North America, the syndrome of intensive care 'burn out' has been described, and in some instances distressing events on the unit can even precipitate suicide attempts (Tomlin, 1977).

Because of the sustained, intimate contact between intensive care nurses and their patients a close relationship is inevitably established, particularly with those whose stay in the unit is prolonged. This exposes the nurse to considerable emotional pressures, which are often exacerbated by frequent contact with the patient's anxious relatives. The work of an intensive care nurse is both physically and mentally demanding, involving the ability to utilize complex equipment, as well as diagnose acute life-threatening events and administer appropriate emergency treatment. Morever, many are reluctant to seek advice, fearing that this might be interpreted as incompetence. Clinicians are also subjected to stress and it has been suggested that their frustration at being unable to help an individual patient may precipitate excessive criticism of colleagues, over-zealous treatment or even avoidance of the unit altogether.

Maintenance of staff morale is therefore crucial. Important aspects to be considered include the provision of adequate numbers of appropriately qualified personnel, close co-operation and discussion of management decisions with medical staff, consistent unit policies and comprehensive teaching in all aspects of intensive care. It is generally considered inappropriate for nurses to be allocated to care for the same patient on successive days. It is now recognized that working in an environment devoid of natural light increases stress amongst all members of staff (Wilson, 1972).

REFERENCES

Baxter S (1974) Psychological problems of intensive care. *British Journal of Hospital Medicine* **11**: 875–885.

Bellamy PE & Oye RK (1984) Adult respiratory distress syndrome: hospital charges and outcome according to underlying disease. *Critical Care Medicine* **12**: 622–625.

Cullen DJ (1977) Results and costs of intensive care. *Anesthesiology* **47**: 203–216.

Department of Health and Social Security (1970) *Intensive Therapy Unit.* Hospital Building Note (HBN) 27.

Downs JB (1984) Crisis and challenge. *Critical Care Medicine* **12**: 843–845.

Fedullo AJ & Swinburne AJ (1983) Relationship of patient age to cost and survival in a medical ICU. *Critical Care Medicine* **11**: 155–159.

Intensive Care Society—*Standards for Intensive Care Units.* London: Biomedica.

Jennett B (1984) Inappropriate use of intensive care. *British Medical Journal* **289**: 1709–1711.

Keene AR & Cullen DJ (1983) Therapeutic intervention scoring system: update 1983. *Critical Care Medicine* **11**: 1–3.

Kerr JH, Coates DP & Gale LB (1985) Use of 'bollards' to improve patient access during intensive care. *Intensive Care Medicine* **11**: 33–38.

Knaus WA, Draper EA, Wagner DP & Zimmerman JE (1985) APACHE II: a severity of disease classification system. *Critical Care Medicine* **13**: 818–829.

Ledingham IMcA (1977) Care of the critically ill. In Ledingham IMcA (ed.) *Recent Advances in Intensive Therapy*, pp 1–7. Edinburgh: Churchill Livingstone.

Thibault GE, Mulley AG, Barnett GO et al (1980) Medical Intensive Care: indications, interventions and outcomes. *New England Journal of Medicine* **302**: 938–942.

Tomlin PJ (1977) Psychological problems in intensive care. *British Medical Journal* **ii**: 441–443.

Turnbull AD, Graziano C, Baron R et al (1979) The inverse relationship between cost and survival in the critically ill cancer patient. *Critical Care Medicine* 7: 20–23.
Wilson LM (1972) Intensive care delirium. The effect of outside deprivation in a windowless unit. *Archives of Internal Medicine* 130: 225–226.

2
Applied Cardiovascular and Respiratory Physiology

In all critically ill patients the immediate objective is to preserve life and prevent, reverse or minimize damage to vital organs such as the brain and kidneys. This is achieved by optimizing cardiovascular and respiratory function in order to maximize delivery of oxygen to the tissues. Subsequently, it is hoped that the underlying abnormality will resolve either spontaneously, e.g. postoperatively and in some viral illnesses such as Guillain–Barré syndrome, or as a result of specific treatment aimed at the underlying disease, such as the administration of antibiotics to a patient with pneumonia. Occasionally, when the aetiology of the acute illness is unknown, this 'breathing space' may allow a diagnosis to be made so that specific therapy can be started.

OXYGEN DELIVERY

This is defined as the total amount of oxygen delivered to the tissues per unit time.

It is dependent on the volume of blood flowing through the microcirculation per unit time (i.e. the cardiac output, $\dot{Q}_t$) and the amount of oxygen contained in that blood (i.e. the arterial oxygen content, C_aO_2) (Table 2.1). Oxygen is transported in combination with haemoglobin and dissolved in plasma, the amount combined with haemoglobin being determined by its oxygen capacity (usually taken as being $1.34\,\text{ml}\,O_2$ per g Hb) and its percentage saturation with oxygen (SO_2), while the volume in solution depends on the partial pressure of oxygen (PO_2) (see Table 2.1). For most practical purposes, except when hyperbaric oxygen is administered, the amount of dissolved oxygen is sufficiently small to be ignored.

Table 2.1 The concept of oxygen flux.

Oxygen flux = cardiac output × arterial oxygen content

Oxygen flux = cardiac output × $[(\text{Hb} \times SO_2 \times 1.34) + (P_aO_2 \times 0.003)]$

For representative values in a normal adult, and ignoring the small amount of dissolved oxygen:

$$1000\,\text{ml}\,\text{min}^{-1} \simeq 5000\,\text{ml} \times \frac{15}{100}\,\text{g}\,\text{ml}^{-1} \times \frac{99}{100} \times 1.34$$

Since oxygen consumption is normally approximately $250\,\text{ml}\,\text{min}^{-1}$ there is an excess of supply over demand which provides a margin of safety if oxygen consumption increases or oxygen delivery falls.

9

In the normal, healthy adult approximately 1000 ml of oxygen is delivered to the tissues each minute (see Table 2.1) and, since the normal oxygen consumption ($\dot{V}_{O_2}$) is 250 ml min^{-1}, only one-quarter of the available oxygen is utilized, leaving 750 ml min^{-1} to spare. Normal arterial blood, in which the haemoglobin is fully saturated, contains 20 vol % of oxygen, and since one-quarter, or 5 vol %, is extracted by the tissues, this leaves 15 vol % in mixed venous blood which is, therefore, 75% saturated with oxygen. Thus, the normal arteriovenous oxygen content difference is 5 ml per 100 ml of blood.

There are, however, several important limitations to the application of the concept of oxygen flux in clinical practice and these will be enumerated as they arise. The first is that some organs, notably the heart, have a very high oxygen requirement relative to their blood flow and may, therefore, receive insufficient supplies of oxygen even when overall oxygen flux is apparently adequate.

CARDIAC OUTPUT

Those factors which determine the volume of blood delivered to the tissues, that is the cardiac output, will be considered first. It is often useful to consider the cardiac output per square metre of body surface area: the cardiac index. In this way, comparisons can be made between patients, and the normal limits can be more closely defined, the normal range for cardiac index being 3–4 l min^{-1} m^{-2}. Maintenance of an adequate cardiac output is obviously crucial to the survival of the critically ill and requires consideration of both the heart rate and the determinants of the stroke volume (Fig. 2.1).

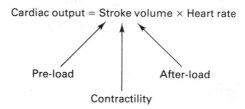

Fig. 2.1 The determinants of cardiac output.

Heart rate and rhythm

The heart rate is largely dependent on the balance of sympathetic and parasympathetic nervous activity and, in health, is directly related to the metabolic rate. At rest, vagal tone predominates and maintains the heart rate at about 70 beats per minute. If both the sympathetic and parasympathetic supply to the heart are interrupted, a rate of approximately 100 beats per minute results.

Extreme bradycardias and tachycardias can cause cardiac output to fall. As heart rate increases, the duration of systole remains essentially unchanged, whereas diastole, and thus the time available for ventricular filling, becomes progressively shorter; stroke volume therefore eventually falls. In the normal heart this occurs at rates greater than about 160 beats per minute, but in those with cardiac pathology, especially when this restricts ventricular filling (e.g. mitral stenosis), stroke volume may fall at much lower heart rates. Furthermore, tachycardias cause marked increases in myocardial oxygen consumption (MVo_2) and this may precipitate ischaemia in areas of myocardium with restricted coronary perfusion. It is therefore most important to control tachydysrhythmias; but it must be recognized that the majority have some underlying cause, such as hypokalaemia, which must be diagnosed and treated before instituting specific therapy. When heart rate falls, on the other hand, a point is reached at which the increase in stroke volume is insufficient to compensate for the bradycardia and again cardiac output falls.

Alterations in heart rate are often caused by disturbances of rhythm (e.g. atrial fibrillation, complete heart block or nodal rhythm) in which atrial transport is lost, thereby further reducing ventricular filling and stroke volume. In this situation, catastrophic reductions in cardiac output may occur and urgent treatment is then required (see also Chapter 9).

Stroke volume

Three factors determine the stroke volume; they are pre-load, myocardial contractility and after-load.

Pre-load

This is defined as the tension of the myocardial fibres at end-diastole, just prior to the onset of ventricular contraction, and is therefore related to their degree of stretch (Fig. 2.2). The main factor influencing pre-load is the

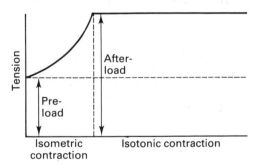

Fig. 2.2 'Pre-load' is the tension of the myocardial fibres prior to the onset of systole and depends on the degree to which they are passively stretched. During isometric contraction the tension in the contractile elements increases; the tension required to open the aortic valve and eject blood from the ventricle is the 'after-load'.

venous return. Starling's law of the heart states that the force of myocardial contraction is directly proportional to the initial fibre length. Therefore, as the filling pressure, and thus the end-diastolic volume, of the ventricle increases, stroke volume rises (Fig. 2.3).

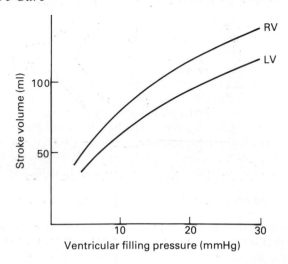

Fig. 2.3 In normal subjects the left ventricular function curve (LV) is displaced downwards because the left ventricle is less compliant and is working against a higher after-load.

If, however, the ventricle is overstretched, excessive dilatation and thinning of the myocardium may cause stroke volume to fall (Fig. 2.4). Furthermore, pulmonary oedema may develop if left atrial pressure rises. This will occur more readily if capillary membrane permeability is increased and/or colloid osmotic pressure is low (usually due to a reduction in serum albumin). The gradients across the pulmonary capillaries, and thus the development of pulmonary oedema, are also influenced by other factors, such as the hydrostatic and oncotic pressures within the interstitial spaces, which

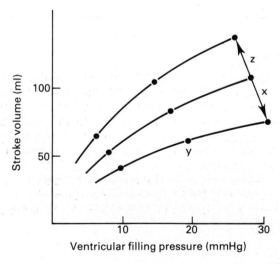

Fig. 2.4 Starling curve; as pre-load is increased stroke volume rises. If the ventricle is overstretched, stroke volume will fall (x). In myocardial failure, the curve is depressed and flattened (y). Increasing contractility shifts the curve upwards and to the left (z).

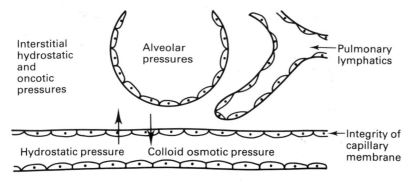

Fig. 2.5 Some factors involved in the genesis of pulmonary oedema.

cannot be quantified. Finally, excess fluid is removed by the pulmonary lymphatics so that frank pulmonary oedema only occurs when this mechanism is overwhelmed or impaired (Fig. 2.5) (Robin et al, 1973).

Achieving the optimal pre-load improves cardiac output by increasing stroke volume without affecting the main determinants of myocardial oxygen requirements, i.e. heart rate and after-load (Table 2.2). Consequently, MV_{O_2} increases only slightly and manipulation of pre-load is therefore the most efficient way of improving cardiac output.

Table 2.2 The determinants of myocardial oxygen consumption.

Heart rate After-load	} major effect
Ventricular wall tension Contractility	
Pre-load Stroke volume	} least effect

Myocardial contractility

The state of myocardial contractility determines the response of the ventricles to changes in pre-load and after-load. Unfortunately, contractility is often reduced in intensive care patients either as a result of pre-existing myocardial damage, e.g. ischaemic heart disease, or due to the acute disease process itself. Changes in myocardial contractility alter the slope and position of the Starling curve in such a way that worsening ventricular performance is manifested as a depressed, flat curve (see Fig. 2.4). Thus, for a given pre-load, stroke volume is less and increasing the filling pressures leads to only limited improvement. Under these circumstances, the body can maintain cardiac output only by increasing the heart rate. As the latter increases there is a marked rise in MV_{O_2}.

After-load

This is defined as the myocardial wall tension developed during systolic ejection (see Fig. 2.2). In the case of the left ventricle it is determined by the resistance imposed by the aortic valve and the peripheral vasculature and is a significant determinant of left ventricular performance. After-load is also influenced by the elasticity of the major blood vessels. Decreasing after-load can increase the stroke volume achieved at a given pre-load (Fig. 2.6), whilst at the same time ventricular wall tension and MVo_2 are reduced. The reduction in wall tension may produce an increase in coronary blood flow, thereby improving the myocardial oxygen supply/demand ratio. An increase in after-load, on the other hand, can cause a fall in stroke volume and is a potent cause of increased MVo_2. Right ventricular after-load is normally negligible since the resistance of the pulmonary circulation is very low. However, in patients with stenosis of the pulmonary valve or pulmonary hypertension, right ventricular after-load may become the dominant influence on overall cardiac performance.

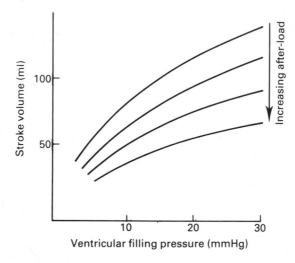

Fig. 2.6 The effect of changes in after-load on the ventricular function curve.

The second limitation of the concept of oxygen delivery is that it only takes into consideration the absolute level of cardiac output and does not provide any information regarding the relative flow to individual organs (e.g. isoprenaline reduces total peripheral resistance but does so mainly by increasing skin and muscle blood flow at the expense of more vital organs such as the kidneys) (see p. 148).

OXYGEN CONTENT

As mentioned previously, it is the oxygen content of the arterial blood (C_ao_2) which is important for the well-being of our patients since it is this, in conjunction with the cardiac output, which determines oxygen delivery. As discussed above, oxygen content is dependent on the amount of haemoglobin present per unit volume of blood, its oxygen capacity and its percentage saturation with oxygen (see Table 2.1). It is for this reason that maintenance of an 'adequate' haemoglobin concentration is essential in critically ill patients. However, tissue oxygenation is also dependent on blood flow. This in turn is determined not only by the cardiac output and its distribution (see above) but also by the viscosity of the blood. The latter depends largely on the packed cell volume (PCV) and it has been shown in dogs with haemorrhage that oxygen transport through the coronary circulation is maximal at a haematocrit of approximately 25%, whereas for the systemic circulation the optimal value is 45% (Jan et al, 1980).

Oxyhaemoglobin dissociation curve (Fig. 2.7)

The saturation of haemoglobin with oxygen is determined by the partial pressure of oxygen (Po_2) in the blood, the relationship between the two being described by the oxyhaemoglobin dissociation curve (Fig. 2.7). The sigmoid

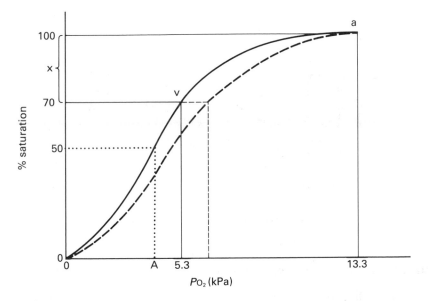

Fig. 2.7 The oxyhaemoglobin dissociation curve. The curve will move to the right (–––) in the presence of an acidosis (metabolic or respiratory), pyrexia or an increased red cell 2,3-DPG concentration. For a given arteriovenous oxygen content difference, the mixed venous Po_2 will then be higher. Furthermore if mixed venous Po_2 is unchanged the arteriovenous oxygen content difference increases and more oxygen is off-loaded to the tissues. a = arterial point; v = venous point; x = arteriovenous oxygen content difference; A = the P_{50} which is normally 3.6 kPa (27 mmHg).

shape of this curve is clinically important for a number of reasons. Firstly, falls in arterial Po_2 (P_aO_2) may be tolerated provided that percentage saturation remains above 90%. Secondly, increasing P_aO_2 to above normal has only a minimal effect on oxygen content unless hyperbaric oxygen is administered (when the amount of oxygen in solution in plasma becomes significant). Lastly, once on the steep 'slippery slope' portion of the curve, a small decrease in P_aO_2 can cause large falls in oxygen content, while increasing P_aO_2 only slightly can lead to useful increases in oxygen saturation.

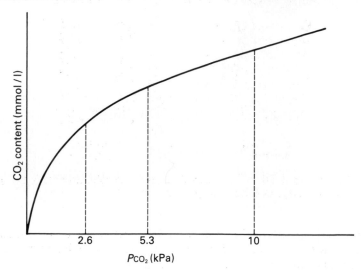

Fig. 2.8 The carbon dioxide dissociation curve. Note that in the physiological range this is essentially linear.

In contrast, the carbon dioxide dissociation curve is virtually linear over the range normally encountered in clinical practice so that alterations in P_{CO_2} cause proportional changes in carbon dioxide content (Fig. 2.8).

The arterial oxygen tension is influenced by the efficiency of pulmonary gas exchange and the mixed venous P_{O_2} ($P\bar{v}_{O_2}$).

PULMONARY VENTILATION AND GAS EXCHANGE

Alveolar ventilation and dead space

The volume of effective alveolar ventilation per unit time ($\dot{V}_A$) is determined by the expired minute volume ($\dot{V}_E$), reduced by the amount 'wasted' in terms of gas exchange (the physiological, or total, dead space, V_D). The latter consists of 'anatomical' dead space (the conducting airways) and alveolar dead space (ventilated alveoli which are either not perfused or relatively underperfused; see below under ventilation/perfusion inequalities), i.e.

$$\dot{V}_A = \dot{V}_E - V_D \qquad 2.1$$

For a single breath, this can be rewritten as:

$$\dot{V}_A = V_T - V_D \qquad 2.2$$
(where V_T is the tidal volume)

In practice, however, V_D varies in proportion to the tidal volume. This is due to the 'cone front effect' (Fig. 2.9). Because gas flow in the large airways is laminar, the leading front is conical, with the gas in the centre moving more rapidly than that towards the periphery; indeed, gas close to the walls of the conducting airways may be stationary. This reduces the effective volume of

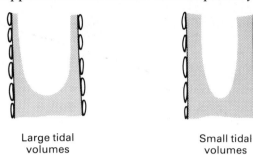

Large tidal
volumes

Small tidal
volumes

Fig. 2.9 The 'cone front effect'; as tidal volume falls the volume of stationary gas
increases, thereby reducing the effective dead space.

the dead space. As tidal volume falls, the amount of stationary gas increases
and dead space is reduced (Briscoe et al, 1954). In clinical practice it is
therefore preferable to refer to the V_D/V_T ratio.

Calculation of V_D/V_T:
Since no gas exchange takes place in the conducting airways and there is
essentially no carbon dioxide in inspired air, all the carbon dioxide in the
mixed expired gas must originate from gas exchanging areas of the lung.
Therefore:

$$\dot{V}_E \times F_E CO_2 = \dot{V}_A \times F_A CO_2 \qquad\qquad 2.3$$

(where $F_E CO_2$ and $F_A CO_2$ are the fractional concentrations of CO_2 in mixed
expired and alveolar gas respectively).
Then, substituting from equation 2.1 for V_A

$$\dot{V}_E \times F_E CO_2 = (\dot{V}_E - V_D) \times F_A CO_2 \qquad\qquad 2.4$$

Substituting partial pressures for fractional concentrations and V_T for $\dot{V}_E$

$$V_T \times P_E CO_2 = (V_T - V_D) \times P_A CO_2 \qquad\qquad 2.5$$

Finally, in an 'ideal' alveolus, $P_A CO_2$ can be assumed to be identical to $P_a CO_2$,
and rearranging the equation:

$$V_D/V_T = \frac{P_a CO_2 - P_E CO_2}{P_a CO_2} \qquad\qquad 2.6$$

This is the Bohr equation. In normal subjects the V_D/V_T ratio is less than 0.3.

Relationship between alveolar ventilation and arterial carbon dioxide
tension:

The amount of CO_2 excreted per unit time ($\dot{V}CO_2$) is clearly determined by the
volume of the expired gas and the concentration of CO_2 in that gas, i.e.

$$\dot{V}CO_2 = \dot{V}_E \times F_E CO_2 \qquad\qquad 2.7$$

Substituting in equation 2.3

$$\dot{V}CO_2 = \dot{V}_A \times F_A CO_2 \qquad\qquad 2.8$$

Substituting partial pressure for fractional concentration and rearranging

$$\dot{V}_A = K \times \frac{\dot{V}_{CO_2}}{P_A CO_2} \qquad \textbf{2.9}$$

(where K is a constant)

As before, $P_a CO_2$ can be substituted for $P_A CO_2$ and therefore rearranging gives

$$P_a CO_2 \propto \frac{\dot{V}_{CO_2}}{\dot{V}_A} \qquad \textbf{2.10}$$

If $\dot{V}_{CO_2}$ remains constant, $P_a CO_2$ is determined solely by the alveolar ventilation (i.e. the tidal volume and the dead space), while for a given level of alveolar ventilation, $P_a CO_2$ is proportional to CO_2 production.

The alveolar air equation:

Derivation:

The amount of oxygen taken up through the lungs per unit time (the oxygen consumption, $\dot{V}_{O_2}$) must be given by the difference between the volume of oxygen breathed in and the volume breathed out. Thus:

$$\dot{V}_{O_2} = (\dot{V}_A \times F_I O_2) - (\dot{V}_A \times F_A O_2) \qquad \textbf{2.11}$$

(where $F_I O_2$ and $F_A O_2$ are the fractional concentrations of oxygen in inspired air and expired alveolar gas respectively).

Rearranging gives

$$F_A O_2 = F_I O_2 - \frac{\dot{V}_{O_2}}{\dot{V}_A} \qquad \textbf{2.12}$$

Substituting for $\dot{V}_A$ from equation **2.8**

$$F_A O_2 = F_I O_2 - (F_A CO_2 \times \frac{\dot{V}_{O_2}}{\dot{V}_{CO_2}}) \qquad \textbf{2.13}$$

$\dfrac{\dot{V}_{O_2}}{\dot{V}_{CO_2}}$ is, of course, the inverse respiratory exchange ratio R and thus

$$F_A O_2 = F_I O_2 - \frac{F_A CO_2}{R} \qquad \textbf{2.14}$$

Fractional concentrations can be converted to partial pressures

$$P_A O_2 = P_I O_2 - \frac{P_A CO_2}{R} \qquad \textbf{2.15}$$

In clinical practice it is usual to measure $F_I O_2$ and multiply this by the barometric pressure to obtain $P_I O_2$. Furthermore, $P_A CO_2$ is considered to be identical to $P_a CO_2$ and R is usually assumed to be 0.8. Thus,

$$P_A O_2 = (F_I O_2 \times PB) - \frac{P_a CO_2}{0.8} \qquad \textbf{2.16}$$

(where PB = barometric pressure)

Composition of alveolar gas (Fig. 2.10):

Room air contains 20.93% oxygen so that the F_1O_2 is 0.21 and, for a normal barometric pressure of 101 kPa (760 mmHg), the P_1O_2 is 21.2 kPa (159 mmHg). There is virtually no CO_2 in inspired air, and the amount of water vapour is relatively small, so that the remainder is largely nitrogen. However, by the time the inspired gases reach the alveoli they are fully saturated with water vapour at body temperature (37°C) (which has a partial pressure of 6.3 kPa (47 mmHg)) and carbon dioxide has been added at a partial pressure of approximately 5.3 kPa (40 mmHg). The P_AO_2 is thereby reduced to approximately 13.4 kPa (100 mmHg).

Thus, the clinician can influence P_AO_2 by altering the F_1O_2, the barometric pressure (i.e. administering hyperbaric oxygen) or the P_aCO_2.

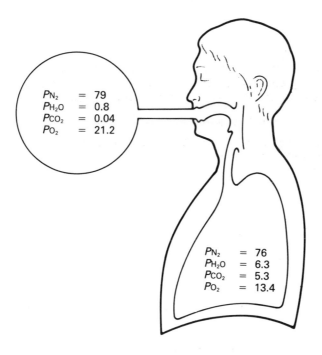

Fig. 2.10 The composition of inspired and alveolar gas (partial pressures in kPa).

Pulmonary gas exchange

If lung function was perfect, alveolar gas would equilibrate completely with arterial blood and P_aO_2 would equal P_AO_2. Even in normal individuals, however, a small pressure gradient exists between the oxygen in the alveoli and that in the arterial blood (the alveolar–arterial oxygen difference, $P_{A-a}O_2$) and this difference increases with age. Any disease of the lung parenchyma will interfere with oxygen transfer and cause an abnormal increase in $P_{A-a}O_2$. Three causes of the $P_{A-a}O_2$ can be identified.

Causes of hypoxaemia

Diffusion defects

A very small (0.133 kPa, 1 mmHg) pressure gradient probably exists between oxygen in the alveoli and that in end-pulmonary capillary blood. However, this is probably not an important cause of hypoxaemia, even in diseases such as fibrosing alveolitis in which the alveolar-capillary membrane is considerably thickened, except possibly during exercise (when pulmonary capillary transit time is markedly reduced) or when P_AO_2 is very low. Because carbon dioxide is so much more soluble than oxygen its excretion is not influenced by diffusion defects (West, 1982).

Right-to-left shunts

Normally, a small amount of venous blood bypasses the lungs via the bronchial and Thebesian veins. Although this amounts to only 2% of the total cardiac output it is one cause of the normal $P_{A-a}O_2$. In some diseases of the lung, such as lobar pneumonia, and in certain cardiac lesions, such as Fallot's tetralogy, a much larger proportion of the cardiac output passes to the left side of the heart without taking part in gas exchange, thereby causing significant arterial hypoxaemia. This hypoxaemia cannot be corrected by administering oxygen to increase P_AO_2, because blood leaving normal alveoli

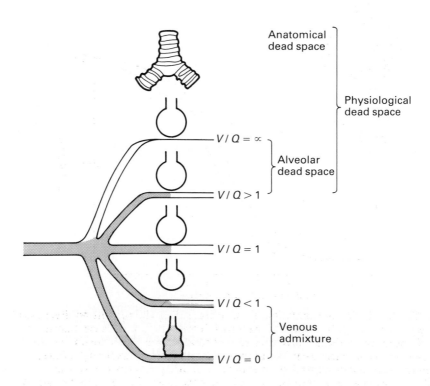

Fig. 2.11 Ventilation/perfusion relationships.

is already fully saturated and further increases in Po_2 will not significantly affect its oxygen content. When this fully saturated blood is mixed with the shunted blood, arterial oxygen content, and therefore P_aO_2, falls proportionately. On the other hand, because of the shape of the carbon dioxide dissociation curve (see Fig. 2.8), the high Pco_2 of the shunted blood can be compensated by overventilating patent alveoli, thus lowering the CO_2 content of the effluent blood. Indeed, many patients with acute right-to-left shunts hyperventilate, causing the P_aco_2 to be lower than normal.

Ventilation/perfusion inequalities (Fig. 2.11) (West, 1977a)

In a perfect lung each alveolus would be perfused with a quantity of blood exactly equal to its volume of ventilation, i.e. the ventilation (V)/perfusion (Q) ratio would be unity ($V/Q = 1$). If alveoli are ventilated but not perfused ($V/Q = \alpha$), or if ventilation is excessive relative to their perfusion ($V/Q > 1$), then a proportion of this ventilation is wasted, and behaves as alveolar 'dead space'. On the other hand, if an alveolus is well-perfused but poorly ventilated ($V/Q < 1$), complete oxygenation of the blood in contact with that alveolus is impossible. Finally, alveoli which are perfused but not ventilated ($V/Q = 0$) behave as true shunts.

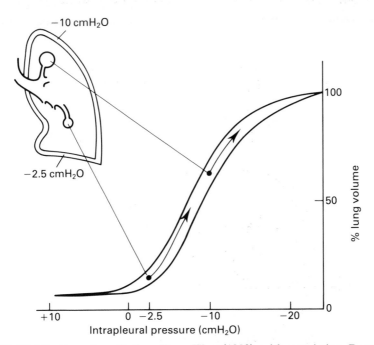

Fig. 2.12 Distribution of ventilation. From West (1983), with permission. Because of the weight of the lungs, intrapleural pressure is less negative at the base than at the apex. Consequently, there is less expansion of basal alveoli, which are on the steep portion of their compliance curve. For the same change in intrapleural pressure, therefore, these alveoli expand more than those at the apex. Hence, alveolar ventilation increases from the apex to the base of the lungs. © 1983, the Williams & Wilkins Co., Baltimore.

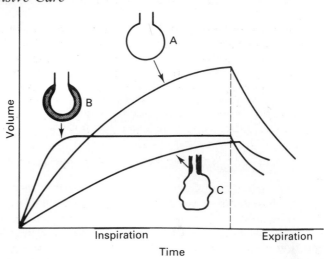

Inspiration   Expiration

Time

Fig. 2.13 Time constants. From West (1983), with permission. 1 time constant = compliance × resistance. For a normal alveolus (A): 0.6 sec = $0.2\,l/cmH_2O$ × $3\,cmH_2O\,l^{-1}\,sec^{-1}$ and by definition an alveolus is 95% filled in 3 time constants, i.e. 1.8 sec. A non-compliant alveolus (B) will have a short time constant, whereas the time constant will be prolonged in those with airway narrowing (C). © 1983, the Williams & Wilkins Co., Baltimore.

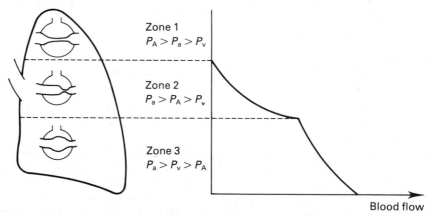

Fig. 2.14 Distribution of blood flow. From West (1983), with permission. Because of a hydrostatic effect the pressure in the pulmonary vessels increases from the apex to the base of the lungs. Consequently, in zone 1, alveolar pressure exceeds both pulmonary arterial and venous pressures; the vessels are therefore collapsed and there is no blood flow (in fact, zone 1 does not exist in normal subjects). In zone 2, pulmonary artery pressure exceeds alveolar pressure, which in turn is greater than pulmonary venous pressure. Flow is therefore determined by the difference between alveolar and arterial pressures; since the former remains constant, flow increases progressively from the top to the bottom of this zone. In zone 3, both arterial and venous pressures exceed alveolar pressure. Flow therefore depends on the differences between these two pressures. Because of distension of the capillaries, blood flow increases slightly down this zone. A further zone, zone 4, may exist at the bases in which blood flow falls again due to compression of extra-alveolar vessels by poorly inflated lung tissue. © 1983, the Williams & Wilkins Co., Baltimore.

Distribution of ventilation (West, 1977b). Even in normal subjects, inspired gas is not evenly distributed throughout the lungs. Studies using inhaled radioactive xenon have demonstrated that ventilation increases from the upper to the lower regions of the lungs. The explanation for this is illustrated in Fig. 2.12. Furthermore, especially in diseased lungs, ventilation may be unevenly distributed due to variations in the time constants of individual respiratory units (Fig. 2.13). Finally, although air is moved through the conducting airways by convection, gas transfer in distal lung segments occurs by molecular diffusion. This diffusion may be incomplete, particularly in abnormal lungs, and may further contribute to an uneven distribution of ventilation.

Distribution of perfusion (West et al, 1964). In the normal lung, blood flow also increases downwards, but does so to a rather greater extent than ventilation (Fig. 2.14). Normally, the overall V/Q ratio is approximately 0.8. This has an effect equivalent to a right-to-left shunt of less than 3% of the cardiac output and causes an $P_{A-a}O_2$ of no more than 0.7 kPa (5 mmHg).

Diseases of the lung parenchyma interfere with the distribution of both ventilation and perfusion, causing an increased 'scatter' of V/Q ratios. This produces an increase in alveolar dead space and hypoxaemia. As discussed above, the former can be compensated by increasing overall ventilation. In contrast to the hypoxia resulting from a true right-to-left shunt, that due to areas of low V/Q can be partially corrected by administering oxygen and thus increasing P_AO_2, even in poorly ventilated areas of lung.

The three-compartment model of pulmonary gas exchange (Riley and Cournand, 1949)

In clinical practice it is often convenient to consider the lungs as if they consisted of three compartments—physiological dead space, perfectly matched V/Q, and venous admixture (Fig. 2.15). The dead space compartment (wasted ventilation), therefore, includes both the anatomical and the alveolar dead space, the latter consisting of 'true' dead space and lung units with V/Q ratios > 1 (see Fig. 2.11). Venous admixture combines all sources of 'wasted blood flow' (i.e. diffusion defects, right-to-left shunts and V/Q ratios < 1 (see Fig. 2.11)) and treats them as if a given proportion of the cardiac output bypassed the lungs altogether. Venous admixture is, then, expressed as a percentage of the cardiac output ($Q_s/Q_t\%$, where Q_s is the flow per unit time through the shunt and Q_t is the total flow, i.e. the cardiac output). Both total dead space and venous admixture can be calculated relatively easily in clinical practice and, by administering 100% oxygen to correct any hypoxaemia due to V/Q inequalities, the relative contribution of true right-to-left shunt and V/Q inequalities to the total venous admixture can be determined. However, this information is of limited clinical relevance and administration of high concentrations of oxygen, even for short periods, may adversely affect lung function. This is because alveolar nitrogen, which is not absorbed, is replaced by oxygen, which is rapidly taken up by pulmonary capillary blood, thereby rendering alveoli unstable and liable to collapse.

$Q_s/Q_t\%$ can be calculated from the shunt equation (Fig. 2.16).

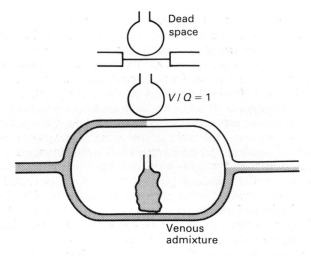

Fig. 2.15 The three-compartment model of pulmonary gas exchange.

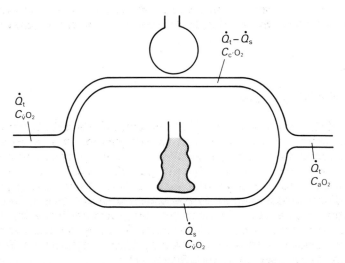

Fig. 2.16 Derivation of the shunt equation. The total amount of oxygen entering the systemic circulation per unit time must be equal to the sum of the amount leaving the ideal alveolus and the amount in the shunted blood. Thus:

$$\dot{Q}_T \times C_aO_2 = [(\dot{Q}_T - \dot{Q}_S) \times C_{c'}O_2] + [\dot{Q}_S \times C_{\bar{v}}O_2]$$

This can be rearranged to give

$$\frac{\dot{Q}_s}{\dot{Q}_t} = \frac{C_{c'}O_2 - C_aO_2}{C_{c'}O_2 - C_{\bar{v}}O_2}$$

$\dot{Q}_t$ = total flow (i.e. the cardiac output)

$\dot{Q}_s$ = flow through the shunt

$(\dot{Q}_t - \dot{Q}_s)$ = flow through ideal alveolus

C_aO_2 = arterial oxygen content

$C_{\bar{v}}O_2$ = mixed venous oxygen content

$C_{c'}O_2$ = end-capillary oxygen content in the ideal alveolus

Oxygen contents can be derived from oxygen saturation and the haemoglobin concentration (see Table 2.1). In the case of arterial and mixed venous blood, oxygen saturation can be derived from the Po_2 using a standard equation. Many automated blood gas analysers will perform this calculation, usually assuming that the oxyhaemoglobin dissociation curve is normally positioned. Some will then proceed to calculate oxygen content, either assuming a normal haemoglobin or using a value entered by the operator. There are significant errors involved in obtaining oxygen contents in this way and it is preferable to use a direct method such as spectrophotometry or a Lex O_2 Con fuel cell analyser (see Chapter 4). If a pulmonary artery catheter is not in place, true mixed venous blood cannot be obtained; however, some authorities suggest that, since in general one is only interested in changes in venous admixture, central venous blood is adequate. Of course it is not possible to obtain end pulmonary capillary blood; it is usual, therefore, to calculate P_AO_2 from the alveolar air equation (see equation **2.16** above) and assume that equilibration in the ideal alveolus is complete so that $P_{c'}O_2 = P_AO_2$. Percentage saturation of haemoglobin with oxygen is then calculated using a standard formula to represent the dissociation curve. Lastly, $C_{c'}O_2$ is derived from the haemoglobin concentration.

The V_D/V_T ratio can be calculated from the Bohr equation (**2.6** above). This requires measurement of P_aCO_2 and collection of expired gas for analysis of F_ECO_2.

MIXED VENOUS $Po_2(P_{\bar{v}}o_2)$

If $P_{\bar{v}}o_2$, and thus mixed venous oxygen content, falls then the effect of a given degree of venous admixture on arterial oxygenation will be exacerbated. When P_aO_2 remains constant, $P_{\bar{v}}o_2$ falls if more oxygen has to be extracted from each unit volume of blood arriving at the tissues. This will occur if cardiac output, and thus oxygen delivery, falls and/or oxygen requirements increase. Thus, worsening arterial hypoxaemia does not necessarily indicate a deterioration in pulmonary function but may instead reflect a fall in cardiac output and/or a rise in oxygen consumption. Similarly, an increase in carbon dioxide production, if not compensated by greater alveolar ventilation, will cause P_aCO_2 to rise (see equation **2.10** above).

The $P_{\bar{v}}o_2$ is also influenced by the position of the oxyhaemoglobin dissociation curve (see Fig. 2.7). Thus, if the arteriovenous oxygen content difference remains constant, a shift of the curve to the right, which occurs with acidosis, hypercarbia, pyrexia and a rise in red cell 2,3-diphospho-glycerate levels, may cause $P_{\bar{v}}o_2$ to rise. Moreover, if $P_{\bar{v}}o_2$ remains unchanged, more oxygen will be unloaded at tissue level. A shift of the curve to the left, on the other hand, will cause a fall in $P_{\bar{v}}o_2$. It might be argued, then, that under certain circumstances an acidosis may be beneficial in terms of tissue oxygenation provided that it is not sufficiently severe to interfere with cardiac function. It is probable, though, that shifts of the dissociation curve are of limited clinical significance. The position of the curve is conventionally described by specifying the partial pressure of oxygen at which haemoglobin is 50% saturated with oxygen (the P_{50}) (see Fig. 2.7).

LUNG VOLUMES (Fig. 2.17)

Normally one breathes in and out from the resting end-expiratory position with a tidal volume of approximately 500 ml. A maximal inspiration, followed by a maximal expiration, is the vital capacity (VC) and comprises the V_T, the inspiratory reserve volume (IRV) and the expiratory reserve volume (ERV).

At the end of a forced expiration intrapleural pressure becomes positive, overcoming the elastic forces which normally keep the distal airways patent, so that the terminal airways collapse. The amount of gas thereby trapped in

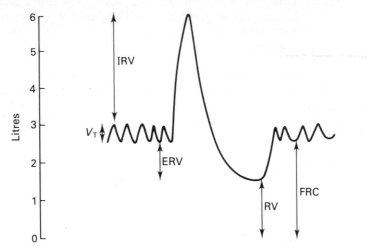

Fig. 2.17 Lung volumes: V_T = tidal volume; IRV = inspiratory reserve volume; ERV = expiratory reserve volume; RV = residual volume; FRC = functional residual capacity.

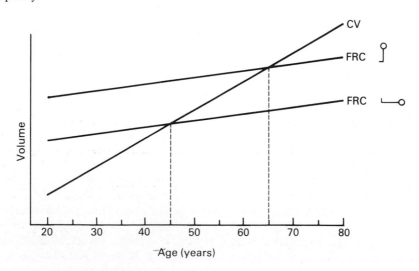

Fig. 2.18 Alterations in closing volume and functional residual capacity with age and changes in posture.

the lungs is called the residual volume (RV). The volume of gas remaining in the lungs at the end of a normal quiet expiration is the functional residual capacity (FRC) and consists of the ERV plus the RV.

The closing volume (CV) is defined as the lung volume at which airway closure first begins. Figure 2.18 shows the rise in CV and the smaller increase in FRC which occurs with age, as well as the influence of positional changes on FRC (Leblanc et al, 1970). It can be seen that under certain circumstances, CV encroaches on FRC, i.e. airway closure occurs during normal tidal breathing. This means that some alveoli will be poorly ventilated or collapsed, causing hypoxaemia.

Compliance and FRC

Compliance is defined as the change in volume produced by a given change in pressure ($\Delta V/\Delta P$). It is possible to determine the compliance of the lungs and the chest wall separately, but in clinical practice it is usual to consider both together. The compliance curve for the lung and chest wall combined is shown in Fig. 2.19.

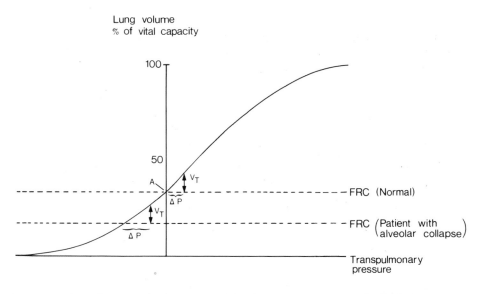

Fig. 2.19 Compliance curve for lung and chest wall combined. Tidal exchange takes place from the resting end-expiratory position (A), at which the tendency for the lungs to collapse is exactly counterbalanced by the tendency for the chest wall to expand. It can be seen that this is also the steepest part of the curve, where small changes in pressure produce large changes in volume (i.e. compliance is greatest). However, as FRC falls the curve becomes flatter, i.e. the lungs become stiffer and compliance falls.

FURTHER READING

Nunn JF (1977) *Applied Respiratory Physiology*. London: Butterworths.
Poole-Wilson PA (1983) Measurement and control of cardiac output. In Tinker J & Rapin M (eds) *Care of the Critically Ill Patient*, pp. 3–18. Berlin: Springer-Verlag.
Rudolph M (1983) Pulmonary ventilation and gas exchange. In Tinker J & Rapin M (eds) *Care of the Critically Ill Patient*, pp. 37–51. Berlin: Springer-Verlag.
Sykes MK, McNicol MW & Campbell EJM (1976) *Respiratory Failure*, chaps 1, 2 & 3. Oxford: Blackwell.
West JB (1983) *Respiratory Physiology—The Essentials*, 2nd edn. Baltimore: Williams & Wilkins.

REFERENCES

Briscoe WA, Forster RE & Comroe JH (1954) Alveolar ventilation at very low tidal volumes. *Journal of Applied Physiology* **7:** 27–30.
Jan K-M, Heldman J & Chien S (1980) Coronary haemodynamics and oxygen utilisation after haematocrit variations in haemorrhage. *American Journal of Physiology* **239:** H326–H332.
Leblanc P, Ruff F & Milic-Emili J (1970) Effects of age and body position on 'airway closure' in man. *Journal of Applied Physiology* **28:** 448–451.
Riley RL & Cournand A (1949) 'Ideal' alveolar air and the analysis of ventilation–perfusion relationships in the lungs. *Journal of Applied Physiology* **1:** 825–847.
Robin ED, Cross CE & Zelis R (1973) Pulmonary edema (first of two parts). *New England Journal of Medicine* **288:** 239–246.
West JB (1977a) Ventilation–perfusion relationships. *American Review of Respiratory Disease* **116:** 919–943.
West JB (1977b) *Ventilation/Blood Flow and Gas Exchange*, 3rd edn, p. 28. Oxford: Blackwell.
West JB (1982) *Pulmonary Pathophysiology—The Essentials*, 2nd edn, pp 25–28. Baltimore: Williams & Wilkins.
West JB, Dollery CT & Naimark A (1964) Distribution of blood flow in isolated lung; relation to vascular and alveolar pressures. *Journal of Applied Physiology* **19:** 713–724.

3
Cardiovascular Monitoring

Appropriate monitoring is essential for rational management of the critically ill patient. Not only does it allow rapid recognition of changes in the patient's condition, but the patient's progress and response to therapy can also be accurately assessed. On the other hand, it must be remembered that invasive monitoring techniques incur a significant risk of complications, many of which may be extremely serious and even life-threatening. It is, therefore, important to use these techniques only when they are essential for successful management of the patient and always to select non-invasive methods where possible.

HEART RATE

As discussed in Chapter 2, this is an important determinant of cardiac output and almost all intensive care patients require continuous electrocardiographic (ECG) monitoring. Not only may changes in heart rate be observed immediately, but dysrhythmias can be detected, diagnosed and treated. Moreover, changes in the ECG pattern may suggest the presence of electrolyte disturbances such as hypo- or hyperkalaemia and hypo- or hypercalcaemia (see Chapter 5) as well as detecting episodes of myocardial ischaemia (ST segment/T wave changes).

BLOOD PRESSURE

Under most circumstances this is a reflection of the adequacy of the cardiac output. However, if the patient is vasoconstricted, with a high peripheral resistance, blood pressure may be normal, or occasionally high, even when cardiac output is low. As well as its value as a guide to cardiac output, the absolute level of blood pressure is important since hypotension may jeopardize perfusion of vital organs, while excessively high pressure can cause bleeding from arterial suture lines or precipitate cerebrovascular accidents.

Traditionally, blood pressure is measured intermittently using a sphygmomanometer cuff and auscultation. Automated instruments are now available, which use a microphone to detect Korotkoff sounds. These automatically record and digitally display blood pressure and heart rate at intervals of between 1 and 15 minutes. Although expensive, they are reliable, accurate and have the advantage of being non-invasive.

When rapid alterations in blood pressure are anticipated, however, continuous monitoring using an intra-arterial cannula is often advisable. An additional advantage of an indwelling arterial cannula is that repeated sampling for blood gas analysis can be performed without repeated puncture

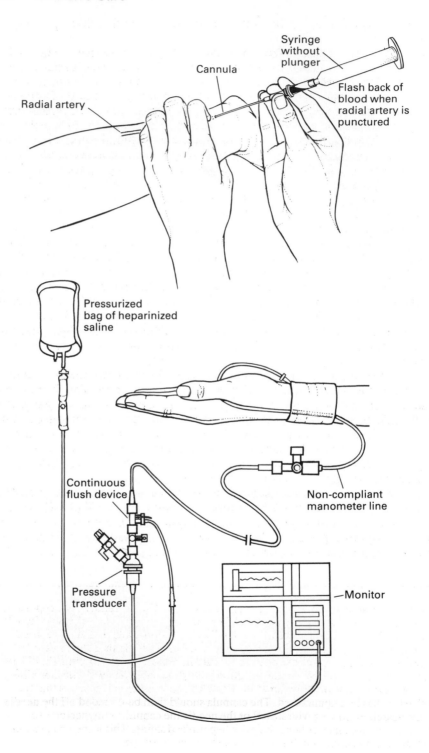

Radial artery

Cannula

Syringe without plunger

Flash back of blood when radial artery is punctured

Pressurized bag of heparinized saline

Continuous flush device

Non-compliant manometer line

Pressure transducer

Monitor

of the artery (which may well be more traumatic than prolonged cannulation).

Usually, the radial artery is punctured percutaneously (Fig. 3.1). Relatively small (20 gauge for adults, 22 gauge for children), parallel-sided cannulae allow blood flow to continue past the cannula, and those made of Teflon FEP are less irritant than, for example, polypropylene or PVC; the use of such cannulae is therefore considered to minimize the risk of thrombosis. Nevertheless, loss of arterial pulsation occurs in a significant proportion of cases and digital ischaemia is the most common complication of arterial cannulation. However, the much feared complication of necrosis of one or more digits is fortunately rare, provided ischaemia is recognized early and the cannula is then removed promptly (Russell et al, 1983). Some feel that cannulation of a larger vessel, such as the femoral artery, carries less risk of occlusive complications since good blood flow continues around the cannula. Femoral artery cannulation has been recommended as a safer alternative to difficult percutaneous radial artery cannulation, or a surgical cut-down, both of which carry an increased risk of complications (Russell et al, 1983). Certainly, cannulation of the femoral artery is relatively easy and this is a useful approach in an emergency, particularly if the patient is hypotensive and other pulses are difficult to palpate. However, some consider that there is an increased risk of infection with the femoral approach (Band and Maki, 1979) although others feel this is insignificant (Thomas et al, 1983) and the overall complication rate is similar for radial and femoral artery cannulation (7.5% and 6.9% respectively) (Russell et al, 1983).

Two other important complications associated with intra-arterial cannulation include accidental injection of drugs and disconnection. The former can cause widespread vascular occlusion with the development of gangrene distally (Zideman and Morgan, 1981), whilst the latter, if unnoticed, can rapidly produce serious hypovolaemia, particularly in children. The risk of these complications can be minimized by clearly labelling the arterial line, by using Luer locks for all connections and by leaving the site exposed at all times so that disconnection is immediately recognized.

It is important that the clinician is aware of some common potential sources of error in intra-arterial pressure measurement (Fig. 3.2). If the arterial trace is 'over-damped' the recorded systolic pressure will be less than the actual systolic pressure. This can occur if the cannula is kinked, or partially obstructed by blood clot, and if there are air bubbles in the

---

Fig. 3.1 Percutaneous cannulation of the radial artery. The arm should be supported, with the wrist extended, by an assistant. The radial artery should be palpated where it arches over the head of the radius and a small skin incision made over the proposed puncture site. In conscious patients a wheal of local anaesthetic should be raised, taking care not to puncture the vessel or obscure its pulsation. The cannula should be inserted over the point of maximal pulsation and advanced in line with the direction of the vessel, at an angle of approximately 30°. 'Flash back' of blood indicates that the radial artery has been punctured. The cannula should then be threaded off the needle into the vessel. Following withdrawal of the needle the cannula is connected to a non-compliant manometer line filled with heparinized saline. This is then connected via a transducer and continuóus flush device to an oscilloscope.

(a)

(b)

(c)

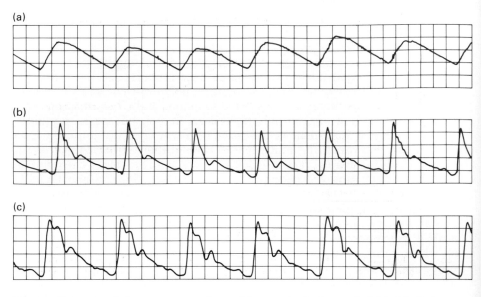

Fig. 3.2 Intra-arterial pressure recordings: (a) excessively damped; (b) 'critically' damped to provide accurate readings; (c) 'under' damped.

manometer line or transducer dome. Conversely, an 'under-damped' trace will 'over-read', particularly at high pressures. Long manometer lines can also introduce inaccuracies since resonant frequencies can develop, again causing the systolic pressure to over-read. The mean arterial pressure is not influenced by either 'damping' or resonance.

PRE-LOAD

As discussed in the preceding chapter, the force with which myocardial fibres contract is dependent on the degree to which they are stretched prior to the onset of systole. This is in turn dependent on the ventricular end-diastolic volume (VEDV) which is directly related to the ventricular end-diastolic pressure (VEDP). The latter can, of course, be measured by direct catheterization of the ventricle, but in clinical practice it is more usual to measure the pressure in the relevant atrium as this is nearly always closely related to VEDP. The relationship between VEDV and VEDP depends on ventricular compliance, so that a stiff ventricle will need a higher EDP to achieve an adequate VEDV—a situation frequently encountered in the critically ill. Also, atrial pressure will not equal VEDP when there is an obstruction, such as a stenosed valve, between the two chambers.

Central venous pressure (CVP)

In the case of the right ventricle the pressure within one of the large veins in the thorax is usually measured—the 'filling pressure' of the right ventricle. This provides a fairly simple method of assessing the adequacy of a patient's circulating volume and the contractile state of the myocardium. It is

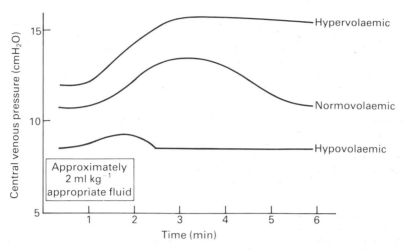

Fig. 3.3 The effects of rapid administration of a 'fluid challenge' to patients with a central venous pressure within the normal range. From Sykes (1963), with permission.

important to realize, however, that the absolute value of the CVP is not as important as its response to a fluid challenge (Fig. 3.3) and it should always be interpreted in conjunction with other monitored values (e.g. heart rate, blood pressure, urine flow and cardiac output) and with clinical assessment (e.g. skin colour, peripheral temperature and perfusion). The hypovolaemic patient will initially respond to transfusion with little or no change in CVP, together with some improvement in cardiovascular status (falling heart rate, rising blood pressure and increased peripheral temperature). As the normovolaemic state is approached the CVP usually rises slightly and stabilizes, while other cardiovascular values normalize. At this stage transfusion should be slowed, or even stopped, in order to avoid overloading the patient (resulting in an abrupt and sustained rise in CVP, usually accompanied by some deterioration in the patient's condition).

The CVP may be read intermittently using a manometer system (Fig. 3.4), or continuously using a transducer connected to an oscilloscope, as illustrated in Fig. 3.1, for intra-arterial pressure monitoring. Whichever method is used, there are several common pitfalls when interpreting CVP measurements, many of which also apply to interpretation of other pressure measurements obtained in the critically ill. These are:

1 *Catheter blocked.* This will result in a sustained high reading which often does not correlate with the patient's overall clinical state. One should check that respiratory oscillations are present and that venous blood can be easily aspirated. A chest x-ray may be taken to confirm satisfactory positioning of the catheter.

2 *Pressure recorded not referred to level of right atrium.* The recorded pressure is a combination of the pressure within the right atrium and a hydrostatic pressure caused by any difference in vertical height between the right atrium and the point of measurement. In order to allow meaningful comparisons between patients, and between repeated readings obtained in the same patient, it is essential that the pressure recorded is always related to

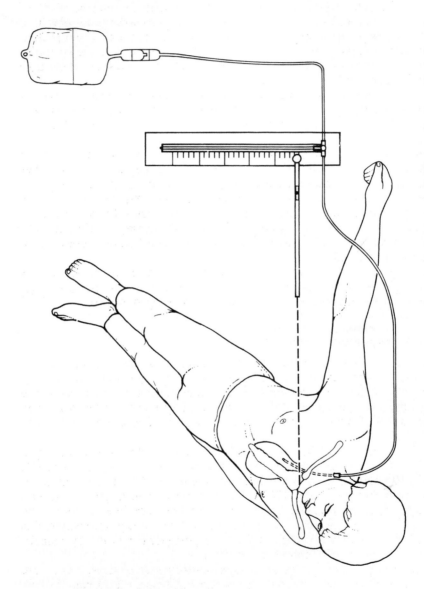

Fig. 3.4 Central venous pressure measurement using a manometer system. The reading must be referred to the level of the right atrium (e.g. the axillary fold or, provided the patient is supine, the sternal notch) using a spirit level.

the level of the right atrium. Failure to adjust the level of the manometer or transducer after changing the patient's position is, therefore, a common cause of erroneous readings. If repeatedly altering the transducer level is considered impractical, an appropriate allowance must be made for the effects of hydrostatic pressure. Various landmarks are advocated to indicate the level of the right atrium (see Fig. 3.4) but it is largely immaterial which of these is chosen as long as it is used consistently and the readings are obtained with the patient in the appropriate position (i.e. sternal notch when patient supine or sternal angle when patient at 45°; the axillary fold or the midpoint between the antero-posterior diameter of the thorax above level of the fourth intercostal space can be used in either position).

3 *Incorrect calibration.* If an electronic transducer and oscilloscope is used, it is important that the system is carefully zeroed and calibrated prior to use and that the calibration and zero are checked if clinically doubtful values are obtained.

4 *One or more infusions in progress through CVP catheter.* If access to central veins proves difficult, then the CVP catheter may be used for other infusions and the pressure measured intermittently. If these infusions continue to be administered by an infusion pump via a Y-piece or 3-way tap while the pressure is read, a falsely high reading will result. Moreover, if the infusions contain inotropic or vasodilator agents, these may be 'flushed' into the patient when the CVP is measured. This can cause sudden episodes of cardiovascular instability.

5 *Catheter tip in right ventricle.* If the catheter is advanced too far it may enter the right ventricle. This may be suspected when an unexpectedly high pressure is recorded, particularly when oscillations are pronounced.

Insertion of central venous catheter

The aim is to position a catheter with its tip in the superior vena cava or the right atrium. Failing this, any large intrathoracic vein is generally satisfactory. This is usually achieved by percutaneous puncture of a central vein such as the internal jugular or subclavian. A few clinicians still prefer to 'cut down' on an arm vein, while, if the chest is open, a cannula may be inserted directly into the innominate vein.

A wide selection of catheters are available for central venous cannulation (Fig. 3.5). The previously popular and easy-to-use catheter-through-needle devices are no longer recommended because the bevel of the needle can shear through the catheter (Peters, 1982). The latter can then migrate centrally, often surprisingly rapidly. Although it is sometimes possible to rescue the catheter using a percutaneous technique guided by an image intensifier, this becomes impossible once it has reached the peripheral pulmonary vessels; even surgical removal is then extremely difficult.

The relatively short and rigid catheter-over-needle devices, which are merely long intravenous cannulae, are particularly simple and easy to use. The longer versions are, however, much less popular. Both have the disadvantage that the needle protrudes beyond the end of the catheter, making it possible to aspirate blood even when the catheter itself is outside the vein. Furthermore, the catheter needs to be fairly sharp and rigid, since it has to be pushed through the skin and subcutaneous tissues. Consequently, it

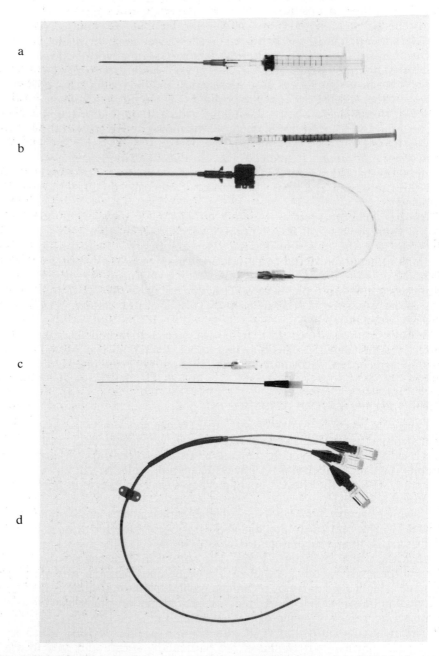

Fig. 3.5 A selection of catheters for central venous cannulation: (a) relatively short, and rigid, catheter over needle; (b) flexible catheter through cannula; (c) guide wire device; (d) triple-lumen catheter.

can damage the vein when advanced and may gradually erode through the vessel wall once in position. These devices are therefore only safe when inserted via the right internal jugular vein, so that the catheter lies in a straight line with its tip in the superior vena cava or right atrium (Peters, 1982).

When other approaches are used, a catheter-through-cannula device is preferable. With these, venepuncture is first performed using a standard intravenous cannula. The needle is then withdrawn and a soft, flexible catheter advanced through the cannula into the vein. The cannula is then removed. The main disadvantage of this technique is that the hole in the vein is larger than the catheter so that there is a risk of bleeding around the puncture site.

Techniques employing a guide wire may be useful in difficult cases and can be used in conjunction with a vein dilator for insertion of large bore catheters (see below for Swan–Ganz catheters). The recently introduced triple-lumen catheters may prove useful in patients who require infusions of irritant drugs (e.g. inotropic agents, concentrated potassium solutions) in addition to CVP monitoring, but in whom there is a shortage of suitable sites for cannulation.

Many approaches to percutaneous cannulation of a central vein have been described, including the antecubital fossa, supra- and infraclavicular approaches to the subclavian vein, the femoral vein and numerous techniques for cannulating the internal jugular vein. However, the general principles of a safe technique are common to all and should be learnt from instruction and demonstration in patients by an expert. The low, anterior approach to the internal jugular vein will be described, since this is probably the safest and surest route to use in an emergency. The infraclavicular approach to the subclavian vein is also popular, but, although ideal for long-term cannulation, probably carries a higher risk of complications (particularly pneumothorax). Other complications of central venous catheterization include vascular perforation, thrombosis, catheter-related sepsis and air embolism (Peters, 1982). Ultrasound-guided puncture has been recommended for difficult cases and to reduce the incidence of complications, particularly for cannulation of the subclavian vein.

If the patient is conscious the procedure must be fully explained and should be carried out with as full sterile precautions as the urgency of the situation allows. (Although generally the operator should 'scrub up' and wear a sterile gown and gloves, in extremely urgent cases, for example cardiac arrest, a 'no touch' technique may be acceptable.)

The patient is placed in the head-down position so that the central veins are distended; this makes cannulation easier and minimizes the risk of air embolism. This position will, however, exacerbate any respiratory difficulty which may be present, particularly if this is due to cardiac failure. The head-down position is also dangerous in patients with raised intracranial pressure.

The skin over the proposed puncture site is cleaned with an antiseptic solution, such as iodine tincture, and sterile towels are placed in position. The patient's head is turned away from the proposed site of entry. Usually, the right side is chosen since this is technically easier for a right-handed operator and on the left there is a danger of damaging the thoracic duct. The apex of the triangle formed by the two heads of sternomastoid, with the clavicle as its

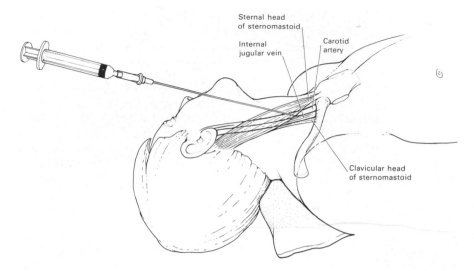

Sternal head
of sternomastoid

Internal
jugular vein

Carotid
artery

Clavicular head
of sternomastoid

Fig. 3.6 Cannulation of the right internal jugular vein with a catheter-over-needle device (see text).

base, is palpated (Fig. 3.6) and a wheal of 2% plain lignocaine raised over this point. The position of the carotid artery should be determined in order to avoid the risk of accidental arterial puncture. A small incision is made in the anaesthetized skin; the cannula, or introducing needle, is inserted through this and directed laterally downwards and backwards so that the vein is punctured just beneath the skin, deep to the lateral head of sternomastoid (Fig. 3.6). If the vein is not encountered, the needle must not be advanced more than a few centimetres because of the risk of a pneumothorax. Failure suggests that either the vein is not sufficiently distended or the cannula is incorrectly positioned. The anatomical landmarks should be checked and the patient can be placed more steeply head-down before the attempt is repeated.

Once the catheter has been inserted and is, to the best of one's knowledge, correctly positioned, venous blood should be easily aspirated; then, the CVP manometer line can be connected. (There is always a risk of air embolism whenever the catheter is open to atmosphere, so necessary periods of disconnection should be as short as possible.) A final check is made by ensuring that, when the infusion bottle is placed on the floor with the giving set tap open, venous blood flows back freely; if it does so, the cannula must be in a large vein. The CVP can then be measured. It is important to check that the fluid level in the manometer falls rapidly and fluctuates with respiration, since this indicates that the tip of the catheter is in an intrathoracic vein.

Finally, a chest x-ray should be taken as soon as possible to verify that the tip of the catheter is centrally placed and to exclude the presence of a pneumothorax (Fig. 3.7). This is particularly important prior to the infusion of large volumes of fluid, especially hypertonic solutions such as might be used for intravenous feeding (Fig. 3.8).

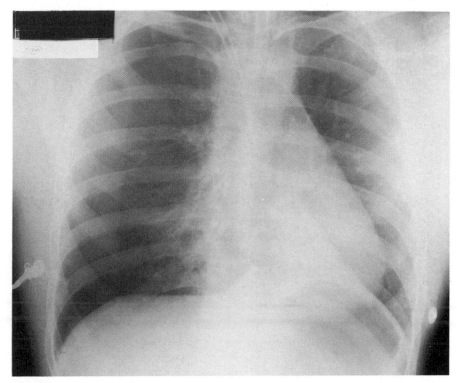

Fig. 3.7 Pneumothorax following insertion of two central venous cannulae via the internal jugular vein. Note also the collapsed left lower lobe (sail shaped shadow behind the heart obscuring the outline of the elevated left hemidiaphragm; the mediastinum is deviated to the left).

Left atrial pressure (LAP)

Under most circumstances the CVP is an adequate guide to the 'filling pressures' of both sides of the heart. However, in many critically ill patients this is not the case and there is a 'disparity in function' between the two ventricles (Pace, 1977). Most commonly, left ventricular performance is worse so that the left ventricular function curve is displaced downward and to the right (Fig. 3.9). This situation is encountered in many patients with clinically significant ischaemic heart disease and has also been reported in multisystem trauma, sepsis, peritonitis, hepatic failure, valvular heart disease and after cardiac surgery. High right-ventricular filling pressures, with normal or low left-atrial pressures, are less common but may occur in situations in which pulmonary vascular resistance (i.e. right ventricular after-load) is raised, such as acute respiratory failure and, even more unusually, right ventricular ischaemia. Moreover, these discrepancies between right and left ventricular performance can be exacerbated by the use of inotropic and vasoactive drugs (Cohn et al, 1969). If there is a disparity in ventricular function after cardiac surgery, then the left atrium can be cannulated directly. However, if the thorax is not open, some other means of determining left ventricular filling pressure must be devised.

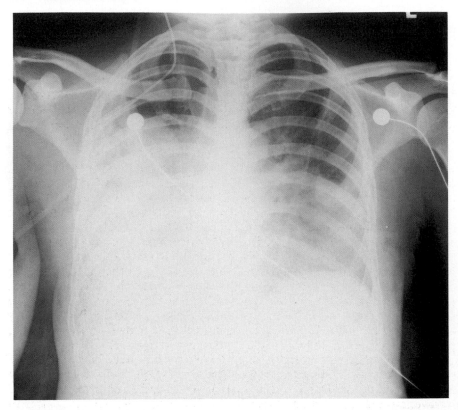

Fig. 3.8 Fluid has been infused into the right pleural space via an incorrectly positioned catheter. There is also bilateral consolidation in the mid and lower zones.

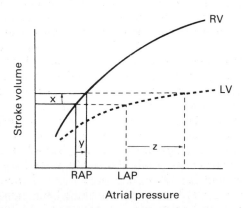

Fig. 3.9 Left (LV) and right (RV) ventricular function curves in a patient with left ventricular dysfunction. Since the stroke volume of the two ventricles must be the same (except perhaps for a few beats during a period of circulatory adjustment), left atrial pressure (LAP) must be higher than right atrial pressure (RAP). Moreover, an increase in stroke volume (x) produced by intravascular volume expansion will be associated with a small rise in RAP (y) but a marked increase in LAP (z).

Pulmonary artery pressures (PAPs)

In 1970, Drs Swan and Ganz described a modified cardiac catheter which incorporated an inflatable balloon at its tip (Swan et al, 1970). This 'balloon flotation catheter' enabled prompt and reliable catheterization of the pulmonary artery, without the need for screening, and minimized the incidence of dysrythmias. Later, a catheter with a slightly increased diameter and larger balloon was introduced which included a proximal lumen for central venous pressure measurement and a thermistor located near the tip. The latter allows determination of cardiac output by the thermodilution technique (see below) (Forrester et al, 1972). Balloon flotation catheters have also been modified for other purposes, including cardiac pacing, pulmonary angiography and continuous monitoring of venous oxygen saturation.

Swan–Ganz catheters can be inserted centrally, through the femoral vein or via a vein in the antecubital fossa. The latter route is perhaps the most comfortable, but it may be difficult to advance the catheter beyond the shoulder region. Furthermore, secure fixation is not easily achieved and involves some degree of immobilization of the arm. On the other hand, the complication rate, particularly the risk of pneumothorax, is less. The left infraclavicular approach to the subclavian vein conforms most closely to the natural curvature of the catheter, and at this site secure fixation is most easily achieved. Catheterization of the right internal jugular vein, however, provides the shortest and most direct route to the right side of the heart.

Because pulmonary artery catheters have to be introduced through a wide bore cannula, a guide wire technique is employed. This involves first making an incision in the anaesthetized skin and puncturing the vein with a standard intravenous cannula. A guide wire with a very flexible, blunt-ended tip is then introduced and the cannula removed. A tapered vein dilator carrying a wide-bore cannula is inserted over the guide wire which is then withdrawn. (If the original skin incision is not sufficiently large, it may prove difficult to push the dilator and cannula through the skin and subcutaneous tissues.) The dilator is then removed and the Swan–Ganz catheter passed through the cannula into the vein. Currently available introducers incorporate a valve mechanism which prevents air embolism and spillage of blood following removal of the dilator and during insertion of the catheter. These cannulae can be left in situ to provide an extra central venous access point and to minimize haemorrhage around the puncture site. A plastic sleeve is provided with some introducer kits which protects a length of catheter, thereby maintaining its sterility. This can subsequently be manipulated, without the risk of contamination, should the catheter become misplaced.

Before the Swan–Ganz catheter is inserted, the balloon should be inflated with the recommended volume of air in order to check for leaks and to ensure that inflation is symmetrical. It should be confirmed that the thermistor is functioning and the various lumens should be flushed with heparinized saline. The technique must be learnt under supervision, since complications are generally inversely related to operator experience.

Passage of the catheter from the major veins, through the chambers of the heart, into the pulmonary artery and the wedge position is monitored and guided by the pressure wave forms recorded from the distal lumen (Fig. 3.10). The catheter should not be advanced too rapidly since redundant loops may

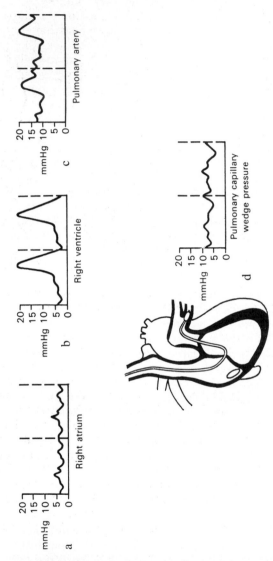

Fig. 3.10 Pressure waveforms as a Swan–Ganz catheter is passed through the chambers of the heart into the 'wedge' position. (a) Once in the thorax, marked respiratory oscillations are seen. The catheter should be advanced further towards the lower superior vena cava/right atrium—oscillations become more pronounced. The balloon should then be inflated and the catheter advanced. (b) In the right ventricle—there is no dicrotic notch and the diastolic pressure is close to zero. The patient should be returned to the horizontal, or slight head-up, position before advancing the catheter further. (c) In the pulmonary artery—a dicrotic notch appears and there is elevation of the diastolic pressure. The catheter should be advanced further with the balloon inflated. (d) Reappearance of a venous waveform indicates that the catheter is 'wedged'. Stop advancing. The balloon should be deflated to obtain pulmonary artery pressure, and then inflated intermittently to obtain pulmonary capillary wedge pressure.

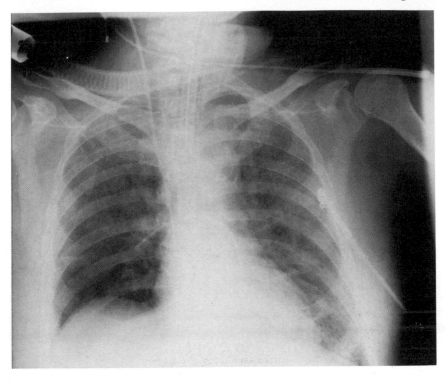

Fig. 3.11 Swan–Ganz catheter correctly positioned in a patient with adult respiratory distress syndrome. (Note the typical alveolar pattern and air bronchograms.)

form in the right atrium or ventricle, with a risk of knotting. X-ray control can be used if difficulty is encountered, but this is rarely necessary. However, a chest x-ray should always be obtained to check the position of the catheter (Fig. 3.11). Once in position, the balloon is deflated and pulmonary artery systolic, end-diastolic pressure (PAEDP) and mean pressure (PAP) can be obtained. The balloon is then inflated intermittently with the recommended volume of air (0.8–1.5 ml) thereby propelling the catheter distally where it will impact in a medium-sized pulmonary artery and record pulmonary capillary wedge pressure (PCWP) (see Fig. 3.10). All intravascular pressures should be measured relative to atmospheric pressure and should therefore be obtained at end-expiration. In patients receiving a positive end-expiratory pressure (PEEP) (see p. 242), the recorded pressure will be incremented by an amount proportional to the level of PEEP. However, this effect is difficult to quantify in the individual patient and depends on a number of factors, including lung compliance.

When the pulmonary artery catheter is in the wedge position, there is a continuous column of fluid between its distal lumen and the left atrium (Fig. 3.12). PCWP is therefore usually closely related to LAP. However, the measurement of PCWP is prone to errors and misinterpretation.

It is clearly essential to establish that a genuine PCWP reading has been obtained (Fig. 3.13). When the catheter 'wedges', a venous waveform should appear, respiratory oscillations should be apparent and the PCWP should be

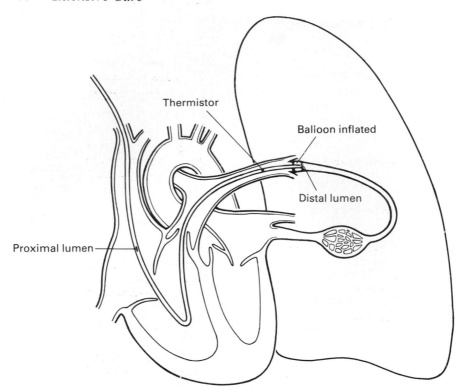

Thermistor

Balloon inflated

Distal lumen

Proximal lumen

Fig. 3.12 Balloon flotation pulmonary artery catheter in the 'wedged' position. There is now a continuous column of blood between the tip of the catheter and the left atrium; pulmonary capillary wedge pressure is therefore usually closely related to left atrial pressure.

less than PAEDP. Some authorities check that it is possible to withdraw 'arterialized' blood. Occasionally, when the balloon is inflated, a PCWP trace is obtained only intermittently. This 'transitional waveform' can occur when the fluctuations in pulmonary artery pressure cause the catheter to 'wedge and unwedge' in a branch of the pulmonary artery. The recorded PCWP may be higher than PAEDP if the balloon is overinflated, or inflates eccentrically, and when the waveform is abnormal, for example large 'V' waves in mitral regurgitation or 'cannon waves' in complete heart block.

Once a genuine PCWP has been obtained, a number of potential causes of misinterpretation remain. The assumption is that PCWP = LAP = LVEDP = LVEDV. As discussed above, the relationship between LVEDP and LVEDV depends on the compliance of the ventricles. The latter is altered in many critically ill patients and some have found PCWP to be a poor predictor of LVEDV. Furthermore, LAP may not accurately reflect LVEDP in the presence of mitral valve disease, left atrial myxoma or severe left ventricular dysfunction. Finally, PCWP will only be equivalent to LAP when there is a continuous column of blood between the catheter tip and the left atrium (see above). This will not be the case when the intervening pulmonary vessels are collapsed by intra-alveolar pressures in excess of pulmonary venous pressure.

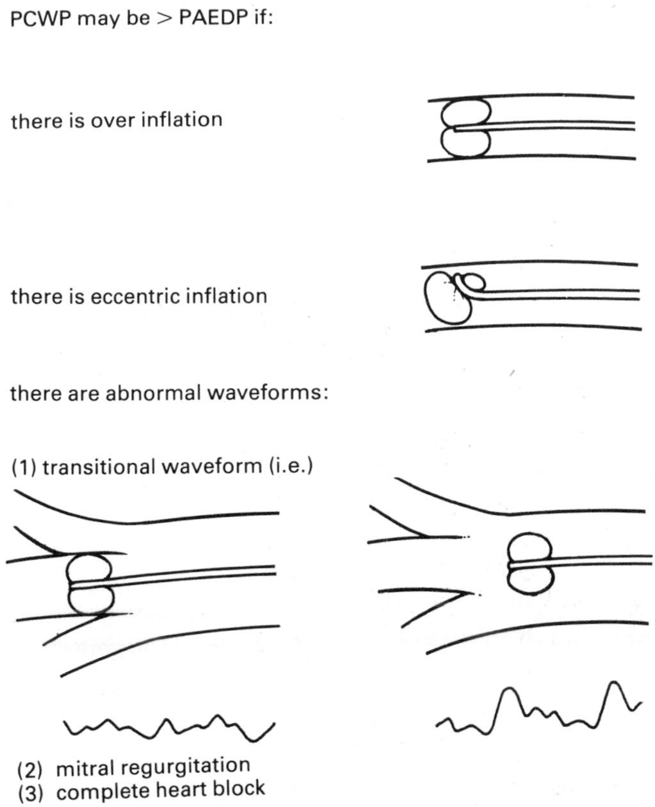

PCWP may be > PAEDP if:

there is over inflation

there is eccentric inflation

there are abnormal waveforms:

(1) transitional waveform (i.e.)

(2) mitral regurgitation
(3) complete heart block

Fig. 3.13 Criteria for a true pulmonary capillary wedge pressure and some causes of inaccurate readings (see text).

This can occur in ventilated patients requiring high inflation pressures or PEEP, particularly if they are hypovolaemic and/or the catheter is in the upper zones of the lungs (West's zones 1 and 2, see above) (Lozman et al, 1974; Kane et al, 1978). Fortunately, because the catheter enters the right ventricle anteriorly through the tricuspid valve and leaves it to enter the pulmonary artery in a posterior direction, the curve on the catheter usually causes it to enter a posterior branch of the pulmonary artery which is supplying the right lower lobe (see Fig. 3.11).

If it proves impossible to obtain a satisfactory PCWP, e.g. if the balloon ruptures, it has been suggested that PAEDP provides a reasonable guide to LAP. However, there is normally a gradient of 1–3 mmHg between PAEDP and PCWP, and this is increased in the presence of pulmonary hypertension, in those with tachycardias and during rapid transfusion (Lappas et al, 1973). In general, PAEDP is an unreliable index of left ventricular filling pressures in the critically ill. It must be emphasized, however, that, as with CVP measurement, the response of PAEDP and PCWP to a fluid challenge is of more significance than the absolute value.

There are a large number of complications associated with the use of Swan–Ganz catheters (Pace, 1977), some of which may be very serious and

Table 3.1 Some complications of Swan–Ganz catheters.

Dysrhythmias	During passage of catheter through right ventricle. Usually benign. Can often be prevented with lignocaine.
Sepsis	At insertion site. Septicaemia. Endocarditis
Knotting	Catheter coils in right ventricle.
Valve trauma	Catheter withdrawn with balloon inflated. Valves repeatedly closing on catheter.
Thrombosis/embolism	
Pulmonary infarction	Catheter remains in 'wedge' position.
Pulmonary artery rupture	Usually fatal. Balloon inflated when catheter already 'wedged'.
Balloon rupture/leak/embolism	

even fatal (Table 3.1). Dysrhythmias are more common when the larger thermodilution catheters are used. It is important to inflate the balloon to the recommended volume in order to conceal the tip of the catheter and prevent it irritating the endocardium during its passage through the right ventricle. Although fatal ventricular tachycardia has been reported (Sise et al, 1981), these dysrhythmias are usually transient and consist of a few benign ventricular premature contractions which stop as soon as the catheter enters the pulmonary artery. If troublesome, they can usually be suppressed with intravenous lignocaine, although in some very unstable patients it may be safer to abandon the procedure. In order to avoid knotting, the catheter should not be advanced by more than 30 cm without observing a change in waveform. Heart valves can be severely damaged if the operator withdraws the catheter without deflating the balloon, while in the longer term, valve cusps can be progressively traumatized by repeated closure against the catheter. Pulmonary infarction may be related to thrombus formation in and around the catheter, but will also occur if the catheter 'wedges' for any length of time. The latter can be avoided by continuously displaying the pulmonary artery pressure so that the spontaneous appearance of a 'wedge' pressure (often caused by softening and migration of the catheter) can be detected and remedied immediately. Although rare (approximately 21 cases in the world literature), pulmonary artery rupture may be fatal due to intractable lung haemorrhage. This complication appears to be commoner in the elderly, particularly in those with pulmonary hypertension, and is due either to continuous impaction of the catheter with erosion of the vessel wall, or rapid inflation of a distally placed balloon.

Despite this rather formidable list of potential hazards, in practice haemodynamic monitoring using the Swan–Ganz catheter has an acceptably low morbidity and mortality (Sise et al, 1981), the majority of complications being closely related to user inexperience. Pulmonary artery catheters should preferably be removed within 72 hours since, after this time, the incidence of infective complications increases (Sise et al, 1981).

AFTER-LOAD

For most practical purposes, in the absence of disease of the aortic or pulmonary valves, changes in after-load are a consequence of alterations in vascular resistance. Unless pulmonary hypertension is present, the resistance of the pulmonary circulation is not an important determinant of cardiac output and changes in after-load are mediated largely by alterations in total peripheral resistance. Although the latter can be calculated relatively easily if blood pressure, central venous pressure and cardiac output are known, it is usually possible to make a reasonable clinical assessment of peripheral vascular tone. For example, vasoconstriction may be indicated by cold, blue, poorly perfused skin and, occasionally, hypertension, whilst in low resistance states the skin is pink and warm.

CARDIAC OUTPUT AND MYOCARDIAL FUNCTION

As discussed in Chapter 2, cardiac output is a major determinant of oxygen delivery and as such is one of the most clinically relevant haemodynamic variables. Indeed, if an accurate, relatively cheap and non-invasive method of measuring cardiac output were available, this variable would probably be determined much more frequently than is currently the case. In the future, this may be achieved by further development of some of the non-invasive techniques described below, but at present the only quantitatively accurate methods of measuring cardiac output are invasive. Consequently, except in the most seriously ill, cardiac output is usually inferred from indirect indices, such as blood pressure, urine output and peripheral perfusion (see below). Moreover, the interpretation of cardiac output determinations, except when they are unquestionably low, can be extremely difficult. Thus, in some critically ill patients tissue perfusion is inadequate despite a normal, or increased, cardiac output (see Chapter 10). These measurements must, therefore, always be interpreted in conjunction with other monitored variables and in this respect an assessment of the balance between tissue oxygen supply and demand is particularly important. This, and other relevant information, such as the systemic vascular resistance, can be derived as outlined in the next chapter to produce a 'physiological profile'. In some respects, therefore, an assessment of end-organ function may provide a better guide to the adequacy of the circulation than isolated cardiac output determinations.

Non-invasive techniques

Over the years, there have been many attempts to develop a clinically viable, non-invasive technique for the determination of cardiac output. These have included the use of impedance cardiography, transcutaneous aortovelography, echocardiography and various radio-isotope techniques.

Impedance cardiography

Two electrical conductors are placed around the subject's neck, with another pair positioned around the lower chest wall. The outer electrodes are supplied with a current, while the inner pair detect voltage changes produced by the alterations in thoracic impedance caused by ventricular ejection. Stroke volume can then be calculated from the magnitude of the voltage fluctuations. This method tends to overestimate the absolute value of cardiac output. Furthermore, other factors such as sweating, lung volume and oedema fluid also influence thoracic impedance and this further limits the accuracy of the technique, particularly in the critically ill. Thus, although impedance cardiography is repeatable and can be used to quantify changes in cardiac output, for absolute determinations it is less precise than invasive methods.

Transcutaneous aortovelography (Hanson and Bilton, 1978)

The velocity and acceleration of blood flow in the ascending aorta can be measured using an ultrasound Doppler probe positioned in the suprasternal notch. Although this technique can be used as a qualitative guide to changes in stroke volume and myocardial performance, it cannot provide an accurate quantitative measure of cardiac output.

Although the above techniques have been available for a number of years, neither has become established in clinical practice. In the future, either echocardiography or radio-isotope methods may prove to be more useful.

Echocardiography

Using two dimensional echocardiography it is possible to locate the anterior and posterior walls of the ventricles and to visualize their movements during the cardiac cycle. In this way, dyskinetic segments may be detected and some assessment can be made of the contractile state of the myocardium. Unfortunately, attempts to calculate stroke volume from the change in distance between the ventricular walls during the cardiac cycle have proved less successful. However, using multiple beams or a moving single beam, it may eventually be possible to visualize the ventricle in three dimensions. Using computer analysis of the images, it might then be possible to obtain reasonable estimates of stroke volume. Echocardiography may also be useful in the critically ill as a means of detecting pericardial effusions and demonstrating diseased valves.

Radio-isotope techniques

These involve the detection of intravenously administered radio-isotopes using a gamma camera; the exact methodology and the information obtained depend on the characteristics of the radio-isotope used. If the isotope remains within the circulation, e.g. technetium-99m tagged to albumin, its first passage through the heart can be recorded by a camera counting over the praecordium. An 'indicator dilution curve' will be produced and cardiac output can be derived in the manner outlined below. Alternatively, the number of counts can be recorded in systole and diastole, the difference being used to calculate the change in ventricular volume during systolic ejection. If, on the other hand, the isotope is taken up by the myocardium (e.g. thallium-201), the ventricular muscle can be visualized directly. Although these techniques are non-invasive, they do expose the patient to radioactivity, thus limiting the number of occasions on which the investigation can be performed. Moreover, they are expensive and relatively inaccurate.

Invasive techniques

Direct Fick method

Fick's principle states that if a substance is added at a constant rate to a column of flowing liquid, then the flow of that liquid is equal to the amount of substance entering the stream, divided by the difference between the concentration of the substance either side of the entry point. The principle is also valid for the removal of a substance and can therefore be applied to the consumption of oxygen by the body. Thus:

$$Q_\mathrm{T} = \frac{\dot{V}_{O_2}}{(C_aO_2 - C_{\bar{v}}O_2)}$$

Conceptually, it may be easier to appreciate that the amount of oxygen consumed by the body can be calculated from the product of the flow of blood to the tissues and the amount of oxygen extracted from each unit of blood. Thus:

$$\dot{V}_{O_2} = Q_\mathrm{T} \times (C_aO_2 - C_{\bar{v}}O_2)$$

and this can be rearranged in order to derive Q_T as above. Indeed, this formula is commonly used clinically to calculate $\dot{V}_{O_2}$.

To obtain cardiac output by the direct Fick method, the oxygen content of arterial and mixed venous blood has to be measured as described below. Oxygen consumption is usually determined by collecting expired gas in a Douglas bag over a timed period. The volume of gas in the bag is measured most accurately using a wet gas meter. The concentration of oxygen in inspired and expired gas is determined using, for example, a paramagnetic analyser (see Chapter 4). If the subject is breathing air the inspired oxygen concentration is, of course, known to be 20.98% and need not be measured. Often, the inspired volume is not measured directly but is derived using a standard formula. $\dot{V}_{O_2}$ is then calculated from

$$\dot{V}_{O_2} = (\dot{V}_I \times F_IO_2) - (\dot{V}_E \times F_EO_2)$$

In practice, there are a number of difficulties which limit the clinical application of this method and it is in fact rarely used in intensive care units, except occasionally for research. Firstly, as well as being relatively complicated and time-consuming, the technique is invasive, requiring both a catheter in the pulmonary artery and arterial puncture. Secondly, the principle on which the method is based applies only under steady-state conditions, when respiratory $\dot{V}_{O_2}$ is identical to tissue $\dot{V}_{O_2}$. This is extremely difficult to achieve clinically, particularly in artificially ventilated subjects. Finally, determination of $\dot{V}_{O_2}$ becomes progressively less accurate as F_IO_2 increases.

Various alternative means of measuring $\dot{V}o_2$ are available which overcome some of these difficulties and may be more appropriate for clinical use. For example, a pneumotachograph can be used to measure inspired and expired volumes continuously (see Chapter 4). This can be combined with continuous determination of F_Io_2 and F_Eo_2 (see Chapter 4) to obtain $\dot{V}o_2$. $\dot{V}co_2$ can also be determined if F_Eco_2 is measured (F_Ico_2 can be assumed to be zero), allowing calculation of the respiratory quotient. An expensive, but clinically viable and accurate system, uses a mass spectrometer to measure inspired and expired concentrations of O_2 and CO_2, together with a tracer gas (argon) dilution technique to determine $\dot{V}_E$. An associated microprocessor calculates and displays $\dot{V}o_2$ and $\dot{V}co_2$ continuously (Roberts et al, 1983).

Indicator dilution techniques

These are based on a modification of the Fick principle in which a substance is added to the central circulation as a bolus, rather than continuously. The appearance and disappearance of this substance is then recorded at a distal site. The cardiac output is calculated from the total amount of indicator injected divided by its average concentration and the time taken to pass the recording site.

Dye dilution. In this technique a bolus of dye (usually of indocyanine green) is injected into the pulmonary artery. Its subsequent passage through the systemic circulation is recorded at a downstream site (usually the radial artery) by continuously aspirating blood through a densitometer. This records the changing concentration of dye, thus describing an 'indicator dilution curve' as shown in Fig. 3.14. (It is essential that the dye mixes completely with

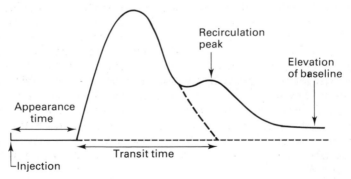

Fig. 3.14 Indicator dilution curve obtained using indocyanine green.

the blood and this might not occur if dye was injected into, for example, the right atrium with sampling from the pulmonary artery.) The amount of dye injected is known while the transit time and average concentration can be determined by analysing the dilution curve. As illustrated in Fig. 3.14, recirculation of dye causes a second peak which interferes with accurate determination of transit time. This is overcome by plotting the curve logarithmically, so that the exponential disappearance of dye becomes a straight line which can be extrapolated to the baseline. The average concentration of dye is determined by integrating the area under the curve.

Unfortunately, dye accumulates in the circulation, causing a progressive elevation of the baseline and this limits the number of times the measurement can be performed. The technique is less accurate when cardiac output is low since the curve is flat, the recirculation peak is more evident and the shape of the curve is difficult to define. Finally, the densitometer has first to be calibrated by mixing a sample of the patient's blood with a known amount of dye.

Thermodilution. Many of the problems associated with dye dilution can be overcome by using cold liquid as the indicator (Forrester et al, 1972) and thermodilution cardiac output determination is now used extensively. In practice, a modified Swan–Ganz catheter, with a lumen opening in the right atrium and a thermistor located a few centimetres from its tip, is inserted as described above. A known volume of liquid, at a known temperature, is injected as a bolus into the atrium. Subsequently, the injectate, which is completely mixed with blood during its passage through the right atrium and ventricle, passes into the pulmonary artery where the fall in temperature is detected by the thermistor (Fig. 3.15). The dilution curve is usually analysed by a computer which provides a direct read-out of cardiac output. Withdrawal of blood is not required and, because the cold is rapidly dissipated in the tissues, there is no recirculation peak and no elevation of the baseline. Measurements can therefore be repeated as often as required. Furthermore, the method is more accurate than dye dilution in low flow states, and the catheters are precalibrated.

The larger the volume of the injectate, and the lower its temperature, the greater is the signal to noise ratio. This increases accuracy and may be particularly important in ventilated subjects in whom pulmonary artery temperature fluctuates during the respiratory cycle (Versprille, 1984). Therefore, although it is possible to use as little as 5 ml of room temperature injectate, it is more usual to inject 10 ml of ice-cold 5% dextrose. The injectate is normally stored in a thermos flask containing iced water. Its temperature is either assumed to be 0°C, or it is measured by a thermistor placed just beyond the syringe. In all cases it is important to avoid warming the injectate by handling the barrel of the syringe. Inevitably, the injectate absorbs heat during its passage through the catheter and the necessary corrections are therefore incorporated in the formulae used to calculate cardiac output. For similar reasons the first of each series of measurements should be rejected since the injectate will include warm fluid from within the catheter lumen.

Accuracy is also dependent on a smooth injection; it is therefore usual to record the shape of the dilution curve on moving paper and to reject uneven curves. Although the use of a 'gun' for injection may reduce wear and tear on the operator, it probably does not significantly increase accuracy. The mean of three consecutive cardiac output determinations, not differing by more than 10%, should be calculated and used as the 'true' value of cardiac output. The repeatability of the method should be within ± 10%, but with care, greater accuracy can probably be achieved (Forrester et al, 1972). Although repeatability can be improved by timing injections to coincide with the same point in the respiratory cycle, values obtained in this way are probably not a true reflection of overall cardiac output. To obtain a truly accurate value for

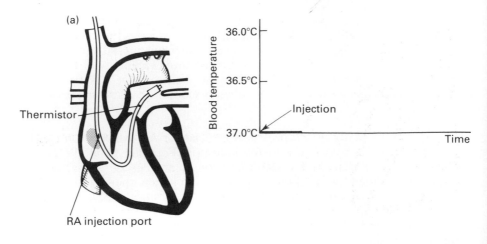

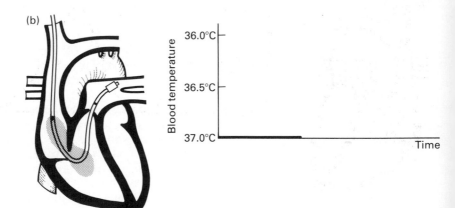

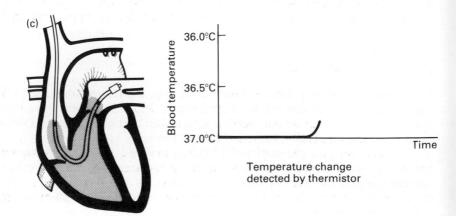

Temperature change
detected by thermistor

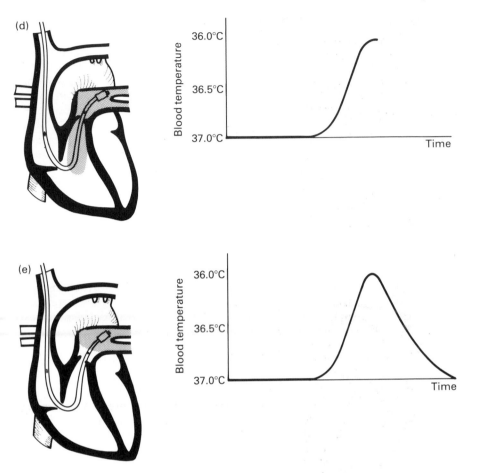

Fig. 3.15 Thermodilution method for cardiac output determination. Notice the absence of a recirculation peak and that there is no elevation of the baseline.

mean cardiac output it may be necessary to perform a series of four measurements spread equally through the ventilatory cycle (Versprille, 1984).

Other invasive techniques

In patients undergoing cardiac surgery, an extractable electromagnetic flow probe can be placed around the aortic root. Clearly, this technique is only applicable to those in whom direct access to the aortic root is possible, but even in such patients the method is rarely used.

Left ventricular angiography can be used to visualize dyskinetic segments and to calculate ejection fraction. Some assessment can then be made of myocardial performance. However, it is not suitable for bedside use in the critically ill and, as with radio-isotope methods, accurate calculation of stroke volume is not possible.

INDICES OF TISSUE PERFUSION

As mentioned above, it is possible to gain a fairly accurate idea of tissue perfusion, and by implication cardiac output, from an examination of the skin. When perfusion is reduced the skin is cold, pale and blue with an increased capillary filling time. Conversely, a patient with warm, pink peripheries probably has an adequate cardiac output. More objective evidence can be obtained by monitoring peripheral temperature and urine output. Measuring peripheral temperature, e.g. from the tip of the great toe, is cheap, non-invasive and provides a good guide to the level of tissue perfusion, provided it is related to a reference value (Henning et al, 1979). Often, the core temperature is measured simultaneously in which case an increased core–peripheral temperature difference is indicative of impaired perfusion. This temperature gradient may be a more reliable indicator of outcome than either cardiac index or arterial blood pressure (Henning et al, 1979). Others recommend that the toe temperature should be related to room temperature.

A fall in peripheral temperature is often the first indication of a deterioration in cardiovascular function, and may occur before changes in other variables such as heart rate, blood pressure or central venous pressure. This is because vasoconstriction is an early compensatory response to reductions in circulating volume or myocardial performance and initially maintains other cardiovascular parameters within the normal range.

A decrease in urine flow is another sensitive indicator of a fall in cardiac output and if oliguria develops, measures aimed at improving kidney perfusion are urgently required in order to prevent acute renal failure.

Finally, the patient's conscious level and mental function is one of the best indicators of the adequacy of circulatory function and tissue oxygenation.

FURTHER READING

Poole-Wilson PA (1983) Measurement and control of cardiac output. In Tinker J & Rapin M (eds) *Care of the Critically Ill Patient*, pp 3–18. Berlin: Springer-Verlag.
Swan HJC & Ganz W (1983) Techniques for investigating cardiovascular function. In Tinker J & Rapin M (eds) *Care of the Critically Ill Patient*, pp 933–944. Berlin: Springer-Verlag.

REFERENCES

Band JD & Maki DG (1979) Infections caused by arterial catheters used for hemodynamic monitoring. *American Journal of Medicine* **67**: 735–741.
Cohn JN, Tristani FE & Khatri IM (1969) Studies in clinical shock and hypotension. VI. Relationship between left and right ventricular function. *Journal of Clinical Investigation* **48**: 2008–2018.
Forrester JS, Ganz W, Diamond G et al (1972) Thermodilution cardiac output determination with a single flow-directed catheter. *American Heart Journal* **83**: 306–311.

Hanson GC & Bilton AH (1978) Clinical experience with transcutaneous aortovelography: preliminary communication. *Journal of the Royal Society of Medicine* **71:** 501–506.

Henning RJ, Wiener F, Valdes S & Weil MH (1979) Measurement of toe temperature for assessing the severity of acute circulatory failure. *Surgery, Gynecology and Obstetrics* **149:** 1–7.

Kane PB, Askanazi J, Neville JF et al (1978) Artifacts in the measurement of pulmonary artery wedge pressure. *Critical Care Medicine* **6:** 36–38.

Lappas D, Lell WA, Gabel JC, Civetta JM & Lowenstein E (1973) Indirect measurement of left-atrial pressure in surgical patients—pulmonary capillary wedge and pulmonary artery diastolic pressures compared with left atrial pressure. *Anesthesiology* **38:** 394–397.

Lozman J, Powers SR, Older T et al (1974) Correlation of pulmonary wedge and left atrial pressures. A study in the patient receiving positive end expiratory pressure ventilation. *Archives of Surgery* **109:** 270–277.

Pace NL (1977) A critique of flow-directed pulmonary arterial catheterization. *Anesthesiology* **47:** 455–465.

Peters JL (1982) Current problems in central venous catheter systems. *Intensive Care Medicine* **8:** 205–208.

Roberts MJ, Boustred ML & Hinds CJ (1983) A multipatient mass spectrometer based system for the measurement of metabolic gas exchange in artificially ventilated intensive care patients. *Intensive Care Medicine* **9:** 339–343.

Russell JA, Joel M, Hudson RJ, Mangano DT & Schlobohm RM (1983) Prospective evaluation of radial and femoral artery catheterization sites in critically ill adults. *Critical Care Medicine* **11:** 936–939.

Sise MJ, Hollingsworth P, Brimm JE et al (1981) Complications of the flow-directed pulmonary-artery catheter: a prospective analysis in 219 patients. *Critical Care Medicine* **9:** 315–318.

Swan HJC, Ganz W, Forrester J et al (1970) Catheterization of the heart in man with use of a flow-directed balloon-tipped catheter. *New England Journal of Medicine* **283:** 447–451.

Sykes MK (1963) Venous pressure as a clinical indication of adequacy of transfusion. *Annals of the Royal College of Surgeons* **33:** 185–197.

Thomas F, Burke JP, Parker J et al (1983) The risk of infection related to radial vs femoral sites for arterial catheterisation. *Critical Care Medicine* **11:** 807–812.

Versprille A (1984) Thermodilution in mechanically ventilated patients. *Intensive Care Medicine* **10:** 213–215.

Zideman DA & Morgan M (1981) Inadvertent intra-arterial injection of flucloxacillin. *Anaesthesia* **36:** 296–298.

4
Respiratory Monitoring

Clinical assessment is of the utmost importance when managing patients with respiratory problems. The use of accessory muscles of respiration, tachypnoea, tachycardia, sweating, pulsus paradoxus and inability to speak are all signs of severe respiratory distress and, together with a subjective assessment of the degree of exhaustion, are often the best guides to the need for artificial ventilation. Carbon dioxide retention may be suspected in a patient with a bounding pulse, warm, vasodilated peripheries, a tremor of the outstretched hand and impaired conscious level, but the presence or absence of cyanosis is an unreliable guide to the adequacy of oxygenation. The final decision as to when to wean a patient from artificial ventilation is also often largely based on clinical judgement, although many objective criteria have been described (see Chapter 13).

Clinical examination of the patient can be supplemented by measurements of tidal volume (V_T) and vital capacity (VC) and these, together with the pulse rate, blood pressure and respiratory rate, should be recorded at regular intervals so that the patient's progress can be observed and any deterioration detected immediately. The most sensitive indicator of increasing respiratory difficulty is a rising respiratory rate which may be accompanied by tachycardia and hypertension. Tidal volume, on the other hand, is less sensitive, while minute ventilation rises initially and falls precipitously only at a late stage when the patient is exhausted. Vital capacity is often a better guide to deterioration and is particularly useful in patients with respiratory inadequacy due to neuromuscular problems.

MONITORING LUNG VOLUMES

Wright's respirometer

Tidal volume, minute volume and vital capacity can be measured most easily in the clinical setting using a Wright's respirometer (Fig. 4.1). Access to the airway is required but this is easily achieved in intubated patients by attaching the device to the catheter mount. In ventilated subjects, the respirometer can be connected to the expiratory limb of the ventilator. In the spontaneously breathing, unintubated patient a mouthpiece can be used or a mask can be closely applied to the patient's face. There is therefore inevitably some degree of interference with the patient's airway and this has the disadvantage of interrupting the oxygen supply, as well as potentially altering the respiratory pattern.

The Wright's respirometer is a delicate instrument which is easily damaged if dropped. Because of the inertia of the vane, and the resistance of the device, this respirometer under-reads at low flows. On the other hand, at high flows, the momentum of the vane causes the instrument to over-read.

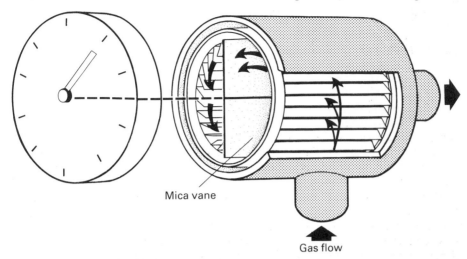

Fig. 4.1 Wright's respirometer. Gas flowing into the device is channelled through a series of tangential slits and rotates the lightweight mica vane. The latter is connected to the pointer on the dial by gears. An electronic version is also available.

Accuracy is also affected by condensation of water vapour and, to a lesser extent, by alterations in the composition of respired gas. Nevertheless, in clinical practice the errors are rarely greater than 10%. The dead space and resistance of the device are low and it is therefore well tolerated by spontaneously breathing patients. Electronic versions are also available.

Pneumotachograph

Whereas the Wright's respirometer is a unidirectional device, which measures only expired volumes, the pneumotachograph records flows in both inspiration and expiration (Fig. 4.2). Flow rates are calculated from the

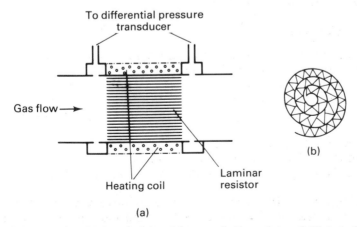

Fig. 4.2 Fleisch pneumotachograph head (see text). From Sykes & Vickers (1973), with permission.

measured pressure difference across the fixed resistance; inspired and expired volumes are obtained by integrating these flows. The best known of these devices is the Fleisch head in which the resistance is formed by a piece of corrugated foil wound into a spiral. This creates a large number of parallel sided tubes which ensure laminar flow. Condensation of water vapour on the foil, which can alter its resistance and create turbulent flow, is prevented by surrounding the device with a heating coil. Mucus traps are also required to prevent obstruction. Although alterations in the composition and temperature of the gas mixture interfere with the measurement, when used carefully an accuracy of $\pm 5\%$ is possible. However, considerable care and attention to detail are required when using these instruments and they have not proved suitable for routine clinical use. Alternatives have therefore been described. These have included the use of a heated wire mesh to provide the resistance, in which case flow is turbulent and sophisticated electronics are required to produce a linear output, and lightweight devices with a variable orifice which are unaffected by water vapour, allow tracheal secretions to pass easily and are relatively insensitive to temperature changes (Osborn, 1978).

Heated wire or thermistor

Another approach to the measurement of inspired and expired volumes is to place a heated wire, or a thermistor, in the gas stream. The magnitude of temperature changes is then dependent on gas flow rates (Yoshiya et al, 1979).

Vortex spirometer

A recently introduced spirometer generates vortices in the gas stream. These are detected and counted by an ultrasonic beam, the number of vortices being dependent on gas flow rate. These 'vortex spirometers' are said to be accurate

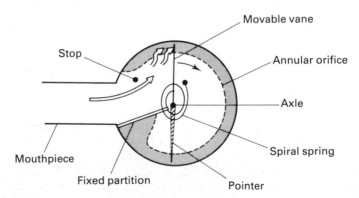

Fig. 4.3 Wright's peak flowmeter. From Sykes & Vickers (1973), with permission. The patient makes a forced expiration. The expired gas is deflected onto the rotating vane which is moved against the resistance offered by the spiral spring. As the vane rotates the annular orifice opens progressively allowing gas to escape to the outside. The maximum deflection of the vane depends on the peak flow rate. The vane is maintained in this position by a ratchet.

over a large range of flows and are largely unaffected by gas composition, humidity or temperature (Westenskow and Tucker, 1981).

ASSESSING AIRWAYS OBSTRUCTION

Clinical evaluation of the severity of airflow obstruction is notoriously inaccurate. The patient's progress, and in particular his response to treatment, can be assessed objectively by serial measurement of the forced expiratory volume in 1 second (FEV_1) using a vitalograph. A more useful indication is obtained by expressing FEV_1, as a percentage of the vital capacity—normally, this value should be greater than 75%. However, the Wright's peak flowmeter (Fig. 4.3) provides a much more convenient means of assessing airways obstruction at the bedside; normal individuals should be able to achieve a peak flow rate of between 300 and 700 l min^{-1}.

'NON-INVASIVE' RESPIRATORY MONITORING

There have been a number of attempts to develop a satisfactory method for continuously monitoring respiratory function which does not intrude on the airway. An example which appears to have potential for use in the spontaneously breathing patient is the inductance plethysmograph (Milledge and Stott, 1977). The inductive element is formed by a coil incorporated in a close-fitting, expanding 'waistcoat'. Changes in thoracic volume alter the inductance of the coil. As with all the non-invasive methods, this device is relatively inaccurate. It has to be calibrated before use, but is then stable for long periods. When using such non-invasive devices, the most valuable information is often obtained by analysing changes in the pattern of respiration. For example, during the onset of acute respiratory failure, as well as the increasing respiratory rate and the later reduction in V_T, the normal breath-to-breath variation in V_T is lost. The reverse trend may be seen during weaning from artificial ventilation.

MONITORING INSPIRED AND EXPIRED GAS COMPOSITION

Oxygen

Most often the inspired oxygen concentration (usually expressed as a fraction of one, F_1O_2) is measured using either a polarographic or a fuel cell method. Determination of the expired oxygen fraction is required less frequently.

Fuel cells produce a voltage which is proportional to the partial pressure of oxygen to which they are exposed. They are unaffected by water vapour, but have a slow response time and are relatively inaccurate. Furthermore, they are depleted by continued exposure to oxygen and this limits their lifespan. Polarographic electrodes also normally have a slow response time, although this can be increased electronically sufficiently to allow breath-by-breath analysis.

Paramagnetic analysers are extremely accurate but they require careful calibration. They are affected by water vapour and, again, the response time is slow. Therefore, they are only suitable for the intermittent analysis of discrete samples of dried gas and consequently their use is generally confined to research.

Mass spectrometers (Gothard et al, 1980) are also very accurate and have the added advantages of a rapid response time and the ability to analyse gas concentrations in the presence of water vapour, thus they are well suited to the continuous analysis of both inspired and expired gas concentrations in ventilated patients. They are, however, expensive, bulky and require considerable expertise during operation and maintenance. These difficulties have limited their introduction into clinical intensive care practice.

Carbon dioxide

Traditionally, the fractional concentration of CO_2 in mixed expired gas ($F_E co_2$) is determined by analysing a Douglas bag collection with an infra-red CO_2 analyser. The $F_E co_2$ has to be measured in order to determine V_D/V_T and $\dot{V}co_2$, as described in Chapter 2.

Continuous breath-by-breath analysis of expired CO_2 (capnography), using either an infra-red analyser or a mass spectrometer, may also provide clinically useful information. Variations in the CO_2 waveform can indicate changes in the production or transport of CO_2, alterations in lung function or apparatus malfunction. Changes in the waveform are not, however, diagnostic and other clinical observations are usually required to determine the underlying cause. Perhaps of more clinical value is the end-tidal CO_2 tension ($P_E' co_2$) which can be considered to reflect $P_A co_2$ and thus $P_a co_2$. $P_E' co_2$ can therefore be used an an immediate guide to the patient's ventilation requirements. However, the discrepancy between $P_E' co_2$ and $P_a co_2$ increases as lung function deteriorates, and changes in $P_E' co_2$ may also be caused by alterations in the distribution of ventilation.

BLOOD GAS ANALYSIS AND ACID–BASE DISTURBANCE

In the early days of intensive care, blood gas analysis was performed using the equilibration technique. This method, developed over 20 years ago by Professor Poul Astrup, was a relatively time-consuming procedure and required some degree of technical expertise. Combined with the reluctance of clinicians to puncture arteries, this meant that blood gas analysis was performed only rarely.

The original Astrup trolleys consisted of a pH electrode and a microtonometer but some of the later versions also included a direct reading 'Clark' electrode for the determination of blood oxygen tension. Subsequently, the equilibration technique was superseded by the commercial development of the direct reading $P co_2$ electrode and all three were then miniaturized sufficiently to be incorporated in a single cuvette, allowing measurements to be performed on one blood sample. Following the introduction of the microprocessor, automation of most of the processes involved became feasible and modern automated blood gas analysers were soon available commercially. At the same time, there was an increasing acceptance of the ease and relative safety of arterial puncture. Consequently, arterial blood gas analysis is now one of the most commonly performed objective tests of respiratory function.

Accuracy of blood gas analysis

Automation of measurement, calculation and display can give a false impression of reliability and accuracy. This may lead to an uncritical acceptance of the results obtained. The clinician must, therefore, be aware of the potential sources of error when performing blood gas analysis and of the ways in which these can be minimized.

Sampling

In the past, it has been recommended that glass syringes should be used to obtain the arterial sample. These were said to have two advantages. Firstly, the plunger moves freely, allowing arterial blood to flow into the syringe under its own pressure. Secondly, glass is an efficient barrier to diffusion of gases out of the sample. In fact, most clinicians find an ordinary plastic syringe, with a continuous negative pressure applied to the plunger, quite satisfactory and in practice diffusion of gases into the wall of the syringe is not a problem (Evers et al, 1972).

On the other hand, continuing metabolism of white blood cells, and to a lesser extent reticulocytes, can cause significant reductions in Po_2 and pH, combined with increases in Pco_2, particularly when the initial oxygen tension is high. If the sample cannot be analysed immediately, metabolism can be slowed by immersing the syringe in iced water, having first sealed the end with a plastic cap (Biswas et al, 1982).

To prevent clot formation within the analyser, the sample must be adequately anticoagulated. On the other hand, excessive dilution of the blood with heparin, which is acidic, will significantly reduce its Pco_2, although dilution probably has little effect on pH or Po_2 (Bradley, 1972). Therefore, heparin, in a concentration of 1000 iu ml^{-1}, should be used and the volume limited to that contained within the dead space of the syringe, i.e. approximately 0.1 ml. Although this will adequately anticoagulate a 2 ml sample, it is not sufficient for the unnecessarily large volumes of blood sometimes presented for analysis.

Even with the most careful technique, air almost inevitably enters the sample. The gas tensions within these air bubbles will equilibrate with those in the blood, thereby lowering the Pco_2 and, usually, raising the Po_2 of the sample. However, provided they are ejected immediately, their effect is insignificant. Nevertheless, errors will arise if bubbles greater than 0.5–1% of the sample volume are not removed, particularly if the sample is stored at room temperature (Biswas et al, 1982).

pH electrodes. Although the traditional pH notation is still used extensively, it is now more usual to refer to the hydrogen ion concentration ([H$^+$]) in nanomoles per litre (nmol l^{-1}). The measurement of pH is particularly prone to error, the commonest cause of erroneous readings being contamination of the electrode with blood proteins.

Pco₂ electrodes. Pco_2 measurements are generally very accurate. When errors do arise they are usually associated with the development of holes in the electrode membrane, or less often, loss of the silver chloride coating on the reference electrode. The membrane can be replaced relatively easily, but in the latter instance a new electrode is required. Since holes in the membrane occur fairly frequently, there is usually no time for protein contamination to become a problem.

Po₂ electrodes. The current output of the oxygen electrode is less for blood than for a gas with an identical Po_2. This discrepancy is called the 'blood gas factor' and is peculiar to oxygen electrodes. It is thought to be due to consumption of oxygen by the electrode from blood immediately adjacent to the tip of the cathode. This generates a gradient of oxygen tension across the sample and causes the electrode to under-read. As with the other electrodes, protein contamination may also cause problems.

Quality control and maintenance

It is essential that on-site equipment, which is used extensively out of hours by both medical and nursing staff, is subject to strict quality control procedures and regular maintenance.

Although automated blood gas analysers are self-calibrating, they should be checked regularly with quality control material, preferably daily. Ampoules containing buffered liquid of known pH and blood gas tensions are available for this purpose. The discrepancy between the measured and the known standard values can then be recorded on a chart such as that shown in Fig. 4.4. Any deviation of these figures outside the predetermined limits

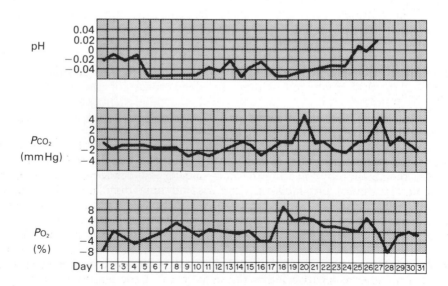

Fig. 4.4 Quality control chart for automated blood gas analyser. 'O' line represents true value for tonometered sample and the continuous line joins the values measured by the instrument. From Cole (1982), with permission.

indicates a significant fault in the relevant electrode. This can then be remedied, e.g. by replacing the membrane. In practice, however, it is more usual to avoid problems by changing the membranes regularly. Although buffered liquids can detect the majority of errors associated with the O_2 and CO_2 electrodes, they may fail to demonstrate protein contamination of the pH electrode. The latter can be detected with tonometered calf serum, although it is usually easier simply to clean the electrode at regular intervals.

For very accurate determination of oxygen tension, the Po_2 electrode should be calibrated with tonometered blood so that the blood gas factor can be calculated. This is expressed as a percentage and can be applied as a correction factor to subsequent measurements. Clearly, it will have a proportionately greater effect on the absolute value of Po_2 at higher oxygen tensions. Furthermore, loss of oxygen into the plastic walls of the cuvette and tubing increases as Po_2 rises; therefore, considerable care is necessary in order to obtain accurate measurements of oxygen tension when Po_2 is high and, if possible, the electrode should be calibrated against blood with a Po_2 close to that to be measured.

Interpretation of blood gases and acid–base status (Flenley, 1978)

The normal values and ranges obtained when blood gas analysis is performed are shown in Table 4.1. As well as direct measurements of hydrogen ion activity (expressed as pH or $[H^+]$), Po_2 and Pco_2, other values relevant to the assessment of the patient's oxygenation and acid–base status are calculated by the microprocessor contained within the analyser.

Table 4.1 Normal values for measurements obtained when blood gas analysis is performed.

H^+	35–45 nmol l^{-1}, 7.35–7.45 pH units
Po_2	10–13.3 kPa (75–100 mmHg)
Pco_2	4.8–6.1 kPa (36–46 mmHg)
Actual HCO_3^-	22–26 mmol l^{-1}
Standard HCO_3^-	22–26 mmol l^{-1}
Base deficit	± 2.5
% saturation	95–100

The total, or actual, bicarbonate concentration is influenced both by alterations in the amount of CO_2, and by metabolic changes in the amounts of acid and alkali in the blood. It is calculated using the Henderson–Hasselbach equation (see below). In order to assess the contribution of metabolic factors, and disregard changes in pH due to alterations in Pco_2, the standard bicarbonate concentration can be derived. This is the amount of bicarbonate that would be present in that particular blood sample if the Pco_2 was 5.3 kPa (40 mmHg), the temperature was 38°C and the blood was fully oxygenated at sea level. The base deficit is simply a convenient figure for calculating the amount of sodium bicarbonate required to correct a metabolic acidosis. It is calculated as the amount of base which one would need to add to, or subtract from, each litre of extracellular fluid to return the pH to a value of 7.4 at Pco_2 of 5.3 kPa (40 mmHg) at 38°C. Most often, the clinician is given the base excess, which will be negative if there is a base deficit (i.e. a metabolic acidosis) and positive if there is a metabolic alkalosis.

Modern automated blood gas analysers will also calculate the saturation of haemoglobin with oxygen using one of the mathematical formulae describing the oxyhaemoglobin dissociation curve. When performing this calculation they usually assume that the curve is normally positioned, although in some the P_{50} can be specified by the operator. Percentage saturation is closely related to the oxygen content of the blood, which, as discussed in Chapter 2, is usually of more clinical relevance than the P_{O_2}. Some analysers will actually calculate oxygen content, either assuming a value for the haemoglobin concentration or by using a value entered by the operator. The calculation also assumes that all the haemoglobin is available to bind oxygen, i.e. there is no met- or carboxyhaemoglobin present.

The interpretation of these results can be considered in two separate parts: disturbances of carbon dioxide homeostasis and acid–base balance, and alterations in oxygenation. In all cases, one must know the history, the age of the patient, the $F_{I}O_{2}$ and any other relevant treatment (e.g. the administration of sodium bicarbonate and the ventilator settings for those on mechanical ventilation).

Disturbances of acid–base balance

All enzyme reactions have optimum values for [H⁺] at which the reaction proceeds most rapidly. Alterations in [H⁺] can, therefore, theoretically lead to a state of 'metabolic chaos' in which some reactions proceed faster than they should, whilst others slow down. The [H⁺] also affects the degree of ionization of various molecules. For example, an alkalosis causes ionized calcium to bind to protein and may precipitate tetany. The distribution of ions across cell membranes is also influenced by the quantity of H⁺ ions in the body and this applies particularly to potassium (see Chapter 5). Severe metabolic acidosis can cause cerebral and myocardial depression (see Chapter 10, p. 146), while the respiratory centre is stimulated initially but is subsequently depressed as the acidosis becomes more severe. A marked metabolic alkalosis may combine with an associated hypokalaemia to depress cardiac function. As discussed in Chapter 2, changes in both [H⁺] and P_{CO_2} cause shifts of the oxyhaemoglobin dissociation curve.

The body therefore resists changes in [H⁺] with a variety of buffer systems, as well as by regulating the excretion of non-volatile acids and bases via the kidney and by adjusting alveolar ventilation to control the arterial carbon dioxide tension.

Buffer systems

A buffer is a mixture of a weak acid (which, in contrast to a strong acid, is only partially dissociated in water) and its conjugate base. In the body, the main buffer systems are carbonic acid/bicarbonate, phosphates and proteins. For the phosphate system:

$$H_2PO_4^- \rightleftharpoons H^+ + HPO_4^{2-}$$

and for the carbonic acid/bicarbonate system:

$$H_2CO_3 \rightleftharpoons H^+ + HCO_3^-$$

At equilibrium the law of mass action applies and states that the product of the concentrations of hydrogen ions and bicarbonate ions divided by the concentration of carbonic acid will remain constant.

$$\text{i.e. } K = \frac{[H^+][HCO_3^-]}{[H_2CO_3]}$$

Henderson rearranged this equation to allow calculation of the hydrogen ion concentration:

$$[H^+] = K \frac{[H_2CO_3]}{[HCO_3^-]}$$

and later Hasselbach modified this equation using the pH nomenclature:

$$pH = pK + \log \frac{[HCO_3^-]}{[H_2CO_3]}$$

Buffer systems are most effective when they are maximally dissociated, that is when the pH is close to their dissociation constant (pK). Protein is an effective intracellular buffer because its pK is similar to the intracellular pH (7.0), whilst the pK of haemoglobin is 7.4. The pK of the phosphate system is 6.8, but that of the bicarbonate system is only 6.1. Nevertheless, the latter is of most interest to clinicians since it is present in large amounts, its components can be measured and it is influenced by renal and respiratory compensatory mechanisms.

$$H^+ + HCO_3^- \underset{\substack{\text{Ionic} \\ \text{dissociation}}}{\rightleftharpoons} H_2CO_3 \underset{\substack{\text{Carbonic} \\ \text{anhydrase}}}{\rightleftharpoons} CO_2 + H_2O \quad \textit{Kidneys}$$
(in solution)

$$\downarrow$$

$$CO_2 \text{ (gas phase)} \quad \textit{Lungs}$$

Alterations in alveolar ventilation can compensate rapidly for metabolic abnormalities, while renal mechanisms operate over a longer time course and can also compensate for respiratory disturbances.

Since $[H_2CO_3]$ is proportional to the P_aco_2 the Henderson equation can be rewritten as

$$[H^+] \propto \frac{Pco_2}{[HCO_3^-]}$$

Pco_2 can therefore be plotted against $[H^+]$ (or pH) and the various acid–base disturbances described in relation to this (Fig. 4.5). Both acidosis and alkalosis can occur, each of which may be either metabolic (primarily affecting the bicarbonate component of the system) or respiratory (primarily affecting Pco_2). Compensatory changes may also be apparent. In clinical practice, arterial $[H^+]$ values outside the range $126\,\text{nmol}\,l^{-1}$–$18\,\text{nmol}\,l^{-1}$ (pH 6.9–7.7) are very rarely encountered.

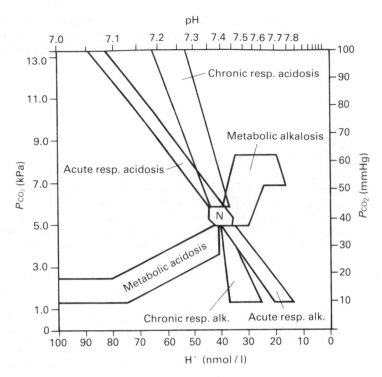

Fig. 4.5 Diagram representing disturbances of acid–base balance (95% confidence limits). The area of normal values is labelled N. From Goldberg et al (1973) *J.A.M.A.* *223:* pp. 269–275, with permission. Copyright 1973, American Medical Association.

Respiratory acidosis

This is caused by retention of carbon dioxide; the P_{CO_2} and $[H^+]$ rise. Sometimes there is a small increase in HCO_3^- (see Fig. 4.5). A chronically raised P_{CO_2} is compensated by renal retention of bicarbonate and $[H^+]$ returns towards normal. A constant arterial bicarbonate concentration is then usually established within 2–5 days. This represents a primary respiratory acidosis with a compensatory metabolic alkalosis. It is worth recognizing that because treatment, such as the administration of diuretics, can exacerbate hypochloraemia and produce further retention of bicarbonate, the $[H^+]$ may be on the low side of normal, even when carbon dioxide retention is the primary abnormality. Common causes of respiratory acidosis include ventilatory failure and COAD (type II respiratory failure—see Chapter 12).

Respiratory alkalosis

In this case the reverse occurs with a fall in P_{CO_2} and $[H^+]$ (see Fig. 4.5), often with a small reduction in bicarbonate concentration. If hypocarbia persists some degree of renal compensation may occur, producing a metabolic acidosis, although some suggest that in practice this is unusual (Flenley,

1983). A respiratory alkalosis is often produced, intentionally or unintentionally, when patients are artificially ventilated; it may also be seen with hypoxaemic (type I) respiratory failure (see Chapter 12) and in those living at altitude.

Metabolic acidosis

This may be due to excessive acid production, most commonly lactic acid during an episode of shock or following cardiac arrest. Another common cause is diabetic ketoacidosis. A metabolic acidosis may also develop in chronic renal failure and following the administration of acid substances. Alternatively, it may be due to the loss of large amounts of alkali, e.g. from the lower gastrointestinal tract or in renal tubular acidosis.

When the aetiology is not clinically obvious, calculation of the 'anion gap' may help to differentiate between the various causes of a metabolic acidosis. This is calculated as the difference between the sum of the bicarbonate and chloride concentrations and the sum of the sodium and potassium concentrations. Normally, the sum of the unmeasured anions (sulphates, phosphates, plasma proteins and anions of organic acids) ranges from 5 to $12 \, \text{mmol} \, l^{-1}$. When the acidosis is due to a loss of base, the 'anion gap' will be normal. Conversely, a metabolic acidosis with an increased 'anion gap' results from a gain of acid, e.g. in ketoacidosis, renal failure, poisoning with methanol, salicylates, or ethylene glycol (antifreeze) and in lactic acidosis.

Lactic acidosis (Editorial, 1973). This may be due to increased production and/or decreased removal of lactic acid. The principal sources of lactic acid are skeletal muscle, brain and erythrocytes; lactate ions are converted to glucose, or oxidized, by the liver and kidney. Two types of lactic acidosis have been identified, designated type A and type B. Type A is more common and is due to inadequate tissue perfusion, cellular hypoxia and anaerobic glycolysis. The ability of the liver to remove the excess lactic acid is often impaired by underperfusion, as well as severe acidosis, and in extreme cases the liver may actually produce, rather than consume, lactate. The clinical picture is usually dominated by the underlying cause and treatment is directed at reversing tissue hypoxia.

Type B lactic acidosis occurs in the absence of tissue hypoxia. Previously, the most common cause was the administration of phenformin to patients with impaired renal or hepatic function. Other causes include diabetic ketoacidosis, severe liver disease, intravenous infusion of sorbitol or fructose, ethanol ingestion, methanol poisoning, acute infections and rare hereditary disorders (e.g. glucose-6-phosphate dehydrogenase deficiency). Renal failure is commonly present, but is probably not a cause in itself. The patient usually presents with marked hyperventilation, which may progress to drowsiness, vomiting and eventually coma. Blood pressure is normal, there is no cyanosis and the patient is well perfused.

Treatment of severe type B lactic acidosis involves removal of the precipitating cause and the intravenous administration of sodium bicarbonate, although it may prove to be extremely difficult to reverse the acidosis and very large amounts of bicarbonate may be required (e.g. 1000 mmol). Therefore, some recommend that the first 2–3 litres are given as an isotonic (1.4%) solution, followed by 8.4% sodium bicarbonate. The large volumes of fluid required may precipitate volume overload and pulmonary oedema. Peritoneal dialysis with bicarbonate-buffered solution has been advocated for resistant cases (Vaziri et al, 1979).

Respiratory compensation for a metabolic acidosis is usually slightly delayed because the blood–brain barrier initially prevents the respiratory centre from sensing the increased blood $[H^+]$. Following this short delay, however, the patient hyperventilates and 'blows off' carbon dioxide to produce a compensatory respiratory alkalosis. As can be seen from Fig. 4.5, there is a limit to this respiratory compensation since values for P_aCO_2 less than about 1.5 kPa (11 mmHg) are in practice never achieved. It should also be noted that respiratory compensation cannot occur if the patient's ventilation is controlled.

Metabolic alkalosis

This can be caused by loss of acid, e.g. from the stomach with nasogastric suction or in high intestinal obstruction, or excessive administration of absorbable alkali. Overzealous treatment with intravenous sodium bicarbonate is frequently implicated. In these causes of metabolic alkalosis the urinary chloride concentration is usually low. Some less common causes of metabolic alkalosis in which urinary chloride is high include hyperaldosteronism, Cushing's syndrome, ingestion of liquorice and severe potassium deficiency. Depletion of the extracellular fluid volume and a reduction in total body potassium are both important precipitating factors in the development of metabolic alkalosis. Contraction of the extracellular compartment causes increased sodium reabsorption in exchange for hydrogen ions. The latter are lost in the urine and bicarbonate reabsorption is increased. Similarly, potassium depletion stimulates the kidneys to retain potassium in exchange for hydrogen ions. Diuretics are frequently implicated in both extracellular fluid volume depletion and hypokalaemia.

Treatment consists of correction of the underlying cause; specific treatment is rarely required. If severe alkalosis persists despite restoring the extracellular fluid volume and correction of potassium depletion, the carbonic anhydrase inhibitor acetazolamide or, occasionally, intravenous hydrochloric acid may be indicated.

Respiratory compensation for a metabolic alkalosis is often slight and it is rare to encounter a $P_aCO_2 > 6.5$ kPa (50 mmHg), even with severe alkalosis.

Interpretation of the acid–base state of the patient, therefore, proceeds as follows:
1 Look at the $[H^+]$ to see whether the patient is acidotic or alkalotic.
2 Look at the standard bicarbonate and the base excess. If the standard bicarbonate is low and the base excess negative (i.e. there is a base deficit) then there is a metabolic acidosis. If the standard bicarbonate is high and the base excess positive then there is a metabolic alkalosis.
3 Look at the PCO_2 to determine whether there is a respiratory component. If

the P_{CO_2} is high then there is a respiratory acidosis; if it is low, a respiratory alkalosis.

4 Although the primary abnormality is often indicated by the direction of the $[H^+]$ change, particularly in severe disturbances, this is not always the case. The nature of the primary abnormality can then only be determined by considering the clinical context in which it has arisen.

Alterations in oxygenation

Having interpreted the acid–base state, one can evaluate oxygenation. When interpreting the P_{O_2} it is important to remember that, as discussed in Chapter 2, it is the oxygen content of the arterial blood that matters and that this is determined by the percentage saturation of haemoglobin with oxygen. The latter is related to the P_{O_2} by the oxyhaemoglobin dissociation curve. The clinical significance of this is discussed in Chapter 2, but it is most important to look at the P_{O_2} in conjunction with the percentage saturation; in general, if the latter is greater than 90%, oxygenation can be considered to be adequate. Remember that $P_a O_2$ is influenced by factors other than pulmonary function, including alterations in $P_{\bar{v}} O_2$ caused by changing metabolic rate and/or cardiac output, and shifts in the position of the dissociation curve (see Chapter 2).

DETERMINATION OF OXYGEN CONTENT

As discussed above, derived values for oxygen content as produced by automated blood gas analysers are not sufficiently accurate even for clinical use. Direct measurement of oxygen content, or its calculation from accurately determined values for haemoglobin and oxygen saturation, is therefore often required, usually in order to derive other important variables such as oxygen consumption and percentage venous admixture.

Originally, direct measurement of oxygen content was performed using the technically difficult and time-consuming Van Slyke manometric technique. This method is no longer used routinely since it is now possible to obtain very accurate measurements of oxygen content with a commercially available fuel cell analyser (Lex O_2 Con, Lexington Instruments Ltd). Using an extremely accurate Hamilton syringe, a known volume of blood (20 µl) is injected into a 'scrubber' containing distilled water. The blood immediately haemolyses and the oxygen is displaced by a gas mixture containing carbon monoxide which is bubbled through the distilled water. The liberated oxygen is carried in the gas stream to a fuel cell which generates a current proportional to the total amount of oxygen. Since the volume of the sample is accurately known the oxygen content per 100 ml of blood can be calculated and displayed by the instrument. Although relatively simple, this method needs considerable care in order to produce good results. The instrument requires meticulous calibration and can easily be damaged by contaminating the fuel cell with blood. It is also essential that the sample is thoroughly mixed before being placed in the Hamilton syringe. This technique is therefore not suitable for use by medical or nursing personnel on-site in the intensive care unit.

In clinical practice, it is more usual to calculate oxygen content from accurately determined values for haemoglobin and oxygen saturation. These can be measured using a photometric technique. The bench oximeters designed for this purpose are relatively robust and easy to operate and can therefore be used on site by doctors who have been instructed in their use. For example, the Radiometer OSM 2 is an automated device which measures the optical absorbence of haemolysed blood at two wavelengths. The absorbance at 505 nm depends on the total haemoglobin concentration, while the ratio of the absorbance at 600 nm to that at 505 nm gives the percentage of oxygenated haemoglobin. Unfortunately, values obtained with this instrument are affected by the presence of abnormal haemoglobins such as carboxyhaemoglobin. It is most unlikely, however, that such abnormal haemoglobins will be present in intensive care patients and, in practice, oxygen contents derived in this way are very accurate. The Instrumentation Laboratories Model 282 is a more sophisticated and slightly more delicate device. It measures absorbances at four separate wavelengths and thus provides values for carboxy- and methaemoglobin as well as oxyhaemoglobin. These values, together with derived oxygen content, are then displayed digitally.

IN VIVO BLOOD GAS MEASUREMENT

There are obvious potential clinical advantages in monitoring blood gases continuously rather than intermittently. The instantaneous detection of changes in blood gas tensions allows rapid evaluation and ajustment of therapy, as well as immediate recognition of deteriorating cardiorespiratory function. The effects of potentially dangerous manoeuvres (e.g. hypoxaemia occurring during endotracheal suction) or accidents such as circuit disconnection are also immediately apparent.

Intravascular blood gas tensions can be monitored continuously using miniaturized electrodes or mass spectrometry, while oxygen saturation can be determined using fibre-optic oximeters. Blood gas tensions and oxygen saturation can also be estimated continuously using transcutaneous techniques.

Electrode systems

Techniques for continuous in vivo determination of oxygen tension are usually based on miniaturized Clark electrodes. In order to facilitate miniaturization, monopolar devices have been developed in which the Ag/AgCl reference electrode is separately applied to the skin. In clinical practice, however, the conventional arrangement of the Clark electrode is most often employed. Usually, these devices incorporate a lumen to allow discrete samples of arterial blood to be obtained intermittently.

Although the linear response of these electrodes is good when compared with bench analysis, they have a tendency to drift and are influenced by changes in body temperature. They therefore have to be calibrated at regular intervals against conventionally analysed arterial samples. Because fresh blood is continuously flowing past the electrode membrane, the blood gas factor is normally small and can be ignored, although in low flow states this may become a significant source of error (Rithalia et al, 1981).

Such electrodes have been widely used to monitor P_aO_2 continuously in neonates, in whom it is essential to control arterial oxygen tension within narrow limits at all times in order to avoid cerebral hypoxia on the one hand, and retrolental fibroplasia on the other. They have also been used for continuous monitoring of venous oxygen tension, and in critically ill adults a sustained fall in $P_{\bar{v}}O_2$ to below 5.3 kPa (40 mmHg) has been found to be a reliable indicator of respiratory or cardiovascular deterioration which was not always clinically obvious (Armstrong et al, 1978). Nevertheless, although a reduction in $P_{\bar{v}}O_2$ implies that tissue oxygenation is impaired, a normal value does not necessarily indicate that oxygenation is adequate. Despite the potential advantages of intravascular Po_2 electrodes, their use has not yet become established in adult intensive care practice.

The development of intravascular electrodes for determination of Pco_2 has been beset by technical problems, mainly the difficulty of miniaturizing glass electrodes and their fragility. These have prevented their introduction into the intensive care unit for long-term monitoring, although they have been used for limited periods in anaesthetized subjects.

Mass spectrometry

As well as being used for the measurement of inspired and expired gas concentrations as outlined above, mass spectrometers have been used to continuously monitor intravascular blood gas tensions. Indwelling, fine-bore, semi-flexible stainless steel catheters (which are impermeable to the analysed gases) are normally employed for sampling. The tip of the catheter is perforated and covered with a gas-permeable membrane, across which blood gases equilibrate. The proximal end is connected to a vacuum system which aspirates these gases into the mass spectrometer. The main advantage of this technique is that several gases can be analysed simultaneously. Clearly, this system will remove gases from the layer of blood adjacent to the membrane, thereby creating a significant 'blood gas factor'. It also requires prior calibration against in vitro blood gas analysis. To date, the cost and complexity of this technique, together with the need for frequent expert maintenance of the apparatus, has limited its introduction into clinical practice.

Fibre-optic spectrophotometry

This technique of in vivo oximetry utilizes an intravascular fibre-optic catheter and is based on the same principles as are employed in the bench oximeters described above. A beam of light consisting of a number of precisely known wavelengths is generated, usually by a light-emitting diode, and transmitted down one of two bundles of optical fibres. Light reflected from the red cells is returned to a photodiode detector along the other bundle of fibres. In this way, the percentage saturation of haemoglobin with oxygen can be measured continuously and accurately in vivo. Although fibre-optic spectrophotometers are generally very stable, the signal may be distorted by deposition of fibrin, or if the tip of the catheter impinges on the vessel wall. The latter can be prevented by enclosing the distal end in a cage.

These devices can be positioned relatively easily in the pulmonary artery and have been used successfully for continuous determination of mixed venous oxygen saturation ($S_{\bar{v}}O_2$). Fibre-optic oximeters have now been incorporated into Swan–Ganz catheters and this may facilitate their introduction into routine clinical practice.

Transcutaneous blood gas measurement (Shoemaker and Vidyasagar, 1981; Eberhard et al, 1981)

Transcutaneous determination of blood gas tensions is an attractive proposition since measurement can be continuous and yet the technique is non-invasive.

Transcutaneous Po_2 ($P_{tc}O_2$). As with continuous intravascular Po_2 determination, most of the initial experience with measurement of $P_{tc}O_2$ was gained in neonates. The principle of the method is based on increasing the diffusion of oxygen from the blood in the subdermal capillary loops to the skin surface, where its partial pressure can be measured with a conventional Clark electrode housed behind a membrane. The oxygen tension gradient from capillary to skin surface is clearly dependent on P_aO_2 but is also influenced by many other factors including skin thickness, tissue blood flow, tissue oxygen consumption and the position of the oxyhaemoglobin dissociation curve. Transcutaneous electrodes therefore incorporate a heating element which is maintained at 44–45°C and warms the underlying skin to approximately 43°C. This increases skin permeability and blood flow, as well as facilitating unloading of oxygen from haemoglobin by shifting the dissociation curve to the right. These effects are, however, to some extent offset by a local increase in oxygen consumption. Nevertheless, provided tissue blood flow is adequate, it is usually possible to obtain a reasonable linear correlation between $P_{tc}O_2$ and P_aO_2.

However, unless the electrode has been calibrated at an appropriate Po_2, the correlation with arterial values can be poor under conditions of hypoxia or hyperoxia. Furthermore, accurate results are very dependent on adequate skin blood flow so that in patients with low cardiac output $P_{tc}O_2$ is a poor indicator of P_aO_2. Although in neonates $P_{tc}O_2$ usually closely reflects P_aO_2, many feel that in adults, even when peripheral perfusion is good, $P_{tc}O_2$ should only be used as an indicator of trends in P_aO_2. Clinically, it has been shown that $P_{tc}O_2$ correlates with P_aO_2 during hyperoxaemia and hypoxaemia, with cardiac output during shock and with oxygen delivery in low flow states and hypoxaemia but not during hyperoxaemia or high output states (Tremper et al, 1980). These authors concluded that monitoring $P_{tc}O_2$ in critically ill adults should be particularly useful since it provides a continuous assessment of oxygen delivery and tissue oxygenation with a response time of less than one minute.

As discussed previously in this section, Clark electrodes consume oxygen and drift. Transcutaneous versions are no exception and require regular calibration against conventionally analysed arterial samples. Although the response time is rapid in infants (10–15 seconds) this increases to 45–60 seconds in adults and the reading will take 5–15 minutes to reach a plateau following application of the electrode. The area of skin underlying the electrode can be damaged by excessive heating; the skin may actually be burnt or tissue oedema can develop causing the electrode to under-read. These problems can be avoided by moving the electrode, which is usually applied to the anterior chest wall, to a new position every three to four hours, although it may be safe to leave small cathode electrodes in place for up to eight hours.

Recently, a polarographic oxygen sensor which can be applied to the conjunctiva has been described and this may in the future prove to be valuable in clinical practice (Fatt and Deutsch, 1983).

Transcutaneous P_{CO_2}. Most of these consist of a conventional glass pH electrode combined with a heating element. Carbon dioxide is, of course, more soluble than oxygen and is produced, rather than consumed, by the tissues. Furthermore, heating the skin increases local CO_2 production and capillary P_{CO_2}. Thus, $P_{tc}O_2$ is consistently higher than P_aCO_2 and the difference between the two varies considerably from patient to patient depending on skin characteristics. However, changes in $P_{tc}CO_2$ do follow the trend of alterations in P_aCO_2, although in shock $P_{tc}CO_2$ can be very high and the discrepancy between P_aCO_2 and $P_{tc}CO_2$ is increased.

Skin oximetry

Oximeters are available which can be applied, for example, to the ear lobe. Again, these are only accurate when peripheral blood flow is adequate and the reading is influenced by pigments both in the skin and the blood (e.g. bilirubin).

OTHER INDICES

In the most severely ill patients, more sophisticated indices of pulmonary function may occasionally prove useful, e.g. in following a patient's progress and response to therapy or deciding when to wean the patient from artificial ventilation.

Alveolar–arterial oxygen difference ($P_{A-a}O_2$)

This can be determined by measuring P_aO_2 and calculating P_AO_2 from the alveolar air equation (Chapter 2). This requires accurate determination of the F_IO_2, barometric pressure and P_aCO_2. The RQ can be assumed to be 0.8. The $P_{A-a}O_2$ has certain limitations as an index of pulmonary function:

1 It is influenced by the P_AO_2 so that even in normal subjects $P_{A-a}O_2$ increases as F_IO_2 rises.
2 It is influenced by the $P_{\bar{v}}O_2$, i.e. it will alter if cardiac output, metabolic rate or the position of the dissociation curve change.

Some feel that it is useful to determine the $P_{A-a}O_2$ with the patient breathing 100% oxygen. This can then be compared with predicted values under these circumstances and with values obtained in the same subject breathing air. However, breathing pure oxygen, even for short periods, can in itself impair lung function and this practice should in general be avoided.

Percentage venous admixture and dead space

Because of the limitations of $P_{A-a}O_2$ just described, it is more satisfactory to calculate percentage venous admixture. Physiological dead space is often calculated at the same time to provide the 'three compartment' analysis of respiratory function as described in Chapter 2.

This three-compartment analysis does not, however, provide any information as to the relative contribution of true shunt and V/Q disturbance to the total venous admixture, nor does it describe the nature of the V/Q inequality. Methods have been developed using the intravenous injection of inert tracer gases of different solubilities which can, when analysed by computer, produce a description of alveolar V/Q distributions. These techniques are not used in clinical practice at present.

Iso-shunt lines

For patients with hypoxaemia due to pulmonary venous admixture, and who are in a reasonably steady state, a series of lines can be plotted relating P_aO_2 to F_iO_2, each line representing the relationship for a particular value of venous admixture. It has been suggested that these 'iso-shunt' lines can be used to limit the frequency of blood gas analysis necessary to control oxygen therapy (Benatar et al, 1973).

The P_aO_2/F_iO_2 ratio

This can be used as a simple index of the severity of lung dysfunction.

Under some circumstances, other indices of respiratory function are sometimes monitored as a guide to management. For example, the maximum inspiratory force (measured as the peak negative pressure achieved when the patient makes a maximal inspiratory effort against a closed valve) has been used to assess a patient's ability to wean from the ventilator (see Chapter 13), while the measurement of FRC and compliance can be of value when adjusting PEEP (see Chapter 13). Changes in compliance can also give some indication of improvement or deterioration in pulmonary function.

Finally, some recent developments in the assessment of disturbances of lung function have included the thermodilution double indicator method for the measurement of extravascular lung water (Noble et al, 1980) and a number of techniques for determining the permeability of the alveolar-capillary membrane (Jones et al, 1982).

COMPUTERIZED MONITORING

Computers, and desk-top or even hand-held calculators, can be used to derive a large amount of relevant physiological data (e.g. vascular resistances, ventricular stroke work, oxygen consumption, oxygen delivery and percentage venous admixture) from measured variables (Shabot et al, 1977). The information produced in this way is now commonly known as a 'physiological profile' and is invaluable when managing complex cardiorespiratory problems. The ability of computers to perform calculations rapidly and reliably has also been utilized in programs designed to calculate, for example, fluid and electrolyte balances, complicated drug dosages (in particular, infusion regimens for inotropic drugs in $\mu g \ kg^{-1} \ min^{-1}$) and regimens for parenteral nutrition.

The storage and retrieval capabilities of computers can be useful for administrative and research purposes, allowing comprehensive patient records to be maintained which can include relevant data concerning diagnosis, treatment, indices of severity of illness (see Chapter 1), complications and outcome. This information allows the director of the unit to monitor its activity, as well as providing a record of morbidity and mortality figures. It can also be used for both retrospective and prospective surveys.

More sophisticated computer applications in intensive care have included monitoring systems which automatically store, manipulate and display patient data (Wiener and Weil, 1978). This data is acquired either directly from the monitoring devices, e.g. intravascular pressure measurements, or entered manually, as is usually the case for laboratory results such as blood gases. The information obtained in this way can be used to calculate important derived variables, such as vascular resistances, and these are then made available to the clinician. Graphical displays of the changes in selected variables over time ('trend plots') can also be produced and displayed on the visual display unit (VDU). All this information can be stored indefinitely on discs and retrieved as required. Although such systems have proved invaluable for research, some remain sceptical about their value for patient care (Cullen and Teplick, 1979) and there is no convincing evidence that earlier expectations of reductions in morbidity, mortality and costs have been fulfilled. Even the use of decision-making algorithms to automate certain aspects of patient care, such as the infusion of blood and administration of vasoactive drugs (Sheppard and Kouchoukos, 1976), appears to be of only limited benefit, although a closed-loop system provided better control of blood pressure in post cardiac surgery patients than could be obtained manually (Sheppard et al, 1975). Closed-loop systems have also been used to control infusions of mannitol to reduce intracranial pressure in head-injured patients.

Finally, computer-assisted learning techniques are proving to be extremely useful for teaching the principles of intensive care medicine to both undergraduates and graduates (Hinds et al, 1982).

FURTHER READING

Adams AP & Hahn CEW (1979) *Principles and Practice of Blood-gas Analysis.* London: Franklin Scientific Projects.

Kenny GNC & Davis PD (1983) Computer techniques in critical care medicine. In Ledingham IMcA & Hanning CD (eds) *Recent Advances in Critical Care Medicine 2*, pp 197–209. Edinburgh: Churchill Livingstone.

Mortimer AJ & Sykes MK (1983) Monitoring of ventilation. In Ledingham IMcA & Hanning CD (eds) *Recent Advances in Critical Care Medicine*, pp 15–28. Edinburgh: Churchill Livingstone.
Spence AA (ed.) (1982) *Respiratory Monitoring in Intensive Care*. Clinics in Critical Care Medicine, vol. 4. Edinburgh: Churchill Livingstone.

REFERENCES

Armstrong RF, Secker Walker J, St Andrew D et al (1978) Continuous monitoring of mixed venous oxygen tension (P_vO_2) in cardio-respiratory disorders. *Lancet* **i:** 632–634.
Benatar SR, Hewlett AM & Nunn JF (1973) The use of iso-shunt lines for control of oxygen therapy. *British Journal of Anaesthesia* **45:** 711–718.
Biswas CK, Ramos JM, Agroyannis B & Kerr DNS (1982) Blood gas analysis: effect of air bubbles in syringe and delay in estimation. *British Medical Journal* **284:** 923–927.
Bradley JG (1972) Errors in the measurement of blood P_{CO_2} due to dilution of the sample with heparin solution. *British Journal of Anaesthesia* **44:** 231–232.
Cole PV (1982) Bench analysis of blood gases. In Spence AA (ed) *Respiratory Monitoring in Intensive Care*. Clinics in Critical Care Medicine, vol. 4. Edinburgh: Churchill Livingstone.
Cullen DJ & Teplick R (1979) The role of computers in the future of intensive care. *Proceedings of the IEEE* **67:** 1307–1308.
Eberhard P, Mindt W & Schafer R (1981) Cutaneous blood gas monitoring in the adult. *Critical Care Medicine* **9:** 702–705.
Editorial (1973) Lactic acidosis. *Lancet* **ii:** 27–280.
Evers W, Racz GB & Levy AA (1972) A comparative study of plastic (polypropylene) and glass syringes in blood-gas analysis. *Anesthesia and Analgesia* **51:** 92–97.
Fatt I & Deutsch TA (1983) The relation of conjunctival P_{O_2} to capillary bed P_{O_2}. *Critical Care Medicine* **11:** 445–448.
Flenley DC (1978) Interpretation of blood-gas and acid-base data. *British Journal of Hospital Medicine* **20:** 384–394.
Flenley DC (1983) Acid-base balance. In Tinker J & Rapin M (eds) *Care of The Critically Ill Patient*, pp 85–97. Berlin: Springer-Verlag.
Goldberg M, Green SB, Moss ML et al (1973) Computer-based instruction and diagnosis of acid–base disorders. A systemic approach. *Journal of the American Medical Association* **223:** 269–275.
Gothard JWW, Busst CM, Branthwaite MA, Davies NJH & Denison DM (1980) Applications of respiratory mass spectrometry to intensive care. *Anaesthesia* **35:** 890–895.
Hinds CJ, Ingram D & Dickinson CJ (1982) Self-instruction and assessment in techniques of intensive care using a computer model of the respiratory system. *Intensive Care Medicine* **8:** 115–123.
Jones JG, Minty BD & Royston D (1982) The physiology of leaky lungs. *British Journal of Anaesthesia* **54:** 705–721.
Milledge JS & Stott FD (1977) Inductive plethysmography—a new respiratory transducer. *Journal of Physiology* **267:** 4–50.
Noble WH, Kay JC, Maret KH & Caskanette G (1980) Reappraisal of extravascular lung thermal volume as a measure of pulmonary oedema. *Journal of Applied Physiology* **48:** 120–129.
Osborn JJ (1978) A flowmeter for respiratory monitoring. *Critical Care Medicine* **6:** 349–351.

Rithalia SVS, Bennett PJ & Tinker J (1981) The performance characteristics of an intra-arterial oxygen electrode. *Intensive Care Medicine* 7: 305–307.

Shabot MM, Shoemaker WC & State D (1977) Rapid bedside computation of cardiorespiratory variables with a programmable calculator. *Critical Care Medicine* 5: 105–111.

Sheppard LC & Kouchoukos NT (1976) Computers as monitors. *Anesthesiology* 45: 250–259.

Sheppard LC, Kouchoukos NT, Shotts JF & Wallace FD (1975) Regulation of mean arterial pressure by computer control of vasoactive agents in postoperative patients. *Computers in Cardiology (IEEE 75 CH 1018-C)* 91–94.

Shoemaker WC & Vidyasagar D (1981) Physiological and clinical significance of $P_{tc}O_2$ and $P_{tc}CO_2$ measurements. *Critical Care Medicine* 9: 689–690.

Sykes MK & Vickers MD (1973) *Principles of Measurement for Anaesthetists.* Oxford: Blackwell Scientific.

Tremper KK, Waxman K, Bowman R & Shoemaker WC (1980) Continuous transcutaneous oxygen monitoring during respiratory failure, cardiac decompensation, cardiac arrest and CPR. *Critical Care Medicine* 8: 377–381.

Vaziri ND, Ness R, Wellikson L, Barton C & Greep N (1979) Bicarbonate buffered peritoneal dialysis. An effective adjunct in the treatment of lactic acidosis. *American Journal of Medicine* 67: 392–396.

Westenskow DR & Tucker SM (1981) Evaluation of a ventilation monitor. *Critical Care Medicine* 9: 64–66.

Wiener F & Weil MH (1978) Computer-based monitoring and data management in critical care. *Methods of Information in Medicine* 17: 252–260.

Yoshiya I, Shimada Y & Tanaka K (1979) Evaluation of a hot-wire respiratory flowmeter for clinical applicability. *Journal of Applied Physiology* 47: 1131–1135.

5
Fluid and Electrolyte Balance and Nutritional Support

FLUID AND ELECTROLYTE BALANCE

A detailed discussion of the basic physiological aspects of fluid and electrolyte balance is outside the scope of this book. This section will therefore consider some aspects of particular importance in the critically ill patient.

The vast majority of intensive care patients are unable to drink and will require intravenous fluid replacement. The average water requirement for a normal adult is between 20 and $60\,ml\,kg^{-1}$ per day, but most intensive care patients are stressed and tend to retain both sodium and water. This is exacerbated by artificial ventilation (see Chapter 13) while in those breathing humidified gases, insensible losses are approximately half the estimated normal $500–900\,ml\,day^{-1}$. Furthermore, normal oxidation of food produces significant volumes of water (0.41, 0.60 and 1.07 ml of water per gram of protein, carbohydrate and fat respectively). Some degree of renal dysfunction is not uncommon and this will further impair the patient's ability to excrete a sodium and water load. Critically ill patients are therefore easily overloaded with salt and water. This is often combined with an increase in capillary permeability and hypoproteinaemia, the combination leading to peripheral and pulmonary oedema. For these reasons some degree of fluid restriction, with minimal sodium intake, is often necessary, particularly in the artificially ventilated patient. Often, an appropriate regimen, initially, is $20\,ml\,kg^{-1}$ of 5% dextrose per 24 hours. Additional sources of fluid and electrolytes, such as the herparinized saline used to flush intravascular catheters and the solutions used as vehicles for intravenous drugs, must also be taken into account.

On the other hand, some patients will be losing abnormally large volumes of fluid and electrolytes, e.g. as diarrhoea or drainage from fistulae. If the patient is pyrexial, sweating or hyperventilating with inadequate humidification, insensible losses will be increased. Urine output may be increased by diuretic therapy or by an osmotic diuresis, as may occur with hyperglycaemia. More rarely, polyuria may result from diabetes insipidus complicating, for example, a head injury.

The situation is therefore complex. Excessive administration of fluid and electrolytes to a critically ill patient may lead to overhydration with 'wet lungs', while in some cases ill-advised fluid restriction, or inadequate replacement of large losses, can cause significant dehydration with the danger of renal damage.

An appropriate intravenous fluid regimen must be devised for each individual patient based on a thorough knowledge and understanding of the factors discussed above, guided by the results of laboratory investigations and, if possible, daily weighing. Plasma urea, creatinine, electrolyte and blood sugar levels should be measured at least once a day, and often more frequently. The total output of fluid as urine, gastric aspirate and from any drains, together with the total intravenous and oral input, should be calculated 12-hourly and the overall fluid balance recorded. If necessary, the intravenous regimen can then be modified accordingly. In difficult cases it may be helpful to measure urinary urea and electrolyte concentrations, as well as the electrolyte content of the gastric aspirate and any drainage fluid, so that the total input and output of each individual constituent can be calculated.

Luckily, the body is generally surprisingly tolerant of our rather crude attempts to control its fluid and electrolyte content, particularly when the kidneys are functioning normally. However, if the basic principles of management are not understood, or careless mistakes are made, serious abnormalities will result. The important constituents to be considered are water, sodium, potassium and magnesium. There may be an excess or deficit of each, either singly or in combination.

Water depletion

Water depletion rarely occurs in isolation since it is usually combined with some degree of sodium loss. Predominant water depletion may occur if intake is inadequate or there are excessive losses of hypotonic fluid caused, for example, by diarrhoea, sweating or hyperventilation. Losses of water are initially distributed evenly throughout the body compartments. Once the deficit is severe enough to cause a decreased circulating volume, aldosterone is released causing renal retention of sodium. Because of the osmotic effect of the increase in plasma sodium concentration, water then leaves the cells and there is loss of tissue turgor. Plasma sodium is increased, plasma urea is slightly increased and plasma osmolality is normal or increased. The PCV rises only in the later stages of water depletion, and the patient is oliguric with a concentrated urine. Treatment is with intravenous 5% dextrose or, if sodium has been lost as well, dextrose–saline.

Water intoxication

This is usually iatrogenic and caused by excessive intravenous administration of hypotonic solutions (e.g. 5% dextrose) in the presence of a reduced ability to excrete water, often caused by increased levels of antidiuretic hormone (ADH) in response to stress or in association with an 'inappropriate' secretion of ADH. Acute, severe water intoxication can cause confusion which may progress to convulsions and coma. Plasma sodium is low, often less than $120 \, \text{mmol} \, l^{-1}$. Mild cases can be treated simply by restriction of intake; in more severe cases twice normal saline can be administered. If renal function is impaired, the latter may be dangerous and dialysis will be required. In some patients with inappropriate ADH secretion fluid restriction alone may be insufficient and in such cases drugs which antagonize ADH, e.g. demeclocycline (demethylchlortetracycline), may prove useful.

Hyponatraemia

A low plasma sodium can be caused not only by water intoxication but also by depletion of total body sodium. Some causes of the latter commonly encountered in intensive care patients are diuretic therapy, renal disease, and fluid losses from the alimentary tract or intra-abdominal drains. Significant sodium depletion will cause a fall in intravascular volume and stimulate release of aldosterone. Urinary potassium excretion therefore increases while sodium ions are retained. Hyponatraemia is often exacerbated by the use of hypotonic intravenous fluids (e.g. 5% dextrose, dextrose–saline) to replace isotonic losses from, for example, the alimentary tract. Usually, the situation can be resolved by the administration of normal saline; very rarely, it may be necessary to use twice normal saline.

A controversial cause of hyponatraemia in the critically ill is the 'sick cell syndrome' (Flear and Singh, 1973). This occurs only in the most severely ill patients and may account for the close association between a low plasma sodium and a poor prognosis. It is postulated that a defect at cellular level causes sodium ions to enter the cell in exchange for potassium ions, which are then lost in the urine. Although plasma sodium is low, total body sodium content is normal. Possible mechanisms include an increase in membrane permeability or a failure of the sodium pump caused by an inadequate supply of energy in the form of adenosine triphosphate (ATP). The aim of treatment is to restore the energy supply to the cells by treating the underlying disease process and improving tissue oxygenation. Occasionally, it may be worth administering an infusion of dextrose, insulin and potassium since this regimen may stimulate cellular uptake of potassium in exchange for sodium, as well as replenishing total body potassium levels. An alternative explanation for this abnormality is that it is simply a response to pure hypokalaemia which causes intracellular hypotonia and a redistribution of water.

Hypernatraemia

As discussed above, hypernatraemia occurs most commonly in situations of predominant water depletion. It may also occur in association with salt retention in acute renal failure and in this situation can be exacerbated by the administration of excessive sodium ions, often as 8.4% sodium bicarbonate given in an attempt to correct a metabolic acidosis. Treatment is with hypotonic intravenous fluids or dialysis.

Hypokalaemia

Potassium depletion is one of the commonest abnormalities of fluid and electrolyte balance encountered in the intensive care unit and is usually related to inadequate replacement of excessive urinary or gastrointestinal losses. There is no known potassium-retaining hormone. For a number of reasons, critically ill patients are particularly prone to the development of hypokalaemia. Elevated levels of aldosterone are found in both cardiac and liver failure as well as part of the stress response, while the administration of steroids and diuretics also increases urinary potassium losses. Enormous quantities of potassium may be lost in the urine during the recovery phases of acute intrinsic renal failure, and severe hypokalaemia may itself lead to tubular dysfunction.

There is a reciprocal relationship between the urinary excretion of hydrogen ions and potassium ions; thus, when hydrogen ions are being reabsorbed by the renal tubules, potassium ions are excreted in order to maintain ionic equilibrium. Likewise, if total body potassium levels are low, this ion is conserved and hydrogen ions are lost in the urine. This leads to a 'hypokalaemic metabolic alkalosis' with a paradoxically acid urine. Sometimes, plasma potassium levels are within the normal range but if there is an unexplained metabolic alkalosis with an acid urine, careful administration of potassium chloride, sometimes combined with dextrose and insulin, will usually correct the alkalosis.

Hypokalaemia may be detected by recognizing the associated ECG changes of ST segment depression, decreased T wave amplitude and U waves (Fig. 5.1). Hypokalaemia can cause supraventricular tachycardias, particularly in the presence of digoxin, as well as more serious ventricular dysrhythmias and, for this reason, must be corrected.

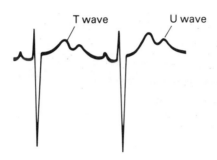

T wave   U wave

Fig. 5.1 Electrocardiographic changes in hypokalaemia—lead V3, showing U waves. These are best seen in the anterior chest leads. Because of T wave flattening and ST depression, the U wave may sometimes be mistaken for a T wave.

Treatment is with potassium chloride by infusion, either alone or combined with dextrose and insulin. Concentrated solutions are extremely irritant and must therefore be administered via a centrally placed catheter. If potassium is given too rapidly, plasma concentrations may reach dangerous levels before equilibration between extra- and intracellular compartments has occurred.

Hyperkalaemia

This is frequently iatrogenic and caused by excessive potassium administration, often when the onset of acute renal failure has been missed. Other causes of hyperkalaemia include acidosis, hypercatabolism and, occasionally, massive blood transfusion (see Chapter 10, p. 144). If suxamethonium is administered to patients with diffuse tissue damage, e.g. muscle trauma, burns, tetanus or paralysis, large quantities of potassium may be released into the circulation. There is a risk of this complication from between 5 and 15 days after the injury, and the danger persists for 2–3 months in patients who have sustained burns or trauma, and for perhaps 3–6 months in those with

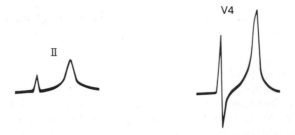

Fig. 5.2 Electrocardiographic changes in hyperkalaemia—leads II and V4. Note tall, peaked, narrow T waves and broad QRS complexes. There is also atrial standstill.

upper motor neurone lesions (Gronert and Theye, 1975). It is of particular importance in patients with renal failure.

The ECG changes associated with hyperkalaemia are peaked T waves and widening of the QRS complexes, followed by bradycardia and asystole (Fig. 5.2). Treatment is therefore urgent. Obviously, potassium administration should be stopped, and in extreme emergencies 10 ml 10% calcium chloride intravenously will temporarily antagonize the cardiac effects of hyperkalaemia. An intravenous injection of 50 ml 50% dextrose containing 20 units soluble insulin will drive potassium into the cells. Alkalinization with sodium bicarbonate and, if possible, hyperventilation will move potassium into the intracellular compartment, as well as enhancing potassium excretion via the kidneys; the former has by far the greater effect on plasma potassium levels. Sodium bicarbonate should be avoided in patients prone to sodium overload, e.g. those with renal failure. Rectally administered sodium or calcium exchange resins have an onset of action within about 30 minutes which should last for up to six hours. In many cases, however, these measures only defer dangerous consequences while arrangements are made for definitive treatment with dialysis.

Hypomagnesaemia

Critically ill patients may develop hypomagnesaemia due to the excessive use of diuretics, the administration of insulin in cases of diabetic ketoacidosis, or large gastrointestinal fluid losses. Hypomagnesaemia may also develop in association with malabsorption and if patients are maintained on parenteral fluids for long periods without supplementary magnesium.

Magnesium is important for normal neuromuscular function and the features of deficiency are similar to those of hypocalcaemia, with tetany and muscle weakness. Treatment is with oral magnesium hydroxide, intramuscular magnesium chloride or, in severe cases, magnesium sulphate by slow intravenous infusion.

Hypermagnesaemia

This occurs most commonly as a result of excessive magnesium administration and/or renal failure. The main adverse effects are on cardiac conduction, with prolongation of the P–R interval and QRS complexes and peaked T waves.

At even higher levels, respiratory paralysis and coma may occur, with cardiac arrest as the terminal event.

NUTRITIONAL SUPPORT

During a period of total starvation, the glycogen stores (150 g and 75 g in muscle and liver respectively) will be depleted within 24–48 hours. Subsequently, energy must be obtained by utilizing triglycerides from fat stores and amino acids derived from protein (mainly muscle but also, to a lesser extent, the viscera). Under these circumstances, a normal, unstressed, 70 kg individual will break down approximately 75 g of protein and 160 g of fat per day, liberating 7500 kJ (1800 kcal) (Cahill, 1970) and producing a negative nitrogen balance of about 12 g day^{-1}. Later, an increasing proportion of the energy requirements is obtained from fat and the negative nitrogen balance falls to approximately 5 g day^{-1}. Critically ill patients are often unable to make this latter adjustment and, combined with an increased metabolic rate (e.g. + 10% following uncomplicated surgery; + 20–50% with major sepsis; + 50–125% in burns (Kinney, 1975)), this can produce a negative nitrogen balance of as much as 35 g day^{-1}.

It has been recognized for many years that there is an increased risk of complications in surgical patients with pre-existing protein/energy malnutrition (Studley, 1936) and that this is largely related to sepsis, presumably associated with inadequate immune responses (Forse et al, 1981) and impaired tissue repair. Institution of nutritional support in the preoperative period may reduce the incidence of sepsis whilst improving healing of wounds and anastomoses. For example, Müller et al (1982) found that preoperative parenteral nutrition significantly reduced both the incidence of major complications and the mortality following surgery in patients with gastrointestinal carcinoma. Furthermore, in patients with enterocutaneous fistulae, both survival rate and the incidence of non-surgical closure of the fistula can be increased by total parenteral nutrition (TPN) (Himal et al, 1974). It is also undoubtedly possible to provide adequate nutritional support for an indefinite period using home TPN in patients with severe irreversible malabsorption (e.g. a 'short-bowel' syndrome) who are otherwise relatively fit.

Although it is known that a patient who loses more than 30% of his initial body weight in the course of an acute metabolic illness has only a remote chance of survival, it has proved more difficult to establish the value of nutritional support during the acute phase of a critical illness. It is not clear, for example, whether under these circumstances TPN can convert a severely catabolic patient to anabolism. Certainly during the first 48–72 hours of the acute episode it is generally unnecessary to feed the patient and during this period TPN may seriously complicate management. Because of the stress response, nutrients are unlikely to be fully utilized, hyperglycaemia is easily provoked and the administration of large volumes of intravenous fluids as TPN can precipitate fluid overload. Nevertheless, nutritional support should be instituted as soon as practicable in order to prevent serious reductions in body cell mass and to ensure adequate supplies of protein and energy for tissue repair and resisting infection. If loss of muscle bulk is allowed to progress, respiratory muscle weakness may compromise the patient's ability to breathe spontaneously. Moreover, malnutrition may be associated with abnormalities of the lung parenchyma as well as an increased susceptibility to pulmonary infection (Askanazi et al, 1982). Larca and Greenbaum (1982) have shown that ventilator-dependent patients who respond to nutritional support by increasing protein synthesis are more likely to wean from respiratory support than those who do not. Generally, in the absence of serious complications, feeding should be initiated within 2–3 days of the acute episode.

Some objective measures of the patient's nutritional state might help the clinician to assess the need for nutritional support. However, although the parameters which can be assessed reasonably easily, such as serum albumin, the triceps skin fold thickness and cutaneous responses to recall antigens (Forse et al, 1981), can define the nutritional status of a population of patients, they are generally relatively insensitive and lack specificity. Fortunately, in the majority of individual cases the need for nutritional support is obvious and such objective tests are usually superfluous.

In the past, many critically ill patients were fed intravenously. This is an expensive technique associated with a significant risk of serious complications and it is now recognized that in the majority of patients enteral feeding, which is relatively cheap and safe, can provide adequate nourishment. However, it is sometimes difficult to provide sufficient protein and energy to achieve an overall positive nitrogen balance, particularly in the hypercatabolic patient.

Enteral nutrition

This method of feeding can be used provided bowel sounds are present and the gastric aspirate is less than $40\,\mathrm{ml\,h^{-1}}$. Rarely, enteral feeding is administered via a gastrostomy or jejunostomy, which may have been fashioned at the time of surgery in a patient undergoing, for example, an oesophago-gastrectomy. In the majority of cases, however, the feed is delivered to the stomach using a nasogastric tube. In patients at risk of regurgitation, e.g. those with gastric atony, it may be advantageous to position the tube in the duodenum or jejunum. Sometimes, it is only possible to achieve this endoscopically.

Fine-bore nasogastric tubes are more comfortable and less likely to cause oesophageal ulceration and stricture than traditional tubes. They can be used in conscious patients, who are able to protect their own airways, and are ideal for long-term use. Some are supplied with a wire introducer, some can be stiffened by placing them in a refrigerator and others have mercury weighted tips. The latter may be easier to position in patients with an endotracheal tube in place. In either case, it is possible when inserting a fine-bore tube to push it past the low pressure cuff of an endotracheal or tracheostomy tube and into the lungs. Unconscious or debilitated patients and those with bulbar palsy may not react to the presence of such a tube in their major airways, and it is most important to check its position before starting the feed. It is usually not possible to aspirate gastric contents through a fine-bore tube, but it may be possible to inject sufficient air to hear this entering the stomach with a stethoscope placed over the epigastrum. An x-ray should then be taken to verify that the tube is correctly positioned.

The majority of intensive care patients are unable to protect their own airways. Some patients are supine and the presence of a nasogastric tube renders the gastro-oesophageal sphincter incompetent, allowing reflux of gastric contents. The presence of a cuffed endotracheal or tracheostomy tube is not a certain barrier to inhalation since liquids may find their way past a low-pressure cuff. In such patients, therefore, fluid must not be allowed to accumulate in the stomach and the nasogastric tube must be of a sufficient size to allow aspiration. Double-lumen nasogastric tubes are available which allow feeding down one lumen and aspiration via the other. It is also easier to be certain of the position of these larger tubes.

The feed should be administered at a constant rate, rather than as boluses, in order to reduce the incidence of diarrhoea. To avoid the risk of regurgitation, the feed can be discontinued every five hours and the stomach aspirated after a one-hour 'rest period'. If large quantities of feed are obtained, gastric stasis is occurring and enteral nutrition should be discontinued. An infusion pump can be used to control the rate of the infusion more accurately and this may further reduce the incidence of diarrhoea in those with impaired gastrointestinal function (Jones et al, 1980). Although the value of 'starter' regimens in reducing gastrointestinal side effects has recently been questioned (Keohane et al, 1984) it is conventional to increase the concentration and volume of feed over 4–5 days. The occurrence of diarrhoea is closely related to concomitant antibiotic therapy (Keohane et al, 1983b, 1984) and this is therefore a common problem in the critically ill. Occasionally, *Clostridium difficile* infection may be responsible, but lactase deficiency is probably a rare cause of diarrhoea (Keohane et al, 1983b). If diarrhoea does occur, some form of roughage, such as Cologel, may be added to the feed and agents such as codeine phosphate or Imodium can be used to reduce gastrointestinal motility.

Other complications of enteral feeding include regurgitation and aspiration, oesophageal ulceration and stricture formation (particularly with large-bore tubes), hyperglycaemia, deficiencies of potassium, phosphate and zinc, as well as mild abnormalities of liver function.

In general, one of the proprietary, low-residue, whole protein feeds should be used. These provide approximately 75 g of protein and 8400 kJ (2000 kcal) in two litres of feed, with a non-protein calorie to nitrogen ratio which is usually less than 200 : 1 (see below). If it is considered necessary, additional energy can be provided by adding, for example, Caloreen or Maxijul to the feed. The majority are lactose-free and contain most of the daily requirements of electrolytes, trace elements and vitamins. Predigested 'elemental' diets have been advocated for those patients in whom luminal nutrient hydrolysis is severely impaired, e.g. exocrine pancreatic insufficiency, obstructive jaundice and short bowel syndrome. However, there is no evidence that these more expensive feeds offer any advantage for the majority of patients. Hyperosmolar feeds may be more likely to produce diarrhoea, although this was not the case in one recent study (Keohane et al, 1984) and it is conventional to use diets which are isotonic with plasma (osmolality in the range 285–300 mosmol kg^{-1}).

Total parenteral nutrition (TPN)

This will be required in those patients in whom enteral nutrition is contraindicated or fails due to gastric stasis, intractable diarrhoea or malabsorption. TPN may also be required when it proves impossible to provide sufficient energy via the enteral route. Probably the most dangerous complication of intravenous feeding is the development of infection and septicaemia. The procedure outlined below is designed to minimize the risk of this and other complications.

The infraclavicular approach to the subclavian vein is the preferred route for insertion of the intravascular catheter, since it allows the patient unrestricted movement of the upper limbs, head and neck, and minimizes movement of the catheter at the skin puncture site. Intravenous feeding is never an emergency and catheter placement should be performed as a planned procedure with full aseptic precautions. A silicone catheter should be used as these are the least thrombogenic and many authorities recommend the use of a subcutaneous 'tunnel'. This may reduce the incidence of catheter-related sepsis (Keohane et al, 1983a), probably because infection originating at the site of exit of the catheter from the skin must travel some distance before gaining access to the blood stream. An alternative is to insert a Hickman catheter surgically. These large-bore silicone catheters seem to be associated with a lower risk of obstruction, and are being used increasingly frequently. The puncture sites should be sprayed with an antiseptic such as povidone–iodine (an alternative is povidone–iodine ointment) and a transparent adhesive dressing applied. This allows frequent inspection of the wound for signs of infection, whilst avoiding the need to disturb the dressing.

Correct positioning of the catheter must be confirmed before intravenous feeding is started. It should be possible to aspirate venous blood freely and a chest x-ray should be performed to ensure that the catheter tip is in the superior vena cava. Usually, an infusion pump is used to ensure that the solution is administered constantly at the required rate throughout the 24-hour period.

Once inserted, the catheter should be used only for intravenous feeding and never for administering drugs, blood or blood products, or for sampling blood. Except under exceptional circumstances, the use of 2- or 3-way taps and Y-connectors must be avoided. Recently, double-lumen Hickman catheters have been introduced which can be used to ensure that one lumen is dedicated solely to the TPN solution, even in those in whom venous access is restricted. In some centres, the various constituents of the appropriate 24-hour feeding regimen are premixed in the pharmacy in a single bag (usually containing 2–3 litres of solution) using an aseptic technique. The giving set is changed with each new feeding bag or at the end of each 24-hour cycle. If facilities for making up a feeding bag are not available, the various constituents of the regimen should be administered simultaneously using 3-way taps or Y-connectors.

The feeding line should be removed if signs of infection (unexplained fever, pus or erythema at puncture sites) or thrombophlebitis develop. On removal, the tip should be sent for culture for both bacteria and fungi.

Selection of the appropriate intravenous feeding regimen

This must provide the patient with protein, energy (carbohydrate with or without fats), electrolytes, water, vitamins and trace elements. Depending on the degree of catabolism, patients will require between 1 and 2 g of protein $kg^{-1} day^{-1}$ (i.e. 7–20 g N_2 per day). In malnourished individuals, the restoration of body cell mass is very slow and appears to be directly related to the total energy intake, provided adequate quantities of protein are also given. However, increasing the protein intake to more than 1.5–2 g kg^{-1} body weight will not accelerate weight gain (Shizgal and Forse, 1980). Surprisingly, it is possible to achieve protein sparing in a previously well-nourished patient following moderately severe trauma, e.g. elective surgery, by administering only amino acids via a peripheral vein. In this way, body cell mass may be preserved until full nutritional support is established either enterally or parenterally. In practice, however, this technique is rarely used.

Energy requirements can be estimated assuming a resting metabolic rate of 126 kJ (30 kcal) $kg^{-1} day^{-1}$ plus another 63 kJ (15 kcal) $kg^{-1} day^{-1}$ in the critically ill. If the patient is pyrexial, another 12.6 kJ (3 kcal) $kg^{-1} day^{-1}$ should be added for each degree centigrade rise in body temperature. Carbohydrate calories are more efficient than lipid calories (Shizgal and Forse, 1980). Approximately 840 kJ (200 kcal)) of the energy requirements should be supplied as carbohydrate for each gram of N_2 in order to achieve efficient utilization of protein, and the two should be administered simultaneously. There is some evidence that in the hypercatabolic patient the optimal calorie to nitrogen ratio falls to about 140 : 1 and that in those who are less catabolic the ratio may be closer to 250 : 1. The administration of excessive quantities of non-protein energy should be avoided since this may lead to the development of generalized fat deposition and a 'fatty' liver.

Protein is administered in the form of solutions containing a mixture of essential and semi-essential amino acids. Often, the nitrogen content is made up with a 'stuffer' of a relatively cheap amino acid, such as glycine. The use of excessive amounts of such 'stuffers' can lead to a rise in blood ammonia levels and a high proportion may be lost in the urine. The body can only utilize L-amino acids and approximately 25% of the total nitrogen content should consist of essential amino acids. A mixture of non-essential amino acids is also required for efficient protein synthesis.

Fructose, sorbitol and alcohol are now no longer used as energy sources. Glucose is the carbohydrate of choice, the only disadvantage being the development of hyperglycaemia. Critically ill patients are generally intolerant of glucose because of high circulating levels of insulin antagonists. Furthermore, exogenously administered steroids and other drugs such as thiazide diuretics, are diabetogenic. Extra insulin is therefore usually required, and potassium may be added as well. Administration of this mixture may reduce the catabolic response (Hinton et al, 1971).

Fat solutions are an excellent source of calories but it can be difficult to incorporate them in a 'feeding bag'. However, because they are iso-osmolar, with a neutral pH, they are non-irritant and can be administered via a peripheral vein. Fat is usually given as the soya bean preparation Intralipid (10% or 20%). It is not essential to administer fat on a daily basis except to provide sufficient energy without administering excessive amounts of glucose and water. Fat solutions do, however, prevent the development of essential fatty acid deficiency and are a source of cholesterol and phosphate (as phospholipids), although the latter may not be readily available. In some cases, it may be sufficient to administer Intralipid once or twice a week via a peripheral vein, although the present trend is to return to administering fat solutions daily. Some patients with hepatic disease or extensive sepsis are intolerant of Intralipid. It is important to ensure that fat solutions are discontinued at least six hours prior to obtaining blood samples and to check that the plasma is not lipaemic. If fat globules are seen, this suggests that the patient is intolerant of fat and there is a risk of contaminating autoanalysers. There is some evidence that Intralipid can interfere with pulmonary function, but in practice this is probably not a significant problem (Askanazi et al, 1982).

Appropriate solutions should be included in the regimen to provide adequate quantities of sodium, potassium, magnesium, calcium and phosphate. Deficiency of the latter is associated with a reduced red cell 2-3, DPG concentration and an increase in the oxygen affinity of haemoglobin. Extra iron may also be required and in long-term intravenous feeding, replacement of trace metals such as copper, manganese and zinc will become important. Hypomagnesaemia may produce latent or overt tetany while zinc deficiency may be associated with impaired wound healing. All water- and fat-soluble vitamins must also be provided, whether by using Parentrovite I and II with vitamin D, vitamin K, vitamin B_{12} and folic acid, or by using some of the newer preparations which contain all of these.

Apart from sepsis and hyperglycaemia, complications of intravenous feeding include fluid overload, metabolic acidosis, electrolyte imbalance and deficiencies of vitamins and trace elements. Careful monitoring is therefore required if these complications are to be avoided. It is clearly important to keep an accurate daily record of fluid balance and the patient should be weighed daily if this is practicable. Urea, electrolytes and blood sugar should also be measured daily. Urine testing for sugar is unreliable. In particular, if, as is usual, the patient is receiving an insulin infusion, blood sugar should be determined by the nursing staff at the bedside using, for example, a reflectometer. Initially, this may be performed hourly, but once a stable regimen is established, the frequency of blood sugar estimations can be progressively reduced to four-hourly. Liver function tests (including estimation of calcium and phosphate), plasma creatinine and a full blood count should be performed twice weekly. A 24-hour collection of urine for determination of urea, electrolyte and creatinine concentrations allows calculation of creatinine clearance and nitrogen balance. The following simplified formula can be used to estimate nitrogen losses:

Nitrogen loss in grams = (mmol urinary urea excreted in 24 h $\times$ 0.028) + 2
(where + 2 represents an approximation of non-urinary urea losses)

Plasma magnesium should be measured once a week, and levels of vitamin B_{12}, folate, iron, total iron binding capacity and zinc should be estimated monthly. Normally, all these investigations should also be performed before feeding begins.

Finally, it has been shown that TPN increases CO_2 production, particularly when glucose is the primary source of non-protein energy (Askanazi et al, 1982) and this may significantly inhibit weaning from ventilatory support in those with borderline respiratory function.

FURTHER READING

Hanson GC (1978) The management of acute disorders of fluid and electrolyte balance. In Hanson GC & Wright PL (eds) *Medical Management of the Critically Ill*, pp 158–188. London: Academic Press.

Shizgal HM (1983) Nutritional failure. In. Tinker J & Rapin M (eds) *Care of the Critically Ill Patient*, pp 483–502. Berlin: Springer-Verlag.

Silk DBA (1983) *Nutritional Support in Hospital Practice.* Oxford: Blackwell.

Willatts SM (1982) *Lecture notes on fluid and electrolyte balance.* Oxford: Blackwell.

REFERENCES

Askanazi J, Weissman C, Rosenbaum SH et al (1982) Nutrition and the respiratory system. *Critical Care Medicine* **10:** 163–172.

Cahill GF Jr (1970) Starvation in man. *New England Journal of Medicine* **282:** 668–675.

Flear CTG & Singh CM (1973) Hyponatraemia and sick cells. *British Journal of Anaesthesia* **45:** 976–994.

Forse RA, Christou N, Meakins JL, MacLean LD & Shizgal HM (1981) Reliability of skin testing as a measure of nutritional state. *Archives of Surgery* **116:** 1284–1288.

Gronert GA & Theye RA (1975) Pathophysiology of hyperkalaemia induced by succinylcholine. *Anesthesiology* **43:** 89–99.

Himal HS, Allard, JR, Nadeau JE, Freeman JB & MacLean LD (1974) The importance of adequate nutrition in closure of small intestinal fistulas. *British Journal of Surgery* **61:** 724–726.

Hinton P, Allison SP, Littlejohn S & Lloyd J (1971) Insulin and glucose to reduce catabolic response to injury in burned patients. *Lancet* **i:** 767–769.

Jones BJM, Payne S & Silk DBA (1980) Indications for pump assisted enteral feeding. *Lancet* **i:** 1057–1058.

Keohane PP, Jones BJM, Attrill H et al (1983a) Effect of catheter tunnelling and a nutrition nurse on catheter sepsis during parenteral nutrition—a controlled trial. *Lancet* **ii:** 1388–1390.

Keohane PP, Attrill H, Jones BJM et al (1983b) The role of lactose and *Clostridium difficile* in the pathogenesis of enteral feeding associated diarrhoea. *Clinical Nutrition* **1:** 259–264.

Keohane PP, Attrill H, Love M, Frost P & Silk DBA (1984) Relation between osmolality of diet and gastrointestinal side effects in enteral nutrition. *British Medical Journal* **288:** 678–680.

Kinney JM (1975) Energy requirements of the surgical patient. In *Manual of surgical nutrition, Committee on pre- and postoperative care, American College of Surgeons.* pp 223–235. Philadelphia: Saunders.

Larca L & Greenbaum DM (1982) Effectiveness of intensive nutritional regimes in patients who fail to wean from mechanical ventilation. *Critical Care Medicine* **10:** 297–300.

Müller JM, Dienst C, Brenner U & Pichlmaier H (1982) Pre-operative parenteral feeding in patients with gastrointestinal carcinoma. *Lancet* **i:** 68–71.

Shizgal HM & Forse RA (1980) Protein and calorie requirements with total parenteral nutrition. *Annals of Surgery* **192:** 562–569.

Studley HO (1936) Percentage of weight loss: a basic indicator of surgical risk in patients with chronic peptic ulcer. *Journal of the American Medical Association* **106:** 458–460.

6
Infection in the Intensive Care Unit

The pattern of hospital-acquired infections has altered dramatically since antibiotics were introduced into clinical practice. In the 1940s, the majority of fatal infections were caused by streptococci (*Strep. pyogenes* and *Strep. pneumoniae*) or *Staphylococcus aureus*. Later, the emergence of resistant strains of *Staph. aureus* caused concern, but in the 1960s these gram-positive organisms were largely superseded as a cause of life-threatening sepsis in hospitalized patients by the gram-negative enteric bacteria. Initially, the dominant organism was *E. coli*, but subsequently other gram-negative bacteria, such as *Klebsiella* spp., *Proteus* spp. and *Pseudomonas* spp. assumed greater importance. More recently an increasing number of these organisms have developed antibiotic resistance, probably encouraged by the widespread use of broad-spectrum antimicrobial agents, many of which are intrinsically more active against gram-positive bacteria. This problem has been compounded by the ability of gram-negative organisms to transfer resistance from one strain to another, for example within the bowel lumen, as 'R' factors or 'plasmids'.

This changing pattern of infection is not, however, solely attributable to the effects of antibiotic therapy; alterations in both the susceptibility of the hospital population and the procedures to which they are subjected have also contributed to this phenomenon. Thus, an increasing number of hospitalized patients survive with impaired immune responses, due either to their disease, e.g. renal failure, diabetes, malignancy or severe trauma, or to therapy with immunosuppressants, cytotoxics or steroids. Furthermore, the risk of infection increases at the extremes of age, in the presence of malnutrition and with the severity of the underlying disease. Cell-mediated immunity (CMI), as measured by the skin reaction to recall antigens, has been shown to be impaired in the critically ill and persistent anergy is associated with a poor prognosis (Bradley et al, 1984). Moreover, the lymphocyte response to mitogens, as well as neutrophil chemotaxis, can be impaired by a number of factors, including surgery, infection, malignancy and malnutrition. It has recently been suggested, however, that in the critically ill this suppression may be selective (Bradley et al, 1984). Some seriously ill patients also become leucopenic and this is recognized as a bad prognostic sign in the presence of infection. Depletion of complement and reduced fibronectin levels (O'Connell et al, 1984) may also predispose to infective complications. Finally, it has been shown that the serum of burned patients can inhibit the lymphocyte response to mitogens and that their leukocyte populations include suppressor lymphocytes (Wolfe et al, 1981).

These highly susceptible patients are now more frequently subjected to invasive procedures, such as intravascular and urethral catheterization, endotracheal intubation or tracheostomy and TPN. These predisposing factors are particularly prevalent in critically ill patients who are therefore very prone to the development of secondary infections, and in whom intractable pneumonia and septicaemia is a common terminal event.

SOURCES AND PREVENTION OF INFECTION

Very often, the source of an infection is the patient's own skin, genitourinary, respiratory or, most importantly, gastrointestinal tract. The causative organism may be either a normal resident or, more often, acquired—e.g. a bacterium introduced into the gastrointestinal tract in the hospital food. Colonization of the stomach with gram-negative organisms is common in critically ill subjects, particularly when gastric pH is elevated by antacid prophylaxis, and under these circumstances regurgitation and aspiration of gastric contents may cause colonization or infection of the respiratory tract (du Moulin et al, 1982). Unfortunately, as mentioned in Chapter 5, the presence of a tracheostomy or an endotracheal tube is not a reliable barrier to such aspiration since liquid readily passes low pressure, high volume cuffs.

The vector in most cases of autogenous infection is the patient's own hands, or those of his attendants. The patient must therefore be prevented from handling infected areas and transferring organisms to vulnerable sites elsewhere, e.g. a tracheostomy stoma. Meticulous hygiene is essential to protect the patient from endogenous infection and will often necessitate frequent changes of bed linen, cleaning of contaminated areas and hand washing.

As well as endogenous sources, the patient is at risk of infection from the environment, his attendants and his fellow patients. The precautions taken to prevent such cross-infection vary from one unit to another and this reflects the lack of evidence as to the efficacy of many of the measures which can be adopted. For example, in some units, clean gowns and overshoes are worn by all staff and visitors who enter the unit. Although this has not been conclusively shown to reduce the incidence of infection, it at least has the advantage of limiting the number of casual visitors and emphasizing the need for personal cleanliness. However, the greatest risk to the patient probably arises from organisms transferred from other patients, or from contaminated areas of the unit such as the sinks, usually on the hands of the staff. In this respect the most important preventive measure is thorough hand washing between patients (Daschner, 1985), although fomites, such as stethoscopes, may also be responsible for transmitting organisms between patients. In some units, disposable aprons, and even gloves, are worn at all times and are changed when moving from one patient to another. In others, such precautions are only employed when a patient is known to harbour resistant organisms. Caps and masks are generally considered to be unnecessary, except when performing aseptic procedures, whilst environmental monitoring is expensive, tedious and probably of little value (Daschner, 1985).

Unit design is an important element in minimizing cross-infection. There must be adequate space around each bed and some single cubicles should be available for barrier, or reverse barrier, nursing. Preferably, these cubicles should be equipped with unidirectional plenum ventilation. Adequate hand-washing facilities are essential and a basin should be provided adjacent to each bed area.

Not only should the staff be trained in the correct procedures for reducing cross-infection, but they must also be motivated to perform them to a high standard at all times. If staffing levels are inadequate, these procedures may be overlooked and movement between patients will increase, particularly in times of stress; as a consequence, the incidence of cross-infection may rise.

Those critically ill patients with endotracheal tubes or tracheostomies in place are particularly liable to develop secondary pulmonary infection. Many of the normal barriers to the introduction of micro-organisms have been bypassed, whilst colonization of tracheostomy wounds, the upper airways and the stomach is common (see above). Moreover, ciliary activity and macrophage function may be impaired, whilst retention of secretions, pulmonary oedema and destruction of the normal bacterial flora by antibiotics all increase the risk of infection. Finally, bacteria may be introduced during endotracheal suction.

The ventilator tubing frequently becomes colonized, usually with organisms from the patient's own respiratory tract, and should therefore be changed daily to avoid proliferation of these bacteria, reinfection of the patient and contamination of the ventilator. Humidifier water can also become contaminated and should be changed regularly, although heating to 60°C should effectively prevent colonization. The ventilators themselves can be potential sources of infection and autoclavable patient circuits are now standard. Some centres use disposable bacterial filters on the inspiratory and expiratory limbs of the circuit, whilst heated filters are incorporated in some ventilators.

All intravascular and urinary catheters must be inserted with full aseptic precautions. Nevertheless, they may become colonized with pathogenic organisms (Pinilla et al, 1983) either because of faulty insertion technique or as a result of inadequate care of the lines and the skin puncture site. Sometimes fibrin deposits at the tip of the cannula become secondarily infected during a septicaemic episode or via a contaminated infusion set. This is particularly likely to occur in patients receiving TPN. All intravenous infusion sets should therefore be changed daily. If signs of infection develop in the absence of an obvious source, or if they persist after apparent eradication of a septic focus, all indwelling catheters should be removed and their tips sent for culture. In this way, the use of antibiotics can occasionally be avoided. Ideally, replacement of indwelling catheters should be delayed to allow elimination of residual organisms, although in practice this is rarely possible.

THE RATIONAL USE OF ANTIBIOTICS

Critically ill patients often receive prolonged courses of the most expensive broad-spectrum antibiotics and, although the use of such agents may be life-saving, there is considerable potential for their abuse. In order to limit the emergence and spread of resistant organisms, antibiotics must be used rationally and sparingly. They should be prescribed only when clearly indicated, prophylactic administration should be carefully controlled and unnecessary treatment of colonization must be avoided.

Unfortunately, it is often extremely difficult to distinguish colonization from infection, particularly in the respiratory tract (Tobin and Grenvik, 1984). Usually, the distinction can only be made on clinical grounds and is based on the presence of the usual signs of infection (pyrexia, leucocytosis, visibly purulent sputum, haemodynamic changes), combined with the recognition of a source of sepsis and a pure, or heavy, growth of a pathogen from the suspected site. If blood cultures are positive, and grow the same organism as has been isolated from the presumed source of infection, it is probable that this is the pathogen. Transtracheal aspiration of sputum via the cricothyroid membrane avoids contamination with organisms in the oropharynx. This technique is safe and sensitive, provided antibiotics have not been administered, but there is a significant incidence of false-positive results. Aspirates obtained via an endotracheal or tracheostomy tube are less likely to be contaminated than expectorated sputum but can still produce false-positive cultures.

Very often, antimicrobial agents have to be administered before the organism has been identified. Under these circumstances, material from all possible sites of infection, as well as blood, should be obtained and sent for culture and drug sensitivities before the first dose of antibiotic is administered. Sometimes, an immediate gram stain will provide a valuable clue as to the probable pathogen. Otherwise, a rational choice of antibiotic should be made on the basis of the organisms most likely to arise from the presumed site of sepsis and the known local patterns of infection. Many hospitals produce policies which guide the choice of antibiotic regimen in particular clinical situations (Table 6.1) and these help to rationalize the use of antimicrobial agents within the hospital environment. Close co-operation with the microbiology department is essential at all times.

Routine cultures of sputum, urine and other available material should be performed at least twice a week and the results of these may then guide the initial choice of antibiotic. Similarly, the tips of all intravascular cannulae

Table 6.1 Suggested antibiotic regimens.

Nature of infection	Possible causative organisms	Recommended antibiotic regimen
Pneumonia Acquired in the community	*Streptococcus pneumoniae* *Haemophilus influenzae* *Mycoplasma pneumoniae* *Legionella pneumophila*	Amoxycillin and erythromycin (can substitute cefuroxime for amoxycillin in those sensitive to penicillin)
	Staphylococcal pneumonia possible	Add flucloxacillin
	Staphylococcal pneumonia confirmed, not responding to flucloxacillin	Add Fucidin to flucloxacillin
	Documented pneumococcal pneumonia	Penicillin
Acquired in hospital	As above plus gram-negative organisms. If mycoplasma or legionnaire's disease a possibility	Cefuroxime Add erythromycin
	Pseudomonas pneumonia and/or septicaemia a possibility	Aminoglycoside and ticarcillin or piperacillin (ceftazidime is an alternative)
Aspiration pneumonia		Cefuroxime and metronidazole

Table 6.1 Continued

Nature of infection	Possible causative organisms	Recommended antibiotic regimen
Intra-abdominal infection		
	Gram-negative enteric organisms, staphylococci and anaerobes (e.g. *Bacteroides fragilis*)	Aminoglycoside (gentamicin, tobramycin or netilmicin) *or* a second- or third-generation cephalosporin combined with Metronidazole
	For *Strep. faecalis*	Add ampicillin (particularly effective for biliary tract infections)
	Pseudomonas aeruginosa a possibility	Add ticarcillin or piperacillin (will also cover *Strep. faecalis*)
Pelvic infections		
	Anaerobes Gram-negative organisms	Metronidazole plus ampicillin or an aminoglycoside
	If clostridial or group A streptococcal infection suspected	Add penicillin to above
	If staphylococcal infection suspected	Add flucloxacillin to above
Urinary tract infections		
	E. coli, *Proteus* spp. *Klebsiella* spp.	Ampicillin or amoxycillin Co-trimoxazole is an alternative Aminoglycoside if organism resistant to above and there is no renal failure
Unusual pathogens		
	Pneumocystis carinii	High-dose co-trimoxazole
	Mycoplasma pneumoniae *Legionella pneumophila*	Erythromycin
	Chlamydia psittaci *Coxiella burnetti*	Tetracycline
	Fungi	Amphotericin (can be combined with 5-fluorocytosine)

should be sent for culture on removal. In some units, nose and throat swabs are also obtained routinely.

In general, if the pathogen has been identified and its drug sensitivities are known, administration of a single antibiotic, if possible with a narrow spectrum of activity, is preferable to the use of combinations. However, the latter may be required for empirical therapy, to prevent the emergence of resistant strains (e.g. in the treatment of tuberculosis) and for the treatment of mixed infections. Furthermore, certain antibiotic combinations are synergistic (e.g. penicillin and gentamicin against *Strep. faecalis*) and may therefore be particularly useful for the treatment of life-threatening infections. On the other hand, the combination of some bacteriostatic and bactericidal agents can be antagonistic, although this is no longer generally considered to be clinically important. Bactericidal antibiotics are probably superior in the treatment of endocarditis, and for neutropenic patients, but there is no evidence that they offer any advantages in other situations. Finally, antimicrobial therapy should not be administered for long periods except under special circumstances.

Pneumonia

The appropriate initial regimen for a patient with pneumonia depends largely on whether the infection was acquired in hospital or in the community. Thus, pneumonias contracted outside the hospital environment can be treated initially with a combination of amoxycillin and erythromycin. The former will cover the common respiratory pathogens, such as *Haemophilus influenzae* and pneumococcus, whilst the latter may be effective against *Mycoplasma pneumonia* and legionnaire's disease. A second-generation cephalosporin, such as cefuroxime, may be substituted for amoxycillin in those allergic to penicillin (although there is some cross-sensitivity) and to broaden the spectrum of activity for pneumonias acquired in hospital. If staphylococcal pneumonia is a possibility, e.g. during an influenza epidemic, flucloxacillin or, possibly, cefuroxime should be used. If this diagnosis is subsequently confirmed and the patient is not responding, the addition of fucidin may prove to be more effective. Penicillin remains the drug of first choice in patients with documented pneumococcal pneumonia. Although cefotaxime, a third-generation cephalosporin, has some antipseudomonal activity, if pseudomonas pneumonia or septicaemia is a possibility it is usually preferable to administer an antipseudomonal penicillin (such as azlocillin, ticarcillin or piperacillin), usually in combination with an aminoglycoside. Alternatively, ceftazidime, which has good antipseudomonal activity, can be used. Aspiration pneumonia can be treated with cefuroxime and metronidazole. In general, aminoglycosides penetrate poorly into lungs and sputum and are therefore rarely used for pulmonary infections.

Intra-abdominal infection

Infections arising from sites within the abdomen will normally require combination therapy to provide an adequate spectrum of activity, at least until the results of cultures and drug sensitivities are available. In this situation, an aminoglycoside is usually administered in combination with metronidazole. There is little to choose between gentamicin and tobramycin, both of which are active against the majority of gram-negative enteric organisms, as well as staphylococci. In order to achieve effective therapy, without the risk of oto- or nephrotoxicity, it is important to monitor blood levels with both these agents. (There is some evidence that netilmicin is a less toxic alternative to the older aminoglycosides.) Amikacin should be reserved for the treatment of documented infection with gentamicin-resistant organisms. Second- or third-generation cephalosporins can be used as alternatives to an aminoglycoside. Metronidazole is given to control infection caused by anaerobic organisms such as *Bacteroides fragilis*, and has superseded clindamycin and lincomycin, both of which were particularly implicated in the causation of pseudomembranous colitis. This combination will not cover *Strep. faecalis* and may be ineffective against some strains of *Pseudomonas aeruginosa*. The addition of ampicillin will provide activity against *Strep. faecalis*, whilst the use of an antipseudomonal penicillin will cover both these organisms. Furthermore, since ampicillin is concentrated in the bile it is particularly effective in the treatment of biliary tract infections.

Pelvic infections

Pelvic sepsis arising from the female genital tract is frequently associated with anaerobic infection and will always require administration of metronidazole, initially in combination with ampicillin or amoxycillin. An aminoglycoside can be substituted for the ampicillin in the most seriously ill or in those who fail to respond. If clostridial infection is suspected, e.g. following a criminal abortion, penicillin should be used, whilst if staphylococcal infection is a possibility, e.g. in tampon-associated toxic shock syndrome, flucloxacillin must be administered.

Urinary tract infections

These often respond well to ampicillin or amoxycillin since they are active against most strains of *E.coli*, *Proteus* and *Klebsiella* and have the advantage of excellent diffusion into the urinary tract. Co-trimoxazole also has good tissue penetration and can be used as an alternative to ampicillin. Provided there is no renal impairment, an aminoglycoside can be effective if culture and sensitivities indicate that such treatment is appropriate.

Prophylactic antibiotics

The use of prophylactic antibiotics is controversial but in general this practice encourages the emergence of resistant strains with which the patient, whose normal bacterial flora is destroyed, then becomes colonized. Situations in which the use of prophylactic antibiotics is generally accepted include cardiac surgery (gentamicin and flucloxacillin), skull fracture with leakage of cerebrospinal fluid (sulphadimidine and flucloxacillin), insertion of prosthetic vascular grafts (flucloxacillin) and in the prevention of gas gangrene following major trauma or amputation of an ischaemic limb (penicillin). Routine prophylactic systemic administration of antibiotics to intensive care patients is not recommended and although instillation of these agents into the lungs does decrease the risk of pulmonary infection, it can lead to the emergence of resistant strains (Klastersky et al, 1974). Recently, however, it has been suggested that routine selective decontamination of the digestive tract with non-absorbable antibiotics can decrease the incidence of infection in multiple trauma patients (Stoutenbeek et al, 1984).

ANTIBIOTIC-ASSOCIATED DIARRHOEA

This is a common complication of antibiotic therapy and can significantly complicate the management of critically ill patients. Mild forms may simply be a consequence of alterations in the bacterial flora, but in some instances there may be a low-grade *Clostridium difficile* infection. Particularly severe diarrhoea occurs in those with pseudomembranous colitis which is caused by the toxin produced by *Clostridium difficile* (George et al, 1978). This condition is usually encountered in patients receiving broad-spectrum antibiotics and was originally described in association with administration of lincomycin and clindamycin. Since then most other antibiotics have been incriminated. The diagnosis is made by growing the organism from the stools or by identifying the toxin. *Clostridium difficile* is always sensitive to vancomycin, which should be administered orally, but metronidazole may also be effective. Sometimes, patients relapse or develop a persistent carrier state.

UNUSUAL PATHOGENS

Clearly, not all the infections seen on the intensive care unit are caused by bacteria. This applies particularly to pulmonary infections which may be caused by tuberculosis, viruses, *Mycoplasma*, *Chlamydia psittaci* (psittacosis), *Coxiella burnetti* (Q fever), protozoans (e.g. *Pneumocystis carinii*) or fungi.

Pneumocystis pneumonia and cytomegalovirus infection characteristically occur in immunocompromised patients (Editorial, 1981), whilst Legionnaire's disease is a recognized complication of impaired immunity, but can also develop de novo. Other viral pneumonias, mycoplasma, psittacosis and Q fever present as primary atypical pneumonia. A rising specific antibody titre confirms the diagnosis, whilst cold agglutinins may be present in those with mycoplasma pneumonia. It may be possible to isolate the causative organism in psittacosis using special culture techniques, although this is dangerous and only performed in special centres. It is possible to visualize *Legionella pneumophila* using fluorescent antibody staining of lung tissue, sputum specimens or bronchial washings. The diagnosis of pneumocystis pneumonia can only be made on lung biopsy and this technique will also demonstrate cytomegalovirus infection.

Pneumocystis carinii pneumonia can be effectively treated, and pre-vented, by the administration of high-dose co-trimoxazole, either orally or parenterally. The antifolate effect of co-trimoxazole may precipitate megaloblastic bone marrow change. Erythromycin is the first choice for treating mycoplasma and Legionnaire's disease and can be used as second-line treatment for Q fever. Tetracycline is the treatment of choice for psittacosis and Q fever and can be used in patients with mycoplasma pneumonia. Rifampicin is an alternative agent for use in psittacosis, and possibly Legionnaire's disease.

Secondary fungal infections usually occur in patients who have received prolonged treatment with broad-spectrum antibiotics, particularly if they are also immunosuppressed. Colonization of skin, nose, throat and tracheostomy wounds is relatively common and rarely requires treatment. However, when fungi are obtained in significant quantities from sputum or urine it can be extremely difficult to distinguish colonization from invasive infection. This distinction is important because, although if necessary colonization can be cleared with topical antifungal agents, invasive disease carries an extremely high mortality and requires prolonged systemic administration of potentially toxic drugs such as amphotericin. Positive blood cultures may indicate significant infection, whilst a rising *Candida* antibody titre also suggests invasive disease. Attempts to detect *Candida* antigen in blood are still being evaluated. Endophthalmitis (hard, greyish-white exudates seen on retinoscopy) is occasionally present and confirms invasive fungal disease. Pulmonary aspergillosis may produce a mycetoma with a characteristic, mobile crescentic translucency seen on the chest x-ray. The serum may contain *Aspergillus* precipitins. If a heavy growth of a fungus, with pus cells, is obtained repeatedly from the sputum of a ventilated patient in the presence of chest x-ray signs of consolidation, treatment for systemic fungal infection is normally indicated. Nevertheless, more invasive techniques will normally be required to establish the diagnosis with certainty (see below).

As well as administering specific antifungal agents, successful treatment depends on removing all possible sources of continuing infection, such as intravascular catheters and prosthetic heart valves. Amphotericin is probably the most effective, and certainly the longest established, antifungal agent, sometimes effecting a cure in disseminated candidiasis and producing a beneficial effect in some cases of aspergillosis. Some degree of renal impairment usually develops soon after commencing amphotericin, but if treatment is continued the glomerular filtration rate (GFR) usually stabilizes at 20–60% of normal. Renal function almost always improves rapidly once treatment is discontinued. Other adverse effects include anaemia, hypokalaemia, thrombocytopenia and hepatic dysfunction. There is some evidence that the combination of amphotericin with the less toxic flucytosine is synergistic and in this way the dose, and adverse effects, of amphotericin may be reduced (Medoff and Kobayashi, 1980). Miconazole is a relatively new agent and its place has yet to be determined. It should not, however, be administered with amphotericin since the combination is chemically antagonistic. If therapy is effective, improvement occurs within a few days, but treatment usually has to continue for several weeks, or even months.

DIAGNOSTIC PROCEDURES IN PNEUMONIA OF UNKNOWN AETIOLOGY (Tobin and Grenvik, 1984; MacFarlane, 1985)

It is sometimes extremely difficult to identify the causative organism in a pneumonia, particularly those due to opportunistic infection in an immunocompromised host. It may not be possible to obtain an adequate quantity of sputum from the lower airways, particularly in those with non-bacterial pneumonia, and expectorated samples are often contaminated with bacteria or fungi during their passage through the upper airways. *Tracheal aspirates* may yield diagnostic material but even these may be contaminated with flora colonizing the upper airways. Oropharyngeal contamination can be avoided by transtracheal needle aspiration via the cricothyroid membrane. The risk of complications with this technique is low, haemorrhage being the main concern, and the diagnostic yield is excellent in bacterial pneumonia, provided no antibiotic has been administered previously.

Diagnostic material can be obtained using *fibre-optic bronchoscopy* with bronchial brushings, bronchioalveolar lavage or transbronchial lung biopsy. Brush biopsies can provide an aetiological diagnosis in approximately one-third of cases, and are particularly advocated for the detection of pneumocystis and fungi. They are less useful in the diagnosis of bacterial pneumonias because the brush can become contaminated in the upper airways, although the use of a 'protected' brush may overcome this problem. Complications of brush biopsy include pneumothorax, haemorrhage and infection. A similar diagnostic yield can be achieved with bronchioalveolar lavage but, again, contamination with upper airway organisms is a problem and it is most suitable for demonstrating parasites and fungi. Complications include hypoxia and infection. It is almost always possible to obtain lung tissue using transbronchial biopsy and an aetiological diagnosis is made in 40–80% of cases. However, the incidence of complications, in particular pneumothorax and haemorrhage, is greatest with this method.

Percutaneous transthoracic needle biopsy also produces a reasonable diagnostic yield but the risks of pneumothorax, pneumomediastinum and haemorrhage are again fairly high.

Open lung biopsy through a small thoracotomy usually enables a histological and microbiological diagnosis to be made. Pneumothorax, haemothorax and infection may all occur, but in experienced hands the morbidity and mortality of this procedure are acceptably low.

The choice of the most suitable technique in an individual patient depends upon a number of factors, including the presumed diagnosis (bacterial, fungal, viral or protozoan), the presence of coagulation disorders, the severity of respiratory failure and the experience of available personnel. For each case the potential benefits and risks must be viewed in the light of these considerations.

FURTHER READING

Cartier F (1983) Opportunistic lung infections in the compromised host. In Tinker J & Rapin M (eds) *Care of the Critically Ill Patient*, pp 899–909. Berlin: Springer-Verlag.
Slack M (1983) Use and abuse of antibiotics. In Ledingham IMcA (ed.) *Recent Advances in Critical Care Medicine 2*, pp 81–96. Edinburgh: Churchill Livingstone.
Stoddard JC (1983) Hospital-acquired infections. In Tinker J & Rapin M (eds) *Care of the Critically Ill Patient*, pp 873–884. Berlin: Springer-Verlag.

REFERENCES

Bradley JA, Hamilton DNH, Brown MW et al (1984) Cellular defense in critically ill surgical patients. *Critical Care Medicine* **12:** 565–570.

Daschner FD (1985) Useful and useless hygienic techniques in intensive care units. *Intensive Care Medicine* **11:** 280–283.

du Moulin GC, Paterson DG, Hedley-Whyte J & Lisbon A (1982) Aspiration of gastric bacteria in antacid-treated patients: a frequent cause of postoperative colonisation of the airway. *Lancet* **ii:** 242–245.

Editorial (1981) Pulmonary problems of the immunocompromised patient. *British Medical Journal* **282:** 2077.

George RH, Symonds JM, Dimock F et al (1978) Identification of *Clostridium difficile* as a cause of pseudomembranous colitis. *British Medical Journal* **i:** 695.

Klastersky J, Huysmans E, Weerts D, Hensgens C & Daneau D (1974) Endotracheally administered gentamicin for the prevention of infections of the respiratory tract in patients with tracheostomy. A double blind study. *Chest* **65:** 650–654.

MacFarlane J (1985) Lung biopsy (editorial). *British Medical Journal* **290:** 97–98.

Medoff G & Kobayashi GS (1980) Strategies in the treatment of systemic fungal infections. *New England Journal of Medicine* **302:** 145–155.

O'Connell MT, Becker DM, Steele BW, Peterson GS & Hellman RL (1984) Plasma fibronectin in medical ICU patients. *Critical Care Medicine* **12:** 479–482.

Pinilla JC, Ross DF, Martin T & Crump H (1983) Study of the incidence of intravascular catheter infection and associated septicaemia in critically ill patients. *Critical Care Medicine* **11:** 21–25.

Stoutenbeek CP, van Saene HKF, Miranda DR & Zandstra DF (1984) The effect of selective decontamination of the digestive tract on colonisation and infection rate in multiple trauma patients. *Intensive Care Medicine* **10:** 185–192.

Tobin MJ & Grenvik A (1984) Nosocomial lung infection and its diagnosis. *Critical Care Medicine* **12:** 191–199.

Wolfe JHN, Saporoschetz AJ, Young AE, O'Connor NE & Mannick JA (1981) Suppressive serum, suppressor lymphocytes and death from burns. *Annals of Surgery* **193:** 513–520.

7

Psychiatric Disturbances*

Patients in intensive care units often experience extreme stress, anxiety and fear of impending death. This can cause serious mental disturbances which, apart from being very distressing for the patient, staff and relatives, may adversely affect the progress of the underlying physical disease. Critically ill patients are often unable to speak, some are unable to communicate at all, and their movement is restricted. Moreover, they are severely deprived of sleep compared with normal, and stages 3 and 4 and REM (rapid eye movement) sleep are severely or completely suppressed (Aurell and Elmqvist, 1985). They also suffer from reduced stimulation, social isolation and physical confinement. Such sensory deprivation is known to induce hallucinations of sound, vision, touch and movement as well as reduced vigilance and an under-estimation of time. Moreover, patients may be subjected to repetitive stimulation (e.g. flashing lights on monitors and infusion pumps, the sound of alarms and ventilators) and occasional serious discomfort or pain. Any impairment of cerebral function, caused, for example, by drugs or metabolic derangement, will exaggerate the psychological response of the patient to these environmental stresses. Finally, certain procedures may be particularly associated with psychiatric disturbances, for example cardiopulmonary bypass and mitral valve surgery, while weaning from mechanical ventilation can be uniquely stressful (Tomlin, 1977).

The most commonly encountered serious mental disturbance is delirium. This usually presents as a sudden global impairment of cognitive processes, with reduced awareness, apathy and drowsiness. Some patients become restless, hyperactive and even violent. Hallucinations and delusions of persecution are common. Characteristically, the severity of the mental disturbance fluctuates, with lucid intervals during the day and deterioration at night. Metabolic disturbances such as dehydration, hyponatraemia, alkalosis, uraemia, hyperchloraemia and hypokalaemia may all predispose to delirium, which is also commoner in the older age groups; children appear to be particularly resistant.

Acute schizophreniform psychotic reactions are seen less frequently. These present as thought disorder, delusions or hallucinations in a patient who is fully conscious and orientated with an intact memory (Kiely, 1976).

Such psychotic reactions have been studied most frequently in patients following cardiopulmonary bypass, but the incidence of serious mental disturbance in this category of patient is now relatively low. This is probably due to a number of factors including shorter bypass times, careful preoperative preparation and attention to environmental factors within the intensive care unit (see below).

*The reader is referred to Baxter (1974) for further information on this subject.

101

Intensive care patients may also exhibit a variety of less severe psychological reactions to their predicament. These range from overwhelming fear, tension and sustained anxiety to severe, often agitated, depression and 'negativism' (Kiely, 1976). Psychological defences to protect 'self' are sometimes manifested as abnormal behaviour patterns. Thus, the patient may exhibit obsessive compulsive behaviour in which he analyses every aspect of his situation and illness in minute detail; alternatively, he may display repression by rejecting his problem and allowing staff a 'free hand'. Some patients become totally dependent, whilst others are wholeheartedly involved in their own treatment, denying any feelings of fear or hopelessness.

Many patients admitted to intensive care units will have pre-existing psychological problems. These will then manifest themselves, sometimes in exaggerated form, as the patient recovers. Although it has been suggested that certain abnormal personality traits or mental diseases may predispose to particular types of physical illness, cases of self-poisoning, drug addiction and alcohol abuse are more obvious examples.

The features of *narcotic addiction* include pin-point pupils and transitory elation which is followed by marked anxiety and restlessness. Anorexia, constipation and extreme weight loss are common, as is loss of libido. Examination may reveal multiple injection sites, sometimes with bruising, abscesses and septic thrombophlebitis. Signs and symptoms of withdrawal include running eyes and nose, sneezing, perspiration, gooseflesh, vague aches and pains, anxiety, restlessness, aggression and dilated pupils. Nausea, vomiting, abdominal pain, diarrhoea, limb cramps, sleeplessness and agitation may also occur.

Alcohol withdrawal is characterized by nervous system excitation which varies from mild sleeplessness and irritability to delirium tremens. In mild cases there is tremor, perspiration, nervousness, dyspepsia, weakness, anorexia, hyperreflexia and insomnia. Severe cases exhibit hypertension, tachycardia, fever, hallucinations (visual, tactile or auditory), disorientation and convulsions. Delirium tremens is characterized by delirium, clouding of consciousness and convulsions. Moreover, alcohol can exacerbate pre-existing psychiatric disorders such as aggressive psychopathy, manic–depressive psychoses and paranoid schizophrenia. Symptomatic alcohol psychoses may occur and include illusions and hallucinations which form the basis for transient paranoid delusions.

PREVENTION

Prevention of these psychological disturbances involves maintaining the patient's contact with reality, together with frequent explanation and reassurance, control of metabolic disturbances and the provision of adequate analgesia and anxiolysis.

In those who are conscious and alert, some form of occupational therapy is required; this may take the form of radio, television or 'talking' books. As normal an environment as possible should be maintained, e.g. darkness and, if possible, uninterrupted sleep at night with natural daylight and wakefulness during the day. Night sedation with, for example, temazepam 10–20 mg orally, is often useful in this respect. It has been suggested, however, that even when conditions for sleep are optimal, critically ill patients are seriously deprived of sleep and that this is due to some fundamental disarrangement of the sleep–wake regulating mechanism (Aurell and Elmqvist, 1985).

It is also important that intensive care units are provided with windows (Wilson, 1972), preferably with a view, and frequent information regarding the time, the day of the week and the season of the year should be provided. It has been suggested that a digital clock/radio and possibly a calendar would be very useful in this respect. The patient should be allowed as much privacy as possible, whilst monitoring and other equipment should be unobtrusively sited, preferably behind the bed, for example on a 'rail system'. Finally, all procedures must be fully explained before they are performed and frequent encouragement regarding the progress of the illness must be provided. It is important to remember that some patients who appear to be unconscious may not be so.

Fortunately, many patients have complete, or partial, amnesia for their time on the intensive care unit, particularly for the periods when they were most seriously ill. This may be at least partly due to the provision of adequate analgesia and sedation which is in any case essential for the patient's comfort. These psychological aspects of patient care are particularly dependent on the nurses who spend many hours at the bedside of one individual patient and have the opportunity to establish a close and understanding relationship.

TREATMENT

Although the patient's inevitable anxiety can usually be safely controlled using benzodiazepines, severe depression is less easily treated. Tricyclic antidepressants are often ineffective, and may be associated with dangerous cardiovascular side effects; some authorities therefore recommend electro-convulsive therapy in the most extreme cases. Psychotic reactions may require treatment with either phenothiazines or butyrophenones. Haloperidol, which has minimal autonomic effects, is probably the agent of choice in the critically ill (Kiely, 1976). A continuous intravenous infusion of 0.8% chlormethiazole may prove useful to control patients during withdrawal from alcohol or other drugs, but large volumes ($60–90\,\text{ml}\,\text{h}^{-1}$) may be required and this can lead to fluid overload. If necessary, symptoms of narcotic withdrawal can be controlled with methadone 10–20 mg which can be repeated 1–2 hours later and should be effective for about 12 hours. Clonidine has recently been suggested as a means of controlling the symptoms of narcotic withdrawal.

RELATIVES

The morale of relatives is also most important and they should receive every possible care and attention. In particular, they should be given frequent, detailed explanations regarding the patient's treatment and progress. As far as possible, free visiting should be allowed since this is beneficial not only to the relatives but also to the patients, helping them to maintain contact with reality. Visitors should be encouraged to talk to, and touch, the patient.

FURTHER READING

Bowden P (1983) Psychiatric aspects of intensive care. In Tinker J & Rapin M (eds) *Care of the Critically Ill Patient*, pp 787–797. Berlin: Springer-Verlag.

REFERENCES

Aurell J & Elmqvist D (1985) Sleep in the surgical intensive care unit: continuous polygraphic recording of sleep in nine patients receiving postoperative care. *British Medical Journal* **290:** 1029–1032.

Baxter S (1974) Psychological problems of intensive care. *British Journal of Hospital Medicine* **11:** 875–885.

Kiely WF (1976) Psychiatric syndromes in critically ill patients. *Journal of the American Medical Association* **235:** 2759–2761.

Tomlin PJ (1977) Psychological problems in intensive care. *British Medical Journal* **ii:** 441–443.

Wilson L (1972) Intensive care delirium. *Archives of Internal Medicine* **130:** 225–226.

8
Prevention of Peptic Ulceration

Acute gastrointestinal haemorrhage associated with peptic ulceration can be a serious and potentially life-threatening complication in critically ill patients. Those with burns (Curling's ulcers), head injuries (Cushing's ulcers), multiple trauma, renal failure, respiratory failure, jaundice, hypotension and severe sepsis are amongst those at greatest risk (Priebe et al, 1980).

Stress ulcers develop acutely and are small, round or oval, with well-demarcated borders and no surrounding oedema. They are usually situated in the fundus of the stomach or the first part of the duodenum and may be multiple. In critically ill patients, damage to the mucosal barrier (e.g. due to ischaemia during an episode of shock) may be combined with hypersecretion of gastric acid, and back diffusion of acid into the stomach wall, to produce ulceration. Cushing's ulcers are associated with markedly elevated circulating gastrin levels, with very high acid production, and their pathogenesis may be peculiar to patients with intracranial pathology.

Most authorities recommend that all critically ill patients, except those receiving enteral nutrition—which appears to protect against gastrointestinal bleeding (Pingleton and Hadzima, 1983)—should receive treatment aimed at preventing stress ulceration. Prophylaxis can be achieved by the regular intragastric instillation of an antacid preparation via a nasogastric tube, or by the administration of an H_2 receptor antagonist. Both methods have been shown to reduce the incidence of significant gastrointestinal haemorrhage in a variety of clinical situations (MacDougall et al, 1977; Halloran et al, 1980; Priebe et al, 1980). It is not certain, however, whether they actually prevent gastric erosions or simply reduce their severity, thereby decreasing the incidence of overt bleeding.

In a recent study (Groll et al, 1986) the incidence of haemorrhage in general intensive care patients was low (8%) and was not affected by cimetidine prophylaxis. Moreover, there is considerable controversy as to which regimen is the most efficacious and practical (Greene and Bollinger, 1984). For example, some have suggested that cimetidine is less effective than antacids in preventing acute gastrointestinal bleeding in the critically ill (Priebe et al, 1980), possibly because they do not provide a 'mucosal barrier'. Furthermore, H_2 receptor blockade inhibits secretion of bicarbonate as well as acid production, possibly rendering the mucosa more sensitive to residual gastric acidity. On the other hand, some studies favour H_2 receptor antagonists (MacDougall et al, 1977), and successful prophylaxis with antacids requires frequent instillation of large volumes in order to maintain gastric pH within acceptable limits as well as to provide continuous protection of the gastric mucosa. This is time-consuming and labour-intensive. The combination of an H_2 receptor antagonist, which will reduce acid secretion, and an antacid, which will neutralize acid and provide a mucosal barrier, might be expected to be particularly effective, but several comparative studies suggest that this is not, in fact, the case (Greene and Bollinger, 1984).

Whichever technique is used, gastric pH must be maintained above 4 and this should be confirmed by regular analysis of the nasogastric aspirate with pH-sensitive paper. Alternatively, pH can be continually recorded using an intragastric electrode. Indeed, in many studies which have purported to show that one or other prophylactic measure was ineffective, gastric pH was either not measured (Groll et al, 1986) or was not increased sufficiently (MacDougall et al, 1977).

Provided the gastric contents are adequately alkalinized there is probably little to choose between the two methods. However, antacids are cheap, effective and free of serious side effects. Although the administration of magnesium-containing antacids often precipitates diarrhoea, whilst aluminium salts tend to cause constipation, these complications can be minimized by using a mixture of the two. Hypermagnesaemia may be produced when large quantities of antacid are administered, particularly in those with renal failure.

The H_2 receptor antagonist cimetidine can also provide satisfactory prophylaxis (Halloran et al, 1980). It does, however, interfere with the metabolism of certain drugs, in particular some of the benzodiazepines, and may be associated with thrombocytopenia, confusion and cardiovascular disturbances. Ranitidine is a more recently introduced H_2 receptor antagonist which has a longer duration of action and may cause fewer side effects than cimetidine, but clinical experience with this agent is as yet limited and more adverse effects may become apparent with increased use.

A reasonable, practical approach to the prevention of stress ulceration is to administer antacids via a nasogastric tube, initially in a dose of 30 ml two-hourly. This can be supplemented with an H_2 receptor antagonist if the gastric pH is not adequately controlled with high doses of antacids, if side effects are troublesome and in particularly high-risk patients. Patients in whom antacids are contraindicated, e.g. those in renal failure, should be given an H_2 receptor antagonist alone, but in reduced dosage. Current evidence supports the use of H_2 receptor antagonists in those with fulminant hepatic failure (MacDougall et al, 1977).

REFERENCES

Greene WL & Bollinger RR (1984) Cimetidine for stress-ulcer prophylaxis. *Critical Care Medicine* **12:** 571–575.

Groll A, Simon JB, Wigle RD et al (1986) Cimetidine prophylaxis for gastrointestinal bleeding in an intensive care unit. *Gut* **27:** 135–140.

Halloran LG, Zfass AM, Gayle WE, Wheeler CB & Miller JD (1980) Prevention of acute gastrointestinal complications after severe head injury: a controlled trial of cimetidine prophylaxis. *American Journal of Surgery* **139:** 44–48.

MacDougall BRD, Bailey RJ & Williams R (1977) H_2-receptor antagonists and antacids in the prevention of acute gastrointestinal haemorrhage in fulminant hepatic failure: two controlled trials. *Lancet* **i:** 617–619.

Priebe JH, Skillman JJ, Bushnell LS, Long PC & Silen W (1980) Antacid versus cimetidine in preventing acute gastrointestinal bleeding. *New England Journal of Medicine* **302:** 426–430.

Pingleton SK & Hadzima SK (1983) Enteral alimentation and gastrointestinal bleeding in mechanically ventilated patients. *Critical Care Medicine* **11:** 13–16.

9
Cardiopulmonary Resuscitation and Management of Dysrhythmias

In the first half of this century, attempts at resuscitation normally consisted of elaborate manoeuvres designed to ventilate the lungs, but these usually achieved only limited chest expansion. For instance, Dr Henry Silvester's technique, described in 1857, was performed with the subject supine and involved lifting the patient's arms 'upwards by the side of the head and then extending them gently and steadily upwards and forwards'. Expiration was achieved by turning the patient's arms and pressing them 'gently and firmly for a few moments against the side of the chest'. This was later superseded by Colonel Holger Nielson's method, described in 1932. The patient was placed in the prone position with the arms flexed and hands placed beneath the head. The operator, positioned by the subject's head, lifted the patient's arms upwards at the elbow, thereby extending the spine and reducing intrathoracic pressure. Expiration was achieved by compression of the lower chest. In the same year, Eve described the 'tilting board' method in which the patient was strapped to a stretcher and rocked. Oscillation of the abdominal contents produced diaphragmatic movement and pulmonary ventilation.

Some have suggested, however, that successful mouth-to-mouth resuscitation had been described much earlier in the Bible. In the second book of Kings, chapter iv, verse 34, there is a description of the revival of an apparently dead child by the prophet Elisha: 'And he went up, and lay upon the child, and put his mouth upon his mouth, and his eyes upon his eyes, and his hands upon his hands; and he stretched himself upon the child; and the flesh of the child waxed warm'. Nevertheless, it was not until 1954 that Elam et al demonstrated that mouth-to-mask respiration with the operator's expired air could produce adequate pulmonary ventilation.

The use of open-chest cardiac massage in humans was reported and discussed by Green in *The Lancet* as long ago as 1906 (Green, 1906). He reviewed 40 cases who had received internal cardiac massage, of whom 17 were initially revived and nine survived long term. Nevertheless, despite Boehm's use of closed-chest cardiac massage in cats in 1878 and Tournade's studies of this technique in dogs in 1934, external cardiac massage (ECM) did not become established in clinical practice until the early 1960s (Baringer et al, 1961). Even then it was only recommended as an alternative to internal cardiac massage when thoracotomy was impractical, partly because it was considered that the risk of serious complications such as haemothorax, haemopericardium and liver lacerations was unacceptably high. Furthermore, although successful resuscitation was undoubtedly possible using ECM, some still suspected that open-chest cardiac massage was a more effective means of sustaining adequate blood flow. Nevertheless, because thoracotomy is a formidable undertaking for the inexperienced, and in view of the substantial risk of direct myocardial damage, most authorities now feel that internal cardiac massage is rarely justified, except when the chest is already open.

Initially, the mechanism by which ECM produced blood flow was speculative. It was suggested that direct compression of the heart between sternum and spine elevated intraventricular pressures above those in the great vessels, thereby generating forward flow through the aortic and pulmonary valves. Cyclical release of sternal pressure allowed chest recoil, reducing intrathoracic pressure and enhancing venous return, while reflux of blood into the aorta and pulmonary artery was prevented by the one-way valves. Later, measurements of intravascular pressures in dogs receiving cardiopulmonary resuscitation (CPR) demonstrated that, as some had already suspected, ECM produced simultaneous and equal pressure increases in both central venous and arterial vessels (Rudikoff et al, 1980). Moreover, the rises in intrathoracic pressure were transmitted fully to the carotid artery but only minimally to the jugular vein, creating a peripheral arteriovenous pressure gradient and antegrade flow. Angiographic studies (Niemann et al, 1979) have shown that aortic flow is produced initially by direct compression of this vessel, and that this is followed by delayed, but simultaneous, opening of the mitral and aortic valves. Flow through the heart persists throughout the period of cardiac compression, and for this reason ECM is most effective when sternal depression is sustained. In fact, lung inflation alone can produce some forward flow, and simultaneous external cardiac compression and positive pressure ventilation produces greater rises in aortic systolic pressure, thereby enhancing forward flow (Rudikoff et al, 1980; Niemann et al, 1979) ('new CPR'). During ECM, backward flow is prevented by competent aortic, mitral, pulmonary and tricuspid valves while transmission of the pressure wave to the venous system is minimized by collapse of the great veins and by valves situated at the thoracic inlet (Rudikoff et al, 1980). The latter probably close when intrathoracic pressure increases rapidly (e.g. during coughing), but remain patent when the increase in pressure is more gradual (e.g. in cardiac failure). Thus, the whole thorax performs as a pump during ECM with flow from intra- to extrathoracic vessels, the heart and lungs acting as a single one-way reservoir of blood. During chest compression, blood is expelled from the thorax into patent arteries and, during this phase, retrograde venous flow is minimized by the presence of valves and by venous collapse at high intrathoracic pressures. Venous return occurs during chest recoil. The cardiac output achieved in this way is probably only a fraction of normal values.

Diagnosis of cardiorespiratory arrest

This is usually straightforward. The patient rapidly loses consciousness, becoming pale, cyanosed and lifeless with absent pulsation in major vessels (carotid and femoral arteries). Heart sounds cannot be heard and respiratory efforts are absent or gasping. The pupils soon dilate and become unresponsive to light. It may be difficult to determine whether the primary event was a respiratory or a cardiac arrest although if a history can be obtained, this may suggest the likely sequence of events. When the primary aetiology is a respiratory abnormality, profound bradycardia and cyanosis often precede cardiac arrest.

TREATMENT

It is vital to call for assistance since it is virtually impossible to perform adequate resuscitation unaided.

Airway and respiration

The first priority is to establish a clear airway. The oropharynx must be cleared of false teeth, vomit, blood and other debris before flexing the neck, extending the head and inserting an oropharyngeal airway. The patient should then be ventilated with added oxygen at a rate of approximately 12 breaths per minute using a face mask and a self-inflating bag. If these are unavailable, then mouth-to-mouth expired air ventilation should be performed, or the lungs can be inflated using a Brook airway (Fig. 9.1).

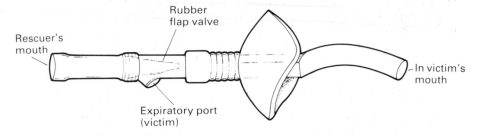

Rubber
flap valve

Rescuer's
mouth

In victim's
mouth

Expiratory port
(victim)

Fig. 9.1 A Brook airway.

Whichever method is used, it is important to ensure that the chest expands with each insufflation. If it proves impossible to achieve adequate ventilation using any of these methods, then endotracheal intubation may be required, although this should normally only be attempted by those experienced in the technique. Prolonged attempts at intubation by unskilled personnel waste valuable time, may exacerbate hypoxia and hypercarbia and can cause structural damage. Nevertheless, the trachea should be intubated as soon as skilled assistance arrives since this secures the airway, ensures effective positive pressure ventilation and protects the lungs from aspiration of stomach contents.

Despite immediate, vigorous, manual ventilation, respiratory acidosis is common during CPR and this may be exacerbated by the administration of sodium bicarbonate, which generates carbon dioxide. This impairs cerebral autoregulation and may contribute to brain ischaemia. Nevertheless, because hypercarbia stimulates the sympathetic nervous system it may be less harmful than a metabolic acidosis. Hypoxia is also common during CPR and is probably due to ventilation perfusion mismatch as a result of alveolar collapse caused by chest compression, combined with reduced lung perfusion. Arterial hypoxaemia is further exacerbated by the fall in $P_{\bar{v}}O_2$ caused by poor tissue perfusion. Finally, lung function may be further compromised during CPR by pre-existing cardiac failure or lung disease, as well as by aspiration of gastric contents. In some circumstances, the application of PEEP during CPR might be expected to improve oxygenation and, although usually associated with a reduction in cardiac output (see Chapter 13, p. 243), could actually enhance forward flow by further augmenting the overall rise in intrathoracic pressure.

Cardiac massage

Some authorities now recommend that, except when cardiorespiratory arrest is due to hypoxia, priority should be given to ECM rather than securing the airway and ensuring adequate ventilation (Gilston and Resnekov, 1971). They argue that in order to prevent ischaemic damage to vital organs, it is more important to re-establish blood flow than to treat hypoxaemia, and that unless the patient was hypoxic prior to cardiorespiratory arrest, the lungs will initially contain reasonable amounts of oxygen. Furthermore, initiation of CPR is not delayed because of aesthetic objections to mouth-to-mouth resuscitation, and immediate ECM or defibrillation may restore effective cardiac activity before myocardial hypoxia has developed. Finally, mouth-to-mouth resuscitation is more difficult to perform effectively than ECM. However, 'chest thumping' is generally not recommended since it is rarely successful, it delays restoration of forward flow and ECM is probably an equally effective means of restoring myocardial activity (Gilston and Resnekov, 1971).

Effective ECM can only be performed on a hard surface. This may be provided by an intensive care or coronary care unit bed, a board placed under the mattress or, failing either of these, by placing the patient on the floor. The heel of one hand should be positioned over the lower third of the sternum and the other hand should be placed over the first. The sternum should be depressed sharply by 2–4 cm by bending at the waist approximately 60 times per minute with the arms straight. For optimal flow, cardiac compression should be forceful and sustained, occupying approximately 60% of each cycle. Traditionally, each lung inflation is followed by 4–6 cardiac compressions. Some authorities now recommend that lung inflation and ECM are performed simultaneously in order to augment the increase in intrathoracic pressure and increase cerebral blood flow ('new CPR', see above) (Chandra et al, 1980). However, 'new CPR' can only be used safely when an endotracheal tube is in place to prevent gastric distension and pulmonary aspiration. Furthermore, because this technique can generate very high intrathoracic pressures, the lung damage associated with CPR may be exacerbated. 'New CPR' can be used when conventional techniques fail to produce adequate forward flow. In some cases, open-chest massage may be required. Abdominal binding and compression of leg veins using the MAST garment (see Chapter 10, p. 142) can also be used to increase intrathoracic pressures and enhance venous return.

Once effective cardiac massage and artificial ventilation have been established, the patient's colour should improve, the pupils may return to normal size, there will be a palpable pulse (although this does not necessarily indicate adequate flow, merely that the pressure wave has been transmitted along a patent, fluid-filled vessel), and the conscious level may improve (head shaking, grimacing). At this stage, an ECG monitor should be attached to the patient, if one is not already in place, and more specific treatment instituted.

Intravenous access

Expansion of the circulating volume is generally not required during CPR, but powerful vasoconstrictors and sodium bicarbonate must be given into a large vein in order to avoid skin necrosis and to ensure rapid delivery to the myocardium. Furthermore, the peripheral veins are often collapsed and difficult to cannulate. It is therefore preferable to insert a cannula into the internal jugular vein. Puncture of the subclavian vein is not recommended in this situation because of the risk of pneumothorax. If it proves impossible to cannulate the internal jugular vein, the external jugular vein may be used as an alternative. It is usually difficult to distinguish between the femoral vein and artery during cardiorespiratory arrest and this approach is therefore generally best avoided. Intratracheal instillation of drugs has been recommended as an alternative when venous cannulation proves difficult, and even as an immediate measure before intravascular access is established. However, some consider this route to be unreliable and 'splash back' of drugs occurs during positive pressure ventilation. Intracardiac injection is traumatic and dangerous (in particular, the left anterior descending coronary artery may be damaged) and should only be used when other routes fail.

Correction of acidosis

Anaerobic metabolism during the period of poor tissue perfusion is associated with increased lactic acid production. Furthermore, metabolism of lactic acid by the liver is impaired by the reduction in hepatic blood flow, and during extreme ischaemia the liver itself contributes to lactate production. Nevertheless, since metabolic acidosis is only deleterious when severe, the routine administration of large quantities of sodium bicarbonate during CPR is inappropriate, particularly following short periods of cardiorespiratory arrest, and may be dangerous. Potential adverse effects of excessive sodium bicarbonate administration include hypernatraemia, with an increased plasma osmolality, hypokalaemia, increased cardiac irritability, impaired myocardial performance, exacerbation of respiratory acidosis and increased affinity of haemoglobin for oxygen. Moreover, sympathomimetic agents may be inactivated when mixed with sodium bicarbonate. As an approximation, about 0.5 mmol of sodium bicarbonate per litre of extracellular fluid (ECF) is required for each minute of CPR in order to neutralize the acidosis. It is therefore not necessary to administer sodium bicarbonate immediately unless the patient is known to have had a pre-existing acidosis, e.g. due to cardiogenic shock. Ideally, subsequent administration of alkali should be guided by frequent acid–base determinations.

Drug therapy

Cardiac arrest is associated with profound vasodilatation, presumably due to extreme tissue ischaemia and acidosis, and this may partly account for the ability of these patients to tolerate enormous doses of sympathomimetics.

This fall in systemic resistance hinders restoration of an adequate blood pressure during CPR and, even though circulating catecholamines are markedly elevated during cardiac arrest, it is usual to administer a powerful vasoconstrictor such as adrenaline, noradrenaline or phenylephrine. It may then be possible to achieve a blood pressure sufficient to perfuse the coronary and cerebral circulations. Some other sympathomimetics (particularly isoprenaline) may also be useful in asystole and to 'coarsen' slow, low-voltage ventricular fibrillation. Inotropic support is often continued following successful resuscitation in order to maintain cerebral and myocardial perfusion.

Calcium chloride is also traditionally recommended for asystole and 'fine' ventricular fibrillation, as well as in cases of electromechanical dissociation, even though ionized calcium levels are usually high following cardiac arrest. (A few patients may have reduced calcium levels due to pre-existing pathology such as renal failure, malabsorption, or hypoparathyroidism, while trauma victims transfused with large volumes of colloids are also sometimes hypocalcaemic.) The correct dose of calcium chloride during CPR is not known and excessive quantities may precipitate digitalis toxicity, arrest the heart in systole ('stone heart'), cause spasm of coronary vessels, exacerbate vasodilatation and depress sinus node function. Moreover, in view of the apparently crucial role of intracellular accumulation of calcium ions in mediating ischaemic cell death, and the possibility that calcium antagonists protect against ischaemic damage, the administration of large quantities of calcium might be deleterious. Finally, accidental mixing of calcium chloride and sodium bicarbonate will precipitate calcium carbonate. Nevertheless, intravenous calcium chloride is a useful means of rapidly reversing the adverse effects of hyperkalaemia (see below). Calcium gluconate contains fewer free calcium ions than calcium chloride and may, therefore, be less effective.

Correction of electrolyte disturbances

Hyperkalaemia is relatively common during CPR, partly due to the release of potassium into the circulation from damaged tissues. It should be treated with glucose/insulin mixtures, calcium chloride and diuretics. In some cases, ventricular fibrillation or tachycardia may have been precipitated by hypokalaemia and this will require aggressive treatment with intravenous potassium chloride.

Treatment of ventricular fibrillation/tachycardia

Ventricular fibrillation (VF) is the commonest cause of cardiac arrest and, because defibrillation is most likely to be successful when performed before the myocardium becomes severely hypoxic, it is worth while administering a 100 J direct current (DC) shock before an ECG is available. 'Coarse' fibrillation (Fig. 9.2b) should be treated with DC shocks of increasing energy up to 400 J. If the VF is slow, and of low voltage, adrenaline and, possibly, calcium chloride should be administered to 'coarsen' the electrical activity before further attempts at defibrillation. Repeated high-energy shocks (>300 J) may be associated with myocardial damage, particularly when the

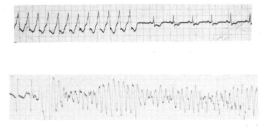

Fig. 9.2 (a) Ventricular tachycardia terminating spontaneously. (b) 'Coarse' ventricular fibrillation.

time interval between successive shocks is short (Doherty et al, 1979). Ventricular tachycardia (VT) (see Fig. 9.2a) should also initially be treated with a DC shock.

When VF or VT is refractory to the above measures, or recurrent, the excitability of the myocardium must be reduced. Traditionally, a bolus dose of 100 mg lignocaine is administered intravenously, followed, if necessary, by a continuous infusion at a rate of 1–3 mg min^{-1}. If necessary, the bolus can be repeated, provided that a total dose of 3 mg kg^{-1} is not exceeded. The main value of lignocaine lies in its ability to prevent ventricular dysrhythmias; its role in assisting defibrillation is less clear. Some authorities therefore recommend the use of intravenous bretylium tosylate in refractory VF since this raises the fibrillation threshold. It should be administered as a bolus of 5–10 mg kg^{-1}, which can be repeated after 30–60 minutes and continued as an infusion. Bretylium can produce hypotension and vasodilatation but does not appear to depress myocardial contractility (Bexton and Camm, 1982). Disopyramide may also be useful for the control of ventricular dysrhythmias, but is less likely to be successful in this situation. It should be administered initially as a bolus of 2 mg kg^{-1} given over 5 minutes intravenously and then continued as a continuous infusion to a total dose not exceeding 800 mg day^{-1}. In some cases, β-blockade or mexiletine may be indicated. Amiodarone is a very powerful antidysrhythmic, useful against both supraventricular and ventricular tachycardias, which can be used to prevent recurrence of VT or VF (Bexton and Camm, 1982). It can, however, produce hypotension when administered intravenously and in the long term is associated with potentially serious side effects such as hepatic dysfunction, pulmonary fibrosis, disturbances of thyroid function and peripheral neuropathy. Its use should therefore be restricted to life-threatening dysrhythmias. When administered intravenously, an electrophysiological effect can probably be obtained within a few hours. A bolus of about 200 mg can be followed by a continuous infusion of approximately 1 g per 24 hours. If possible, oral amiodarone 200–600 mg per day should be started simultaneously.

It is important to remember that hypokalaemia is a potent cause of ventricular ectopic rhythms and if present this should be rapidly corrected. Similarly, persistent dysrhythmias may be related to hypoxia, acidosis or alkalosis, hyperosmolar syndrome, alterations in plasma levels of magnesium or calcium, or to myocardial failure.

If the patient is in asystole, the prognosis is generally poor. It may be possible to convert asystole to ventricular fibrillation by giving adrenaline (or isoprenaline) and calcium chloride. Some recommend the administration of atropine to counter parasympathetic hyperactivity, although this may lower the fibrillation threshold in the presence of increased sympathetic drive. Transvenous pacing should only be considered when cardiac arrest is preceded by complete heart block, or in those with digitalis toxicity.

Patients with extreme bradycardia may respond to intravenous atropine and, if necessary, this can be followed by an intravenous infusion of isoprenaline or salbutamol. In the presence of heart block, a transvenous intracardiac pacing wire should be inserted. Sequential atrioventricular pacing often produces a better cardiac output than ventricular pacing. In some centres, intra-oesophageal or thoracic wall pacing is used when it proves impossible to position a wire transvenously.

Sometimes, myocardial damage is so severe that there is no cardiac output despite the presence of electrical activity on the ECG. In these cases, it is important to exclude cardiac tamponade. Occasionally, the patient may respond to inotropic agents, or calcium, but in general the prognosis in cases of electromechanical dissociation is hopeless.

Abandoning CPR

It is not possible to diagnose brain stem death with confidence during CPR and therefore attempts at resuscitation should only be abandoned when it proves impossible to restore effective myocardial activity. CPR should continue for longer in those who are hypothermic or the victims of near drowning (see Chapter 11). In some patients with terminal disease, CPR is started inappropriately (Hershey and Fisher, 1982) and should then be abandoned as soon as the circumstances are clear. This situation can usually be avoided by establishing that resuscitation would be inappropriate as soon as the nature and extent of the underlying disease have been determined.

POSTRESUSCITATION MANAGEMENT

The complications of external cardiac massage include traumatic injury to the abdominal viscera, in particular rupture of the liver and spleen, damage to the myocardium and chest wall, as well as pulmonary aspiration and impaired lung function. In one study, rib fractures were seen in 34% of those who had received CPR, while myocardial contusion occurred in 1.3% and haemopericardium in 8.1%. Aspiration pneumonia was seen in 1.3% (Nagel et al, 1981). Ruptured liver or spleen will require restoration of the circulating volume followed by surgical repair, although in practice it is unlikely that such complications will be diagnosed at the time, and even then surgery is rarely feasible.

A minority of patients will be resuscitated easily and quickly. They rapidly regain consciousness and resume spontaneous ventilation. They can be extubated immediately and subsequent treatment is aimed at preventing a recurrence. However, many of those who are successfully resuscitated will initially remain unconscious, often with absent or inadequate spontaneous respiratory efforts and hypotension. In these cases, subsequent management is aimed at restoring cardiovascular and respiratory function and minimizing cerebral damage.

Cardiovascular function

It is vital to ensure that cerebral, and coronary, blood flow are adequate following resuscitation and it is therefore essential to restore the systemic blood pressure. This requires manipulation of the circulating volume, guided by the CVP or PCWP as indicated, and, if necessary, the administration of inotropic agents. Metabolic derangements and fluid and electrolyte disturbances must also be corrected. Intra-aortic balloon counterpulsation (IABCP) may be indicated in those with cardiogenic shock or persistent myocardial ischaemia (see Chapter 10).

Respiratory function

The endotracheal tube must be left in place until the patient is conscious and has effective cough, gag and swallowing reflexes. Later, some patients may require a tracheostomy. Controlled ventilation is clearly indicated when respiratory function is impaired, for example in those with pulmonary oedema, aspiration pneumonitis or a significant flail segment. Furthermore, hyperventilation may improve cerebral autoregulation, as well as reducing cerebral acidosis (see Chapter 14). Nevertheless, although it is universally accepted that hypoxaemia and hypercarbia must be avoided at all costs, the role of deliberate hyperventilation, and of prolonged (>48 hours) controlled ventilation when respiratory function is adequate, remains unclear (see Chapter 14) (Gisvold et al, 1984a). A reasonable approach is to initiate controlled ventilation in all patients following a global ischaemic insult and to reassess the situation 4–6 hours later. Suitable patients can then be allowed to breathe spontaneously.

Cerebral function (Hinds, 1985)

Provided there is no pre-existing intracranial pathology, e.g. cerebrovascular disease, and cardiac arrest was not preceded by hypoxia, ischaemic brain damage can probably be prevented by maintaining a cerebral blood flow as low as one-seventh of normal (Gilston and Resnekov, 1971). This can usually be achieved if CPR is correctly performed. Nevertheless, cerebral perfusion is not usually sufficient to sustain normal brain activity during CPR and patients may remain unconscious, sometimes with fixed dilated pupils, and yet recover normal cerebral function. Sometimes, signs of cerebral activity such as frowning, head shaking, struggling and an eyelash reflex may be present during CPR and these suggest that the brain is being adequately oxygenated.

If, however, resuscitation is protracted, cerebral function usually deteriorates progressively due to a gradual reduction in cerebral blood flow and persistent relative ischaemia. Furthermore, cerebral lactic acidosis, which is not corrected by the systemic administration of sodium bicarbonate, impairs autoregulation (the mean perfusion pressure during CPR is less than

50 mmHg and is therefore below the lower limit for autoregulation) and depresses cerebral function.

The ultimate outcome for those patients who are successfully resuscitated could be considerably improved if it were possible to ameliorate the cerebral damage caused by cardiorespiratory arrest and protracted CPR. Clearly, this could be achieved if improved techniques of CPR were developed which maintained normal cerebral perfusion. (Although 'new CPR' may enhance forward flow and systemic blood pressure, it is possible that the potential increase in cerebral blood flow is prevented by a simultaneous rise in intracranial and venous pressures.) It is also possible, however, that events occurring during recirculation may initiate or exacerbate cell damage and that appropriate interventions might therefore limit the degree of brain damage.

Control of seizures

Seizure discharges may exacerbate postischaemic cerebral damage by increasing metabolic demands and precipitating neuronal hypoxia in areas of marginally perfused brain. Moreover, sympathetic nervous activity is increased and this constitutes an extra demand on the patient's limited cardiorespiratory reserve. It is therefore accepted that prophylactic administration of anticonvulsants and aggressive treatment of seizures, both of which are associated with minimal risks, is normally justified (Shapiro, 1984).

Cerebral perfusion

There is evidence that the degree of cerebral damage is influenced by the adequacy of cerebral perfusion following restoration of cardiac activity. Thus, it appears that the brain can recover from quite prolonged periods of normothermic relative ischaemia (up to 20 minutes) provided that cerebral blood flow is subsequently adequate, although a number of other factors are probably also important (Gilston, 1979).

Initially, systemic hypertension, combined with the loss of autoregulation, may cause cerebral hyperperfusion with oedema formation and disruption of the blood–brain barrier. Subsequently, however, hypoperfusion is nearly always the dominant abnormality. This is associated with prolonged, severe depression of cerebral cortical blood flow and an increased cerebrovascular resistance. Possible explanations have included cellular swelling with raised intracranial pressure, intravascular coagulation, increases in viscosity, microvascular endothelial swelling and release of vasoactive metabolites of arachidonic acid, e.g. thromboxane (see Chapter 10, p. 131). It has also been suggested that cerebrovascular spasm may be caused by an influx of calcium ions into anoxic vascular smooth muscle (White et al, 1983). Because autoregulation is impaired, the aim should be to achieve normotension, or slight hypertension, during the postarrest period (Shapiro, 1984); extreme hypertension, which might exacerbate oedema formation and intracranial hypertension, should be avoided.

Based on these findings, suggested therapeutic interventions have included anticoagulation, haemodilution with dextrans or oxygen-carrying blood substitutes, administration of calcium antagonists, prostacyclin, diuretics and steroids, and manipulation of the arachidonic acid cascade. There is little evidence to support the use of steroids, diuretics or anticoagulants in this situation and it appears that cerebral oedema is unusual following global brain ischaemia, except in those who have sustained extensive neuronal damage incompatible with survival (Gisvold et al, 1984a). The value of other measures remains uncertain.

Metabolic factors

It has been suggested that elevated brain glucose levels predispose to cerebral oedema and enhance lactic acid production by increasing the supply of substrate, thereby exacerbating neuronal damage. A number of experimental studies have in fact demonstrated that high blood glucose levels prior to cardiac arrest are associated with a worse neurological outcome (Pulsinelli et al, 1982). The clinical implications of these findings are at present unclear, although it would seem sensible to avoid hyperglycaemia in high risk situations.

Biochemical abnormalities

The rapid depletion of cellular energy stores which follows sudden, complete ischaemia, leads to failure of the ionic pump, membrane depolarization and cellular swelling. There is also an accumulation of calcium ions within the cells. This may initiate a number of harmful reactions (including the release of free fatty acids, particularly arachidonic acid, and the production of free radicals of oxygen) and could be the 'final common pathway' leading to cell death.

The potential of calcium entry blocking drugs as cerebral protective agents is therefore being investigated (White et al, 1983). These may act by preventing cerebrovascular spasm and maintaining cerebral blood flow, or by reducing the calcium-induced liberation of damaging free fatty acids and superoxide radicals (White et al, 1983).

It has also been suggested that barbiturates might protect the brain from ischaemic damage by virtue of their ability to act as 'free radical scavengers'. These agents also reduce brain metabolism, cerebral blood flow, and intracranial pressure and may improve the cerebral oxygen supply/demand ratio. A number of experimental studies have suggested that barbiturate pretreatment and, possibly, early postinsult therapy, is beneficial in focal ischaemia. However, recent studies have failed to confirm earlier work which had indicated that barbiturates might be of value in experimental global brain ischaemia (Gisvold et al, 1984b), and in a randomized clinical trial of thiopentone loading in comatose survivors of cardiac arrest there were no significant differences in outcome between treatment and control groups (Brain Resuscitation Clinical Trial 1 Study Group 1986).

At present, therefore, the clinical use of barbiturates, or other intravenous anaesthetic agents, to ameliorate postischaemic cerebral damage cannot be justified. The role of calcium antagonists and other specific agents remains unclear. Although it seems likely that multiple therapeutic interventions will ultimately be required to achieve a significant beneficial effect, there is a danger that some treatments will counteract the effects of others (Shapiro, 1984). Furthermore, the timing of each intervention in relation to the episode of cardiorespiratory arrest will probably prove to be crucial. Current management of patients following CPR is therefore based on supporting cardiorespiratory function in order to ensure optimum conditions for brain recovery, and the only undisputed therapeutic principles are to restore systemic blood pressure, ensure adequate oxygenation, avoid hypercapnia and abolish seizures.

PROGNOSIS OF CARDIORESPIRATORY ARREST

Not surprisingly, the results of CPR initiated in the community are inferior to those achieved within the hospital environment, probably largely related to delays in initiating resuscitation, combined with lack of skill and interruptions in CPR while the patient is moved. In particular, coma is more frequent in those who suffer a cardiorespiratory arrest outside hospital and the prognosis for cerebral recovery is closely related to the duration of coma. Thus, permanent cerebral damage is extremely unusual when coma lasts for less than six hours and relatively unusual with coma of between 6 and 24 hours duration. Recovery of consciousness is unprecedented when coma persists for more than seven days (Thomassen and Wernberg, 1979).

Even within hospitals, organizational deficiencies and absent or malfunctioning equipment, may significantly delay the institution of effective CPR, and the outcome for those who arrest on general wards is poor (only 3% of patients discharged). The outlook for those who arrest in the intensive care unit or emergency department is, however, considerably better and in one series 19% of patients were discharged home (Hershey and Fisher, 1982). This disparity between survival rates in the two locations was not attributable to differences in the immediate response to CPR since 58% of cases on general wards and 60% of those in the ICU or emergency department were initially successfully resuscitated. Rather, it reflected the severity of the underlying illness in those receiving CPR on the general wards, for many of whom attempted resuscitation was clearly inappropriate (Hershey and Fisher, 1982). The importance of determining whether CPR is indicated for a particular patient before cardiac arrest supervenes has been stressed by a number of authors (Editorial, 1982).

Good prognostic features include a previously normal heart, prompt initiation of effective CPR and cardiac arrest due to primary ventricular fibrillation. Conversely, when cardiac arrest occurs in a patient with progressive myocardial failure, often in asystole, the outlook is grave.

MANAGEMENT OF DYSRHYTHMIAS

Dysrhythmias occurring in critically ill patients are frequently secondary to associated abnormalities such as hypoxia, electrolyte disturbances (particularly hypokalaemia or hypomagnesaemia), sudden alterations in arterial carbon dioxide tension, increased circulating catecholamine levels or sepsis. In some cases, pre-existing cardiac disease or myocardial contusion (see Chapter 11,

p. 161) may contribute to the development of rhythm disturbances. Because of the dangers associated with the use of any antidysrhythmic agents (see below) these abnormalities must be identified and, if possible, corrected before resorting to specific therapy. Subsequent definitive treatment is then only indicated when the dysrhythmia persists and is associated with a significant haemodynamic disturbance. Specific therapy may also be required when persistence of the abnormality is likely to impair cardiac performance (e.g. when the ventricular rate is very rapid) or if the dysrhythmia is of a type conventionally considered to predispose to more serious rhythm disturbances (e.g. 'R on T' ventricular premature contractions (VPCs)). Furthermore, if it is not possible to correct the underlying abnormality immediately (e.g. a patient with atrial fibrillation secondary to pneumonia and septicaemia) it is often futile to attempt to restore sinus rhythm since, even if this is achieved, the dysrhythmia will almost certainly recur. Under these circumstances, the ventricular rate should be controlled and any haemodynamic disturbance minimized.

Critically ill patients are generally intolerant of antidysrhythmics, almost all of which are negatively inotropic, and in general these agents should be avoided. If this is not possible, they should be administered cautiously in reduced dosage. Direct current cardioversion does not impair myocardial function unless excessively high energy shocks (>300 J) are used or administered repeatedly (Doherty et al, 1979) and this is therefore often the most appropriate initial treatment when restoration of sinus rhythm is essential. Similarly, digoxin does not depress the myocardium and remains a valuable agent for use in seriously ill patients.

The choice of the most appropriate antidysrhythmic for a particular patient is often difficult and the various classifications of the available agents are unlikely to be of much help to the practising clinician (Aronson, 1985).

When complex dysrhythmias are encountered and/or the abnormality fails to respond to simple measures, a cardiologist should, if possible, be consulted.

Treatment of specific dysrhythmias

Treatment of ventricular fibrillation and tachycardia is discussed on pp. 112–113.

Sinus bradycardia

As heart rate falls, cardiac output is maintained by an increase in stroke volume, due largely to a rise in end-diastolic volume. If this compensatory mechanism fails, blood pressure falls, ventricular filling pressures rise and coronary perfusion is jeopardized. Sometimes nodal, or ventricular, 'escape' rhythms are seen, in which case the heart rate should be increased, initially by administering atropine intravenously. In persistent cases, repeated administration of atropine may be required. Alternatively, a continuous intravenous infusion of a β-stimulant, such as isoprenaline or salbutamol can be instituted. Provided there is no abnormality of atrioventricular (AV) conduction, atrial pacing is occasionally indicated, but a temporary ventricular electrode should also be inserted in case the atrial system fails or an AV conduction abnormality supervenes. As well as producing haemodynamic improvement, increasing the heart rate may abolish escape rhythms.

Sinus tachycardia

This is nearly always a secondary phenomenon related to hypovolaemia, pyrexia, hypoxaemia, hypercarbia, anaemia, pain or anxiety. These abnormalities must be identified and, when possible, corrected. Specific treatment is therefore usually not required and, because the reduction in heart rate may be associated with a fall in cardiac output, may actually be deleterious. Nevertheless, because tachycardia markedly increases myocardial oxygen requirements (see Chapter 2), it is sometimes prudent to control the heart rate, usually with a β-blocker. This applies particularly to patients with ischaemic heart disease, although β-blockers must be used cautiously, if at all, in those with impaired ventricular performance.

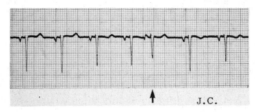

Fig. 9.3 Atrial premature contraction, associated with an inferior myocardial infarction.

Atrial premature contractions (APCs) (Fig. 9.3)

These are usually benign and therefore do not normally warrant intervention. Treatment may be indicated, however, in a patient who has reverted to sinus rhythm following an episode of atrial fibrillation (in this situation closely coupled APCs may precipitate atrial fibrillation), when APCs are not conducted (this may lead to a very slow effective ventricular rate), and in those in whom APCs are known to precipitate a re-entry tachycardia. APCs are usually treated with either disopyramide or quinidine.

Supraventricular tachycardias

Atrial and junctional tachycardias (Fig. 9.4). These are often indistinguishable on the surface ECG, but both can be managed in the same way. The tachycardia, together with impaired or absent atrial transport, can produce haemodynamic deterioration, particularly in those with poor ventricular function. Furthermore, myocardial oxygen requirements increase while coronary blood flow, which occurs mainly in diastole, falls.

Occasionally, carotid sinus massage restores sinus rhythm, or may increase the degree of AV block, enabling atrial and junctional tachycardias to be distinguished from each other and from atrial flutter (Fig. 9.5).

Synchronized direct current cardioversion is usually the most appropriate initial treatment. Verapamil, a calcium channel blocker predominantly

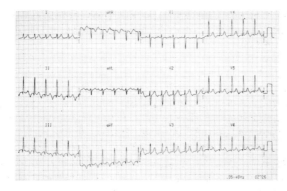

Fig. 9.4 Supraventricular tachycardia.

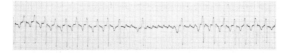

Fig. 9.5 Carotid sinus massage reveals atrial flutter.

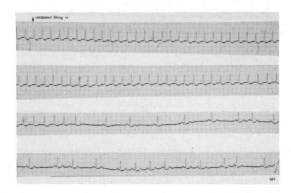

Fig. 9.6 Supraventricular tachycardia terminated by intravenous verapamil.

affecting the AV node, is likely to slow the ventricular rate and may restore sinus rhythm in paroxysmal supraventricular tachycardia (Heng et al, 1975) (Fig. 9.6). It should be administered slowly intravenously in a dose of up to 5 mg, repeated if necessary at approximately 5 minute intervals up to a total dose of 20 mg. However, verapamil can produce marked myocardial depression, with profound hypotension, and should be used extremely cautiously in the critically ill. Moreover, it should never be given with a β-blocker, since the combination is known to cause extreme bradycardia, hypotension (Packer et al, 1982) and even asystole.

Provided the patient is not digitalized, and there is no possibility of digitalis toxicity, digoxin can be used as a safer alternative to verapamil in order to slow the ventricular rate. When a supraventricular tachycardia is likely to have been precipitated by digitalis toxicity, digoxin should be withdrawn and hypokalaemia, if present, corrected. Phenytoin (50–100 mg intravenously every 5 minutes, not to exceed a total dose of 1 g) is a particularly effective antidysrhythmic in this situation. The parenteral formulation of phenytoin is alkaline and very irritant and should therefore be administered via a central vein.

β-Blocking agents are sometimes used to slow the ventricular rate in supraventricular tachycardias, and may occasionally restore sinus rhythm in those with a junctional tachycardia. However, they must be given cautiously when myocardial function is impaired. β-Blockade may also be used to prevent recurrence and sotalol, which also has specific antidysrhythmic properties (Bexton and Camm, 1982), has proved particularly effective in this respect.

If sinus rhythm is restored, disopyramide, a membrane-stabilizing agent with anticholinergic properties (Baines et al, 1976), in a dose of 100–200 mg orally three times a day or up to 600 mg intravenously per 24 hours, can be given to prevent a recurrence. Alternatively, verapamil can be used in a dose of 40–120 mg orally three times a day or as a continuous intravenous infusion of up to 100 mg per 24 hours.

If it proves impossible to restore sinus rhythm, or if the above measures fail to prevent a recurrence, combination drug therapy may be required (e.g. disopyramide and a β-blocker). Alternatively, atrial 'overdrive' pacing may effectively terminate the dysrhythmia.

Atrial flutter. Synchronized direct current cardioversion is nearly always the treatment of choice, particularly since this dysrhythmia usually responds poorly to drug therapy. Intravenous verapamil may slow the ventricular rate, and very occasionally restores sinus rhythm (Heng et al, 1975) while atrial 'overdrive' pacing is sometimes effective, especially after pretreatment with disopyramide. Digoxin is not recommended since very large, potentially toxic doses are often required to control the ventricular rate.

Atrial fibrillation (Fig. 9.7). When atrial fibrillation occurs de novo, synchronized direct current cardioversion is indicated. If cardioversion fails, or the dysrhythmia recurs, it is often safest to digitalize the patient. Digoxin is also used to control the ventricular rate in those with chronic atrial fibrillation. Acute prior administration of digoxin is not an absolute contraindication to DC shock, but low energies (20–50 J) should be used

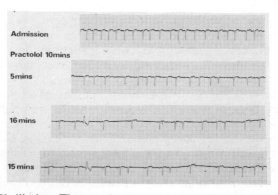

Fig. 9.7 Atrial fibrillation. The ventricular rate is slowed by the administration of a β-blocker.

initially because of the danger of precipitating a ventricular tachydysrhythmia. If necessary,such a dysrhythmia can be treated with lignocaine (see below).

Verapamil can be used to control the ventricular rate, and subsequent administration of disopyramide may then restore sinus rhythm. In this situation, pretreatment with verapamil blocks the AV node and prevents the anticholinergic action of disopyramide from enhancing AV nodal conduction and increasing the ventricular rate. Occasionally, verapamil alone restores sinus rhythm (Heng et al, 1975). β-Blockade is also sometimes used to control the ventricular rate. However, in patients with increased sympathetic drive (e.g. heart failure or thyrotoxicosis) this may be difficult to achieve and there is a danger of administering an overdose of digoxin and/or the β-blocker.

Very occasionally, if atrial fibrillation is poorly tolerated and fails to respond to other therapy, amiodarone (see below) can be used as an atrial stabilizing agent and may cause reversion to sinus rhythm in such patients (Faniel and Schoenfeld, 1983).

Ventricular premature contractions (Fig. 9.8). The significance of VPCs is uncertain, particularly in the absence of ischaemic heart disease. They may be idiopathic and benign or related to associated abnormalities, most commonly

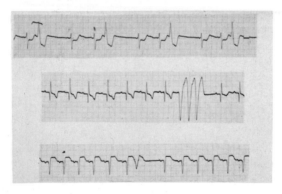

Fig. 9.8 Ventricular premature contractions (VPCs): (a) unifocal trigeminy; (b) salvo of VPCs; (c) R on T VPC.

hypokalaemia. Specific treatment is usually instituted because of concern that they may precipitate VF/VT. Traditionally, a bigeminal rhythm, VPCs occurring more frequently than 5 per minute or in runs of two or more, as well as those which are multifocal or with the R wave superimposed on the T wave, are considered to be 'warning' dysrhythmias which may degenerate into VF/VT, and require treatment. However, the value of such prophylactic measures has been questioned since, although it is possible to reduce the incidence of warning dysrhythmias, and possibly VF/VT, it is uncertain whether this influences the ultimate outcome. Furthermore, following myocardial infarction the frequency of 'warning' dysrhythmias is the same in those who do not develop primary VF as in those who do develop it (Lie et al, 1975). Despite these reservations, most authorities recommend prophylactic treatment for sinister VPCs which persist after correction of associated abnormalities and certainly it is usual to institute such therapy after a recurrence of VF/VT.

Lignocaine probably remains the drug of choice in this situation since it is well tried, generally effective and causes less myocardial depression than some of the newer alternatives such as flecainide (Nathan and Hellestrand, 1984). It can be given as an intravenous bolus dose of $1\,mg\,kg^{-1}$ over 1–2 minutes followed by a continuous infusion at $2-3\,mg\,min^{-1}$. Lignocaine may be associated with dizziness, drowsiness, speech disturbances, tremor and agitation. It is metabolized by the liver and the dose should therefore be reduced in those with hepatic failure or a low cardiac output. In overdose, lignocaine can produce hypotension, fits and conduction disturbances.

Mexiletine is more toxic than lignocaine when administered intravenously, but can be given orally and may be used as maintenance therapy for those who have responded well to intravenous lignocaine. Side effects include skin rashes, nausea and central nervous system disturbances. Disopyramide is sometimes useful but is more negatively inotropic than other agents and may be associated with anticholinergic side effects. Flecainide is poorly tolerated by those with ventricular dysfunction and can even induce dysrhythmias in such patients (Nathan and Hellestrand, 1984).

Idioventricular rhythm (Fig. 9.9). A reduction in the sinus rate, sinus arrest or sino-atrial block may be associated with an idioventricular escape rhythm. Often, the ventricular rate is increased above the expected 40–60 beats per

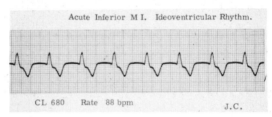

Acute Inferior M I.   Ideoventricular Rhythm.

CL 680   Rate 88 bpm   J.C.

Fig. 9.9 Idioventricular rhythm associated with inferior myocardial infarction.

minute by the effects of the underlying disease, such as a myocardial infarction. This rhythm is often benign but if associated with a haemodynamic disturbance can usually be abolished by increasing the sinus rate.

Disturbances of conduction

First-degree AV block (Fig. 9.10). This is generally benign but may progress to second-degree block, in which case the Wenckebach phenomenon (Mobitz Type I) usually develops.

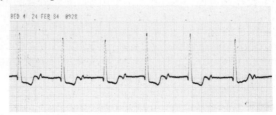

BED 4 24 FEB 84 0928

Fig. 9.10 First-degree AV block.

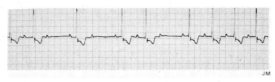

Fig. 9.11 Second-degree AV block—Mobitz Type I.

Second-degree AV block—Mobitz Type I (Wenckebach) (Fig. 9.11). This is commonly associated with an inferior myocardial infarction and is almost always self-limiting. The Wenckebach phenomenon does not usually therefore require treatment. However, if a 2:1 cycle develops it may be associated with haemodynamic deterioration.

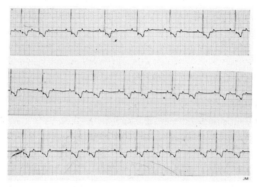

Fig. 9.12 Second-degree AV block—Mobitz Type II.

Mobitz Type II (Fig. 9.12). This often progresses to complete heart block and some authorities therefore recommend insertion of a temporary transvenous pacing wire.

Third-degree AV block (Fig. 9.13). When associated with myocardial infarction, this is caused by ischaemia of the AV node and the conduction disturbance is usually transient. However, when complete heart block accompanies anterior myocardial infarction, it is indicative of a large infarct sufficient to damage the His–Purkinje system. This implies a poor prognosis.

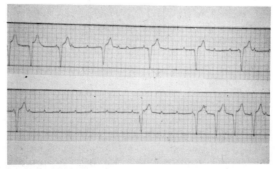

Fig. 9.13 Third-degree AV block.

Treatment involves the administration of drugs to increase the ventricular rate, e.g. atropine (if the ventricular complexes are narrow) or isoprenaline, followed by insertion of a temporary transvenous wire. β-Stimulants should only be used if the patient is hypotensive since they may increase infarct size and precipitate dysrhythmias.

Fascicular block. Prophylactic pacemaker insertion has been recommended for patients with right bundle branch block and left anterior or posterior hemiblock, as well as for those with bifascicular block and a prolonged P–R interval. This is most often indicated in the context of evolving acute myocardial infarction.

In patients with impaired ventricular function, the loss of atrial transport may be poorly tolerated and in these cases atrioventricular sequential pacing may produce haemodynamic improvement (Hartzler et al, 1977).

FURTHER READING

Brownlee WC & Rowlands DJ (1983) Cardiac arrhythmias and their treatment. In Tinker J & Rapin M (eds) *Care of the Critically Ill Patient*, pp 147–161. Berlin: Springer-Verlag.
Gilston A (1983) Cardiopulmonary resuscitation. In Tinker J & Rapin M. (eds) *Care of the Critically Ill Patient*, pp 127–145. Berlin: Springer-Verlag.
Grenvik A & Safar P (eds) (1981) *Brain Failure and Resuscitation (Clinics in Critical Care Medicine)*. New York: Churchill Livingstone.
Jacobson, S (ed.) (1983) *Resuscitation (Clinics in Emergency Medicine)*. New York: Churchill Livingstone.
Safar P (1981) *Cardiopulmonary Cerebral Resuscitation. A Manual for Physicians and Paramedical Instructors*. Laerdal, Stavanger, Norway: World Federation of Societies of Anaesthesiologists.

REFERENCES

Aronson JK (1985) Cardiac arrythmias: theory and practice. *British Medical Journal* **290:** 487–488.
Baines MW, Davies JE, Kellett DN & Munt PL (1976) Some pharmacological effects of disopyramide and a metabolite. *Journal of International Medical Research* **4** (supplement 1): 5–7.
Baringer JR, Salzman EW, Jones WA & Friedlich AL (1961) External cardiac massage. *New England Journal of Medicine* **265:** 62–65.
Bexton RS & Camm AJ (1982) Drugs with a class III antiarrythmic action. *Pharmacology and Therapeutics* **17:** 315–355.
Brain Resuscitation Clinical Trial 1 Study Group (1986) Randomized clinical study of thiopental loading in comatose survivors of cardiac arrest. *New England Journal of Medicine* **314:** 397–403.
Chandra N, Rudikoff M & Weisfeldt ML (1980) Simultaneous chest compression and ventilation at high airway pressure during cardiopulmonary resuscitation. *Lancet* **i:** 175–178.
Doherty PW, McLaughlin PR, Billingham M et al (1979) Cardiac damage produced by direct current countershock applied to the heart. *American Journal of Cardiology* **43:** 225–232.

Editorial (1982) Cardiac resuscitation in hospital: more restraint needed. *Lancet* **i:** 27–28.

Elam JO, Brown ES & Elder JD (1954) Artificial ventilation by mouth-to-mask method. *New England Journal of Medicine* **250:** 749–754.

Faniel R & Schoenfeld P (1983) Efficacy of i.v. amiodarone in converting rapid atrial fibrillation and flutter to sinus rhythm in intensive care patients. *European Heart Journal* **4:** 180–185.

Gilston A (1979) Complete cerebral recovery after prolonged circulatory arrest. *Intensive Care Medicine* **5:** 193–198.

Gilston A & Resnekov L (1971) *Cardio-respiratory Resuscitation.* London: Heinemann Medical.

Gisvold SE, Safar P, Rao G et al (1984a) Prolonged immobilization and controlled ventilation do not improve outcome after global brain ischaemia in monkeys. *Critical Care Medicine* **12:** 171–179.

Gisvold SE, Safar P, Hendrickx HHL et al (1984b) Thiopental treatment after global brain ischemia in pigtailed monkeys. *Anesthesiology* **60:** 88–96.

Green TA (1906) Massage as a means of restoration in cases of apparent sudden death. *Lancet* **ii:** 1708–1714.

Hartzler GO, Maloney JD, Curtis JJ & Barnhorst DA (1977) Hemodynamic benefits of atrioventricular sequential pacing after cardiac surgery. *American Journal of Cardiology* **40:** 232–236.

Heng MK, Singh BN, Roche AHG, Norris RM & Mercer CJ (1975) Effects of intravenous verapamil on cardiac arrythmias and on the electrocardiogram. *American Heart Journal* **90:** 487–498.

Hershey CO & Fisher L (1982) Why outcome of cardiopulmonary resuscitation in general wards is poor. *Lancet* **i:** 31–34.

Hinds CJ (1985) Prevention and treatment of brain ischaemia. *British Medical Journal* **291:** 758–760.

Lie KI, Wellens HJJ, Downar E & Durrer D (1975) Observations on patients with primary ventricular fibrillation complicating acute myocardial infarction. *Circulation* **52:** 755–759.

Nagel EL, Fine EG, Krischer JP & Davis JH (1981) Complications of CPR. *Critical Care Medicine* **9:** 424.

Nathan AW & Hellestrand KJ (1984) Flecainide acetate: a review. *Clinical Progress in Pacing and Electrophysiology* **2:** 43–53.

Niemann JT, Garner D, Rosborough J & Criley JM (1979) The mechanism of blood flow in closed chest cardiopulmonary resuscitation. *Circulation* **60** (supplement 11): 74(abstract).

Packer M, Meller J, Medina N et al (1982) Hemodynamic consequences of combined beta-adrenergic and slow calcium channel blockade in man. *Circulation* **65:** 660.

Pulsinelli WA, Waldman S, Rawlinson D & Plum F (1982) Moderate hyperglycaemia augments ischemic brain damage: a neuropathologic study in the rat. *Neurology* **32:** 1239–1246.

Rudikoff MT, Maughan WL, Effron M, Freund P & Weisfeldt ML (1980) Mechanisms of blood flow during cardiopulmonary resuscitation. *Circulation* **61:** 345–352.

Shapiro HM (1984) Brain resuscitation: the chicken should come before the egg. *Anesthesiology* **60:** 85–87.

Thomassen A & Wernberg M (1979) Prevalence and prognostic significance of coma after cardiac arrest outside intensive care and coronary units. *Acta Anaesthesiologica Scandinavica* **23:** 143–148.

White BC, Winegar CD, Wilson RF, Hoehner PJ & Trombley JH (1983) Possible role of calcium blockers in cerebral resuscitation: a review of the literature and synthesis for future studies. *Critical Care Medicine* **11:** 202–207.

10
Shock

DEFINITION

The word 'shock' probably entered the English language in the late 16th century, derived from the French word 'choc' meaning a sudden or violent blow between two armed forces or warriors. It was not used medically until 1743 in the French text of le Dran's 'A treatise of reflections drawn from experiences with gunshot wounds', when it referred to the physical force involved. Later, in 1831, Latto used the term to describe the effects of cholera on circulatory function. In current medical practice, shock can be defined as 'acute circulatory failure with inadequate or inappropriate tissue perfusion resulting in generalized cellular hypoxia'. The various causes of shock can be classified as shown in Table 10.1.

Table 10.1 Causes of shock.

CARDIOGENIC

OBSTRUCTIVE

		Exogenous losses
	Hypovolaemic	
		Endogenous losses
PERIPHERAL CIRCULATION		Dilatation
	Normovolaemic	Sequestration
		AV shunting

CAUSES

Abnormalities of tissue perfusion may result from 'pump failure', mechanical obstruction, loss of circulating volume, abnormalities of the peripheral circulation or, very often, a combination of these factors.

In cardiogenic shock, cardiac output falls because of an abnormality of the heart itself, most commonly as a result of an acute myocardial infarction. Cardiogenic shock may develop if more than 40% of the left ventricular myocardium is damaged while infarction of more than 70% is usually rapidly fatal. Cardiogenic shock may also occur as a result of an acute ischaemic mitral regurgitation or ventricular septal defect, and may be seen after cardiac

128

surgery or as a secondary complication of other forms of shock. In obstructive shock, the fall in cardiac output is caused by a mechanical obstruction to the circulation, e.g. a pulmonary embolus, or by restriction of cardiac filling, as occurs in tamponade. In hypovolaemic shock, the circulating volume is reduced, venous return to the heart falls and there is a reduction in stroke volume, cardiac output and blood pressure. Hypovolaemia may be due to exogenous losses, such as occurs with haemorrhage and burns, or endogenous losses. In the latter, fluid is lost into the interstitial spaces through leaky capillaries or into body cavities such as the bowel (e.g. intestinal obstruction).

In other situations, e.g. septicaemia and anaphylaxis, abnormalities of the peripheral vessels themselves (dilatation, opening of arteriovenous shunts and sequestration of blood in venous capacitance vessels) may lead to shock due to relative hypovolaemia and a reduction in peripheral resistance. True hypovolaemia nearly always supervenes in these cases because of fluid losses due to an increase in capillary permeability. In septic shock, the primary abnormality may be a disturbance of cellular metabolism.

Septic shock is being diagnosed increasingly frequently; this is due partly to greater awareness of the condition, and partly to a true increase in its incidence. The latter has been caused by the greater number of susceptible patients (older population, the use of immunosuppressive agents and steroids, patients with diseases compromising immunity) combined with the wider use of invasive techniques (intravascular catheters, parenteral nutrition, urinary catheters) and the extensive use of antibiotics.

Toxic shock syndrome occurs most commonly in young menstruating women and is associated with tampon use. It is caused by toxins produced by focal staphylococcal infection.

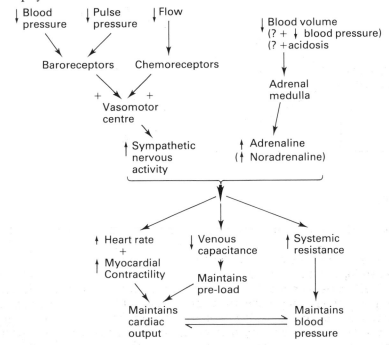

Fig. 10.1 The sympathoadrenal response to shock.

PATHOPHYSIOLOGY (Wilson, 1980)

Sympathoadrenal response to shock (Fig. 10.1)

Hypotension stimulates the baroreceptors, and to a lesser extent the chemoreceptors, causing increased sympathetic nervous activity. Later, this is augmented by the release of catecholamines from the adrenal medulla. The resulting vasoconstriction, together with positive inotropic and chronotropic effects, helps to restore blood pressure and cardiac output. Opioid peptides containing the enkephalin sequence, which are widely distributed throughout the body, particularly within the sympathetic nervous system, have been identified within the same chromaffin cells as catecholamines and are also released into the circulation in shock (Hinds, 1985).

The reduction in perfusion of the renal cortex stimulates the juxtaglomerular apparatus to release renin. This converts angiotensinogen to angiotensin I which is in turn converted to the potent vasoconstrictor, angiotensin II in the lungs. In addition, angiotensin II stimulates secretion of aldosterone by the adrenal cortex causing sodium and water retention. This helps to restore the circulating volume (Fig. 10.2)

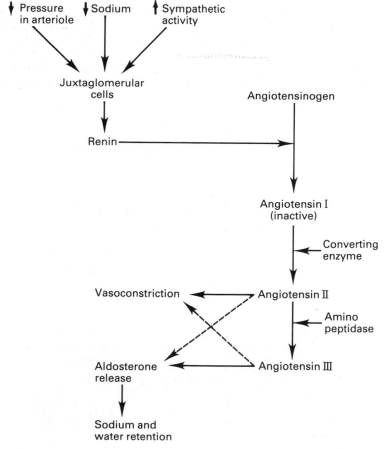

Fig. 10.2 The renin–angiotensin system in shock.

Neuroendocrine response to shock

Pituitary hormones are also released during shock so that circulating levels of adrenocorticotrophic hormone (ACTH), growth hormone (GH) and vasopressin (antidiuretic hormone, ADH) are elevated. β-Endorphin is derived from the same precursor molecule as ACTH (pro-opiomelanocortin); consequently, plasma levels of this peptide also increase in response to stressful stimuli such as shock (Hinds, 1985). It has recently been suggested that this or other endogenous opioid peptides, e.g. the enkephalins, may be partly responsible for some of the cardiovascular changes seen in shock (Hinds, 1985). Cortisol production increases, causing further fluid retention and antagonizing the effects of insulin. This, combined with increased glucagon activity, produces a tendency to hyperglycaemia.

Vasoactive substances (Emau et al, 1984)

Arachidonic acid metabolites. This essential fatty acid can be metabolized via the cyclo-oxygenase pathway to form prostaglandins or, alternatively, via the lipoxygenase pathway to produce leukotrienes (Fig. 10.3).

There are a large number of prostaglandins, each of which has distinct physiological effects. Thus, while some cause vasoconstriction, others are vasodilators, and while some activate platelets, others inhibit their aggregation. Some of the prostaglandins also increase vascular permeability. Those members of the family currently considered to be of particular importance in shock are prostacyclin (PGI$_2$), which is a vasodilator and

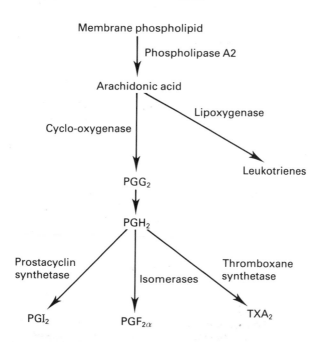

Fig. 10.3 Arachidonic acid metabolites.

inhibits platelet aggregation, thromboxane, which causes pulmonary vasoconstriction and activates platelets, and $PGF_{2\alpha}$, which may be responsible for the early phase of pulmonary hypertension commonly seen in septic shock. Clearly, the net effect of the release of these substances in an individual patient will depend on the relative concentrations of each particular prostaglandin. The role of leukotrienes in shock is less certain but they may be responsible for increased vascular permeability, vasoconstriction and a reduction in cardiac output (Hagmann et al, 1984).

Lysosomal enzymes. These are released not only when cells die but also in response to hypoxia, ischaemia, sepsis and acidosis. As well as being directly cytotoxic, they can cause myocardial depression and coronary vasoconstriction. Furthermore, lysosomal enzymes can convert inactive kininogens, which are usually combined with α_2-globulin, to vasoactive kinins such as bradykinin. These substances can cause vasodilatation and increased capillary permeability as well as myocardial depression. They can also activate clotting mechanisms.

Induced histamine. This substance is distinct from the preformed 'mast cell' histamine which is released in many allergic phenomena, and the effects of induced histamine cannot be prevented by administering conventional antihistamines. Release of induced histamine may make a small contribution to the increase in vascular permeability in septicaemia, but is unlikely to be relevant in shock of other aetiologies.

Endotoxin. This is a complex lipopolysaccharide derived from bacterial cell walls. Its toxic effects are mediated by the phospholipid portion of the molecule known as lipid A. Endotoxin is cytotoxic, damages endothelium, uncouples oxidative phosphorylation and activates complement through both the alternative and classical pathways (Leon et al, 1982).

It appears that all these vasoactive substances are of particular importance in the pathogenesis of septic shock.

Microcirculatory changes

Since shock is a syndrome caused by inadequate tissue perfusion, the final common pathway for the pathophysiological changes is the microcirculation.

In the early stages of septic shock there is vasodilatation, opening of arteriovenous shunts, increased capillary permeability and a defect of oxygen utilization by the tissues. Initially, before hypovolaemia supervenes, or when therapeutic replacement of circulating volume has been adequate, cardiac output is usually high and peripheral resistance low. The supranormal cardiac output is probably a result of intense sympathetic activity occurring in response to baroreceptor stimulation, while the reduction in systemic resistance may be due to opening of arteriovenous shunts in the presence of precapillary vasoconstriction. Although this may in part account for the reduced oxygen extraction often seen in patients with sepsis, flow through the capillary beds is increased in hyperdynamic shock and there is probably also a primary defect in cellular oxygen utilization. Vasodilatation and increased capillary permeability also occur in anaphylactic shock.

In the initial stages of other forms of shock, and when hypovolaemia supervenes in sepsis and anaphylaxis, increased sympathetic activity causes constriction of both precapillary arterioles and, to a lesser extent, the postcapillary venules. This helps to maintain systemic blood pressure. Furthermore, the hydrostatic pressure within the capillaries falls and fluid is sucked from the extravascular space into the intravascular compartment. This 'transcapillary refill', combined with the salt and water retention described above, to some extent restores the circulating volume and promotes flow by reducing viscosity. If shock persists, the accumulation of metabolites, such as lactic acid and carbon dioxide, combined with the release of vasoactive substances, causes relaxation of the precapillary sphincters, while the postcapillary venules, which are more sensitive to hypoxic damage, become relatively unresponsive to these substances and remain constricted. Blood is therefore sequestered within the dilated capillary bed and fluid is forced into the interstitial spaces, causing interstitial oedema, haemoconcentration and an increase in viscosity. In addition, blood becomes more viscous at low flow rates since the streaming effect, which normally channels red blood cells (RBCs) down the centre of vessels, is reduced. Moreover, RBCs become less elliptical and there is a reversible aggregation of erythrocytes and platelets.

This reduction in flow through the microcirculation, combined with the increase in viscosity, renders these patients highly susceptible to procoagulant stimuli. The release of ADP from platelets in response to the presence of particulate matter, noradrenaline, some prostaglandins and thrombin, together with the reduced flow and increased viscosity, leads to platelet aggregation and clot formation within the capillary bed. Moreover, cell damage caused, for example, by the effects of endotoxin and antigen/antibody complexes on the capillary endothelium, leads to the release of tissue thromboplastins. The production of PGI_2, which inhibits platelet aggregation, by the capillary endothelium may be impaired, and factor XII may be activated directly by endotoxin and/or antigen.

Plasminogen is converted to plasmin, which breaks down these clots liberating fibrin/fibrinogen degradation products (FDPs). The cells supplied by capillaries blocked by this process of disseminated intravascular coagulation (DIC) (Hewitt and Davies, 1983) inevitably become hypoxic and eventually die. Tissue ischaemia is further exacerbated as capillaries are compressed by interstitial oedema. This process therefore causes serious damage to vital organs in shock. Finally, because clotting factors and platelets are consumed in DIC they are unavailable for haemostasis elsewhere and a coagulation defect results—hence the alternative name for DIC of 'consumption coagulopathy'. This process occurs earlier and is more severe in septicaemic shock.

The capillary endothelium is damaged by a number of factors, particularly in septic shock, including DIC, microemboli, release of vasoactive compounds, leukocyte aggregation and complement activation (see section on adult respiratory distress syndrome, pp. 220–221). Capillary permeability is thereby increased so that fluid is lost into the interstitial space causing further hypovolaemia, interstitial oedema and organ dysfunction.

Organ dysfunction

The most vital organs of the body, such as the brain and heart, are relatively protected from the ill effects of alterations in blood pressure by their ability, within certain limits, to maintain blood flow at a constant level despite alterations in perfusion pressure (Fig. 10.4). This 'autoregulation' is an intrinsic property of some vascular smooth muscle and is independent of its innervation. It is lost when the vessels become rigid, e.g. due to atheroma, and the limits for autoregulation are reset at higher levels in those with pre-existing hypertension (Fig 10.4). Because sympathetic tone is often high in shocked patients, the autoregulation curve is shifted to the right, i.e. tissue flow will fall at higher pressure than in normal subjects. Later in the evolution of shock, vasoparalysis may occur (see above), and under these circumstances autoregulation may fail, i.e. flow characteristics become passive and pressure-dependent. Furthermore, dilatation of healthy vessels in the presence of atheroma elsewhere may 'steal' blood from areas supplied by diseased vessels. This can cause, for example, symptoms of cerebral ischaemia, particularly in the elderly.

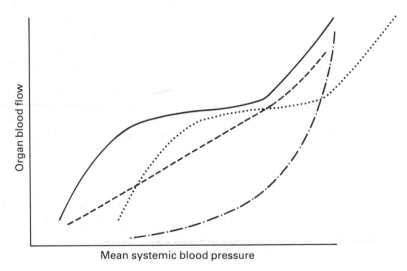

Fig. 10.4 Autoregulation of organ blood flow. Flow to vital organs is normally maintained constant over a wide range of perfusion pressures (———). When vessels are rigid, e.g. due to atheroma, flow is linearly related to pressure (----). Passive flow (–·—·–·) occurs in distensible vessels, e.g. normal arterioles in skin and those in ischaemic areas with toxic arteriolar paralysis. In hypertensive subjects (······) the limits for autoregulation are reset at a higher level.

Heart

In cardiogenic shock, disease of the myocardium is, of course, the primary abnormality. Despite the ability of the coronary circulation to autoregulate, and the reduction in myocardial oxygen consumption which usually occurs when blood pressure falls, heart failure may develop during prolonged severe shock of any aetiology. Myocardial ischaemia, affecting particularly the vulnerable endocardial layer, is almost certainly an important cause of this reduction in cardiac performance. When systemic blood pressure falls below a certain critical level, myocardial blood flow is inevitably reduced, especially when the ability of the coronary circulation to autoregulate is impaired by atheroma. Myocardial ischaemia may be exacerbated by the 'steal' phenomenon just described, a reduction in the distensibility of collateral vessels and obstruction of capillary flow by myocardial oedema. Furthermore, the local effects of cellular hypoxia can cause abnormalities of excitation and contraction with the development of dysrhythmias and impaired myocardial function. Some authorities believe that fragmentation of cellular proteins by lysozymes in the pancreas and splanchnic region can release small molecular weight polypeptides, such as 'myocardial depressant factor' (Lefer and Martin, 1970), which are negatively inotropic. Moreover, lysozymes can themselves cause myocardial depression and coronary vasoconstriction.

Lungs

In the early stages of shock, the reduction in pulmonary blood flow and perfusion pressure leads to V/Q inequalities with an increased dead space, while in hyperdynamic patients V/Q will be low. The patient usually develops a tachypnoea in response to the metabolic acidosis and chemoreceptor stimulation, so that $P_a co_2$ is often reduced while $P_a o_2$ may be either normal or low.

Patients in whom shock is severe and prolonged may develop respiratory failure 12–48 hours after the initial episode. Previously, this was referred to as the 'shock lung syndrome', and it is one cause of the adult respiratory distress syndrome (ARDS) (see Chapter 12). The development of ARDS in shock is almost invariably associated with sepsis and is a rare sequel of pure hypovolaemia, even when this is severe and prolonged. Similarly, sepsis is frequently associated with respiratory abnormalities.

Finally, respiratory failure associated with shock may be caused, or exacerbated, by other factors such as aspiration of gastric contents, fluid overload, lung contusion, thermal inhalation injury, pulmonary infection and oxygen toxicity. (These subjects are discussed elsewhere.)

Kidneys (see Chapter 15)

Oliguria is almost invariable in the shocked patient and may be prerenal, renal or postrenal. Prerenal oliguria will respond to volume expansion and this should be achieved as rapidly as possible in order to prevent progression to established acute renal failure. Postrenal causes, such as urethral damage in trauma victims, must also be excluded. A few patients with septic shock may develop an inappropriate polyuria which occurs despite significant hypovolaemia.

Liver (see Chapter 16)

This organ is to some extent protected from ischaemic damage, not only by its ability to autoregulate but also by its dual blood supply. Nevertheless, under extreme circumstances, hepatic failure may develop. This is often irreversible and is therefore associated with a very poor prognosis.

Splanchnic circulation

The bowel is relatively resistant to the marked ischaemia which it suffers in shock, but eventually mucosal damage, particularly affecting the villi, will occur. The barrier to the absorption of toxic substances from the bowel lumen is therefore lost and endotoxaemia and/or bacteraemia may then further complicate the picture.

Metabolic changes

Once the supply of oxygen to the cells becomes insufficient for continuation of the tricarboxylic acid (TCA) cycle, production of energy in the form of ATP becomes dependent on anaerobic metabolism. Under these circumstances, glucose is metabolized in the normal way to pyruvate but is then converted to lactate instead of entering the Kreb's cycle. The H^+ ions thereby released cause a metabolic acidosis. This pathway is relatively inefficient in terms of energy production. Despite the increased cellular permeability to glucose induced by hypoxia, shocked patients are often hyperglycaemic because of the elevated circulating levels of insulin antagonists such as cortisol, growth hormone, and catecholamines, as well as catecholamine-induced glycogen breakdown. Blood levels of fats and amino acids also rise. Eventually, because of reduced availability of ATP, the sodium pump fails, cells swell due to accumulation of salt and water, and potassium losses increase. In the final stages, release of lysosomal enzymes may contribute to cell death.

CLINICAL SIGNS OF SHOCK

Although many clinical features are common to all types of shock, there are certain important respects in which they differ.

Hypovolaemic shock

Signs of inadequate tissue perfusion in shock include cold, pale and blue skin with increased capillary filling time, oliguria or anuria and, in severe cases, confusion and restlessness due to cerebral ischaemia. Increased sympathetic activity produces vasoconstriction which, although helping to maintain blood pressure, further reduces tissue blood flow and causes tachycardia and sweating. As shock becomes more severe, the skin changes spread further proximally. Hypotension is an unreliable sign, particularly in hypovolaemic shock, since blood pressure may be maintained despite the loss of up to 25% of the circulating volume. On the other hand, such a patient will exhibit all the signs of the compensatory sympathetic activity just described. It is therefore not adequate simply to restore blood pressure in shock and treatment must be continued until the tachycardia has settled, the patient stops sweating, peripheral perfusion is improved and urine flow is adequate.

In the initial stages of shock, the patient is often tachypnoeic, either due to associated chest or lung injury or in an attempt to compensate for a metabolic acidosis. The development of a tachypnoea some time after the onset of shock is often the first sign of the development of ARDS or the fat embolism syndrome.

Cardiogenic shock

The signs of cardiogenic shock are the same as those described for hypovolaemic shock with the addition of the signs of myocardial failure. These may include elevated jugular venous pressure (JVP), basal crepitations, pulsus alternans and a 'triple' rhythm.

Obstructive shock

In massive pulmonary embolus, the signs of shock will be combined with those of right ventricular failure. In cardiac tamponade, the characteristic features of muffled heart sounds and pulsus paradoxus may be detected in addition to the elevated JVP. The latter may exhibit Kussmaul's sign (JVP rises on inspiration).

Anaphylactic shock

In anaphylactic shock, there is sudden collapse with profound vasodilatation. The skin is warm and pink, sometimes with an urticarial rash, and the blood pressure is low. Often, there is also bronchospasm. Later, hypovolaemia will supervene due to loss of protein-rich fluid into the tissues through the 'leaky' capillaries. This is manifested as oedema which is often most obvious in the face, but, more dangerously, may also affect the pharynx and larynx.

Septic shock

Signs of sepsis include pyrexia and rigors, although these are not invariably present and some patients may actually be hypothermic. In the early stages of septicaemia, the patient may be vasodilated, with a high cardiac output; the peripheries are therefore warm and pink with rapid capillary refill and bounding pulses. Blood pressure is often normal initially but falls later. As hypovolaemia develops due to the increased capillary permeability, or if hypovolaemia was previously present due to other causes, vasoconstriction occurs and the patient becomes cold, pale and blue with either a normal or, more often, a low blood pressure.

Following restoration of his circulating volume, such a patient may again become warm and vasodilated with a supranormal cardiac output. Later, myocardial depression may occur and the patient will again exhibit the features of a 'low output' state. Thus, the clinical phases of septic shock are classically described as warm normotensive, warm hypotensive and cold hypotensive. Other signs of septicaemia include confusion, restlessness, tachycardia, tachypnoea, sweating, nausea and vomiting. Oliguria and jaundice are often present. Coma may occur.

As described above, DIC may be a feature of shock of any aetiology but is particularly common in sepsis. Clinical signs are limited to the development of purpuric spots and increased bleeding from wounds and venepuncture sites. Particularly severe DIC classically occurs in meningococcal septicaemia and may be associated with bilateral haemorrhage into the adrenal glands, causing profound hypotension.

The diagnosis of septic shock is often difficult and a high index of suspicion is required if cases are not to be missed or diagnosed too late. Particularly in the elderly, the classical signs may not be present and, for example, mild confusion, tachycardia and tachypnoea may be the only clues, sometimes associated with unexplained hypotension.

MONITORING AND LABORATORY INVESTIGATIONS IN SHOCK

Monitoring of the critically ill has been dealt with in Chapters 3 and 4, but some further aspects of monitoring the shocked patient will be discussed here.

Cardiovascular monitoring

If mistakes are to be avoided, frequent clinical examination is essential, even in the most fully monitored patients. It is usually possible to make some sort of assessment of volume losses in hypovolaemic shock, although such approximations can be grossly inaccurate; in major trauma, for example, losses are often considerably underestimated.

Examination of skin colour, temperature, capillary refill time and the presence or absence of sweating, together with the rate and character of the pulse provides a rapid guide to the severity of shock and the response to treatment. In straightforward cases, e.g. a fit young man with moderate haemorrhage following a road traffic accident (RTA), invasive monitoring may be unnecessary. Clinical assessment combined with frequent blood pressure measurement using a sphygmomanometer may be sufficient, although it is often wise to catheterize the bladder and measure the hourly urine output. An ECG is non-invasive and will allow instant observation of pulse rate and the detection of dysrhythmias. The more seriously ill, and those who fail to respond to initial treatment, will require invasive monitoring, including CVP measurement and intra-arterial pressure recording. As discussed in Chapter 3, measurement of the core to peripheral temperature gradient (or the big toe temperature related to ambient temperature) together with the hourly urine output, provides a good guide to the adequacy of cardiac output and tissue perfusion. In selected cases, e.g. those with myocardial problems or ARDS, a pulmonary artery catheter may be a useful guide to volume replacement and allows direct measurement of cardiac output.

Respiratory monitoring

The respiratory rate must be recorded at frequent intervals and should gradually decrease as the metabolic acidosis resolves. The subsequent development of tachypnoea is an indication that all is not well, and may herald the onset of fat embolism or shock lung. A chest x-ray must always be taken and may initially reveal unsuspected rib fractures, pneumothorax, haemothorax or widening of the mediastinum (suggestive of aortic dissection).

The onset of ARDS will be associated at first with a 'ground glass' appearance on the chest x-ray which may later progress to a mottled appearance with areas of consolidation in an 'alveolar' pattern. Air bronchograms may also be seen (see Chapter 12). Blood gas analysis will then reveal hypoxia with a normal or low P_aCO_2. A rising P_aCO_2, severe hypoxia, increasing tachypnoea and exhaustion suggest that IPPV will be required.

Biochemical investigations

Metabolic acidosis is almost invariably present in shock and provides a guide both to its severity and the response to treatment. A fall in blood lactate levels within a few hours of initiating resuscitation suggests a favourable outcome (Ledingham et al, 1982). A proportion of septic patients will have a metabolic alkalosis. In some, this may be related to identifiable causes such as massive blood transfusion or hypokalaemia, but in others the aetiology is unclear.

Urea and electrolytes should always be measured since they provide a baseline which may be useful in the event of subsequent deterioration. They may also reveal unsuspected problems such as pre-existing renal dysfunction. Likewise, blood sugar levels should always be estimated. Liver function tests will be of importance later since hepatic dysfunction may follow the period of ischaemia, and breakdown of transfused blood and haematomas increases bilirubin levels. The total protein and albumin levels should be measured frequently since the albumin level in particular determines plasma colloid osmotic pressure. The latter can be measured directly using an 'oncometer' and can influence the development of pulmonary oedema (see Chapter 2) (Puri et al, 1980).

Haematological investigations

The haemoglobin concentration (Hb) and packed cell volume (PCV) should always be measured although, because of the variable degree of haemo-concentration which may occur, these measurements do not provide a reliable guide to the extent of blood and fluid losses. They are, however, useful when deciding which solution to use for volume replacement (see below).

Thrombocytopenia and clotting abnormalities may occur, either as a result of transfusion of large amounts of stored blood or the development of DIC. A falling platelet count is often the first indication of the latter and the diagnosis may be confirmed by measuring circulating levels of FDPs.

In septic shock, the white blood count is often raised, although sometimes the patient is leukopenic. A rising white count some time after an episode of shock may indicate the development of sepsis, e.g. an intra-abdominal abscess in a patient with multiple injuries.

Microbiological investigations

In those patients with septicaemic shock, every effort must be made to identify the source of infection and the causative organism. Samples of urine, sputum, cerebrospinal fluid (when indicated) and pus from drainage sites should be sent to the laboratory for microscopy and culture. Blood cultures should also be performed, although not infrequently these are negative even when the clinical diagnosis is beyond doubt. In some cases, it may be possible to detect the presence of endotoxin in the circulation using the '*Limulus* lysate' test, even when blood cultures are negative. This test uses an extract of amoebocytes present in the haemolymph of the horseshoe crab (*Limulus polyphemus*), which forms a solid gel within 24 hours of being exposed to endotoxin. Recently, the technique has been modified by the introduction of synthetic substrates which bypass the gelation steps and release a chromophere. The use of these chromogenic substrates increases the sensitivity and specificity of the method and may allow quantification of endotoxaemia (Scully, 1984). If an organism is isolated, and appropriate antibiotics are administered, the prognosis of septic shock is much improved. It should be remembered that shock may be the result of infection with rickettsiae, viruses or fungi, as well as bacteria.

TREATMENT

GENERAL CONSIDERATIONS

In all forms of shock, the aim of treatment is to restore oxygen delivery to the tissues (see Chapter 2) while at the same time correcting the underlying cause, e.g. by stopping haemorrhage or eradicating infection.

In cases of shock associated with intra-abdominal sepsis, or indeed abscess formation in any site, an aggressive approach to surgical exploration and drainage of pus must be adopted. If there is any doubt about the origin of the septicaemia, all intravascular catheters should be removed and their tips sent for culture. This alone may lead to resolution of sepsis.

In order to identify the source of infection, a thorough clinical examination should first be performed, followed by conventional chest and abdominal x-rays. In difficult cases, more sophisticated imaging techniques may prove useful. For example, portable, real-time ultrasonography is non-invasive and can be used at the bedside to localize fluid collections in chest and abdomen. It can also demonstrate gallstones, obstruction to the biliary tree and pyonephrosis. Once the collection has been identified, the ultrasound image can be used to guide diagnostic and therapeutic needle aspiration. This can be particularly useful in the case of a loculated empyema. Unfortunately, the ultrasound image is distorted by neighbouring gas-filled structures such as stomach and large bowel. Thus, although ultrasound can visualize a right subphrenic abscess satisfactorily, it is less valuable when fluid is suspected in the left subphrenic or paracolic regions. Under these circumstances, a CAT scan may be more useful, although this will involve moving the patient from the intensive care unit and can therefore be hazardous. Again, CAT scanning can be used to guide percutaneous needle aspiration of fluid collections. Gallium-67 citrate and indium-labelled white cells have been used to detect inflammatory foci. However, they do not differentiate a sterile inflammatory response from septic collections, nor is localization sufficiently accurate to allow needle aspiration.

Appropriate antibiotic therapy is vital in sepsis and should be guided by the source of infection, whether this was acquired in hospital or in the community, and known local patterns of sensitivity (see Chapter 6).

It is important to remember that shocked patients may require analgesia since this is easily overlooked in the heat of the moment. Because of the sluggish muscle blood flow, opiates should be administered in small, divided doses intravenously (e.g. papaveretum 5 mg i.v.).

RESPIRATORY CONSIDERATIONS

The first priority in all acutely ill patients is to ensure an adequate airway. This often simply requires insertion of an oropharyngeal airway but in some cases endotracheal intubation may be necessary. The latter also protects the lungs from inhalation of blood, vomit and other debris and is often essential in those with severe facial injuries. Very rarely, emergency tracheostomy may be required.

All shocked patients should receive supplementary oxygen, and those with severe chest and/or head injuries may require immediate intubation and mechanical ventilation. Because of the adverse haemodynamic effects of positive pressure ventilation (see pp. 237–238), it is important (when time allows) to optimize the patient's cardiovascular performance, e.g. by restoring his circulating volume, prior to instituting artificial ventilation. Later, IPPV, often combined with PEEP, may be necessary in those patients who develop ARDS.

CARDIOVASCULAR CONSIDERATIONS

Restoration of blood flow to the tissues requires treatment aimed at improving the cardiac output. As well as controlling heart rate, the three determinants of stroke volume (pre-load, contractility and after-load) must be manipulated appropriately.

Pre-load and volume replacement

The first priority in all forms of shock is optimization of pre-load since, as discussed in Chapter 2, this is the most efficient way of increasing cardiac output. Volume replacement is obviously of primary importance in hypovolaemic shock but is also required in anaphylactic and septic shock because of vasodilatation, sequestration of blood and loss of circulating volume due to the increase in capillary permeability. Low-output, high-resistance septic shock is usually the result of such hypovolaemia, while the myocardial failure described as occurring late in the course of septicaemia is probably rare. Thus, such patients will often respond well to expansion of their circulating volume and are thereby frequently converted to a high output, low resistance state.

In obstructive shock, high filling pressures may be required to maintain an adequate stroke volume, while even in cardiogenic shock careful volume expansion may on occasions lead to a useful increase in cardiac output. On the other hand, patients with severe cardiac failure in whom ventricular filling pressures may be markedly elevated can benefit from measures to reduce pre-load (and after-load), such as the administration of diuretics and vasodilators (see below).

A crude assessment of the extent of the volume deficit is usually possible, although, as mentioned previously, these estimates can be very inaccurate. Blood losses are often under-estimated, particularly when there are scalp and facial wounds since this is a very vascular area and bandaging merely disguises the extent of the haemorrhage. Measurement of Hb, PCV, urea and electrolytes is usually unhelpful. The clinical response to transfusion (slowing heart rate, improved tissue perfusion and rising blood pressure) may be a sufficient guide to the volume required but, often, monitoring of CVP and/or PCWP will be necessary. When interpreting these variables, it is important to appreciate that the compliance of the ventricles is often reduced in shock (see Chapter 3).

The circulating volume must be replaced as quickly as possible (minutes not hours) since rapid restoration of cardiac output and perfusion pressure reduces the chances of serious organ damage, particularly the development of acute renal failure. Thus, in many cases of severe haemorrhagic shock, two or more large-bore intravenous cannulae will be required so that fluid can be transfused rapidly under pressure. Careful monitoring will ensure that despite this aggressive approach, volume overload does not occur.

The clinical use of a 'g' suit (military antishock trousers, MAST) to limit blood loss and reduce venous pooling in victims of massive trauma was first described in Vietnam. Although the application of MAST helps to maintain blood pressure, rapid deflation of the 'g' suit may be associated with profound hypotension. This response has also been described in a patient who sustained a severe compression injury to the lower abdomen and pelvis when his wide leather belt was removed and his tight-fitting jeans were cut off (Scurr and Cutting, 1984).

CHOICE OF FLUID FOR VOLUME REPLACEMENT

Blood

In haemorrhagic shock, it would seem logical to replenish the circulating volume with whole blood as soon as this becomes available. In other forms of shock, e.g. those with full thickness burns, transfusion of packed cells may be required to maintain the haemoglobin concentration at acceptable levels. In extreme emergencies, uncross-matched O-negative blood can be used, but an emergency cross-match can be performed in only 30 minutes and is almost as safe as the standard procedure. There is a trend at present for donor blood to be separated into its various components and it may therefore be necessary to transfuse packed red cells to maintain adequate levels of Hb and use plasma, or plasma substitute, for volume replacement. It has been suggested that limited normovolaemic haemodilution (PCV 25–30%) might improve tissue oxygen delivery since the reduction in oxygen-carrying capacity may be offset by an increase in cardiac output and improved distribution of flow through the microcirculation (Messmer, 1975).

Blood transfusion may be complicated by incompatibility reactions, pyrexia due to contained pyrogens and the transmission of diseases such as viral hepatitis. Recently, the possibility of transmitting acquired immune deficiency syndrome (AIDS) has caused concern, particularly in North America (Editorial, 1984). Other special problems may arise when large volumes of stored blood are transfused rapidly. These include:

1 *Hypothermia*. Bank blood is stored at 4°C; so, if large volumes are transfused, the patient will become hypothermic. Furthermore, peripheral venoconstriction may slow the rate of the infusion, and cold blood transfused rapidly through a centrally placed cannula can induce dysrhythmias. For these reasons, the blood should be warmed, most simply by passing it through a plastic coil placed in a water bath, although dry heaters are also available.

2 *Microembolism*. Stored blood contains microaggregates, consisting mainly of dead platelets and white blood cells. The majority of these are not removed by the filters present in normal giving sets which have a pore size of approximately 120 µm. As mentioned previously, some consider microemboli to be a contributory factor in the development of ARDS and suggest that pulmonary dysfunction in trauma victims may be prevented, or ameliorated, by removing these microaggregates with 40 µm filters (Reul et al, 1973). Others have suggested, however, that hypoxaemia in trauma victims is more dependent on the nature and severity of the injury than massive blood transfusion (Collins et al, 1978) and the value of routine filtration remains unproven. Nevertheless, the disadvantages of such filters are few (mainly the cost and slowing the rate of transfusion) and many still recommend their use, particularly when large volumes of blood are administered. It has been suggested that fine-screen filtration reduces the incidence of febrile reactions to transfused blood by removing the majority of the leukocytes (Schned and Silver, 1981). Fresh blood should not be filtered since this will remove functioning platelets and possibly viable clotting factors.

3 *Coagulopathy*. Stored blood has essentially no effective platelets and is deficient in clotting factors. Consequently, with large transfusions, a coagulation defect may develop. This should be treated by replacing clotting factors with fresh frozen plasma (FFP). The administration of platelet concentrates is less often required. Very occasionally, cryoprecipitate can be used to correct a proven deficiency of factor VIII.

4 *Metabolic acidosis/alkalosis*. Stored blood is now preserved in citrate/ phosphate/dextrose (CPD) which is less acidic than the acid/citrate/dextrose (ACD) solution used previously. Metabolic acidosis attributable solely to blood transfusion is unusual and in any case rarely requires correction. Patients will often develop a metabolic alkalosis 24–48 hours after a large blood transfusion, probably largely due to metabolism of the citrate, and this will be exacerbated if the preceding acidosis has been corrected with intravenous sodium bicarbonate.

5 *Hypocalcaemia*. Stored blood is anticoagulated using citrate, which binds the calcium ions required for clotting. When this blood is transfused rapidly, the excess citrate may reduce total body ionized calcium levels, causing myocardial depression. This is uncommon in practice but if necessary can be corrected by administering 10 ml of 10% calcium chloride intravenously. Routine administration of calcium is not recommended.

6 *Increased oxygen affinity*. As mentioned in Chapter 2, the position of the

oxyhaemoglobin dissociation curve is influenced by the concentration of 2,3-DPG in the red cell. In stored blood, the red cell 2,3-DPG content is reduced so that the curve is shifted to the left. The oxygen affinity of haemoglobin is therefore increased and oxygen delivery is impaired. This effect is less marked with CPD blood. Red cell levels of 2,3-DPG are substantially restored within 12 hours of transfusion.

7 *Hyperkalaemia.* Potassium levels rise progressively when blood is stored. However, when the blood is warmed prior to transfusion, the cells begin to metabolize, the sodium pump becomes active and potassium levels fall. Hyperkalaemia is rarely a problem with massive transfusions.

SAGM blood. Recently, additive solutions have been developed which are nutrient media allowing red cell storage without the presence of plasma. In this way, plasma extraction from donor blood is maximized, the shelf-life of the red cell suspensions is prolonged and transfusion is facilitated by the reduction in viscosity. The most commonly used additive is SAG (saline, adenine, glucose) to which mannitol (M) is now added to reduce spontaneous lysis. One possible disadvantage of these suspensions is that macroaggregates may form progressively, and ways of minimizing this problem are currently being investigated.

In view of these complications of blood transfusion, and in particular the risk of transmitting disease, as well as the expense, many centres are attempting to reduce their use of stored blood. It is now recognized that previously fit patients who have suffered an episode of haemorrhagic shock can survive with extremely low haemoglobin concentrations, provided their circulating volume, and thus their ability to maintain an adequate cardiac output, is maintained. However, it is controversial whether a modest degree of anaemia (Hb $10 \, g \, dl^{-1}$, PCV 30%) is advantageous because of improved flow through the microcirculation or is disadvantageous because tissue oxygen delivery can only be maintained by an increased cardiac output or hypervolaemia (Messmer, 1975). Because of these considerations, as well as the trend towards 'component' therapy mentioned previously, the use of crystalloid solutions, plasma, plasma substitutes and oxygen-carrying solutions is assuming greater importance in the management of shock.

Crystalloid solutions

Although crystalloid solutions (e.g. Ringer–lactate) are cheap, convenient to use and free of side effects, the use of large volumes of these fluids should in general be avoided. They are rapidly lost from the circulation into the interstitial spaces and volumes of crystalloid 2–4 times that of colloid are required to achieve an equivalent haemodynamic response (Rackow et al, 1983; Virgilio et al, 1979). Moreover, volume expansion is transitory, colloid osmotic pressure (COP) is reduced (Virgilio et al, 1979; Rackow et al, 1983), fluid accumulates in the interstitial spaces and pulmonary oedema may be precipitated (Rackow et al, 1983). In one study of patients undergoing intra-abdominal vascular surgery, pulmonary function on the first postoperative day was significantly worse in the group receiving crystalloid than in those given colloid (Skillman et al, 1975). Nevertheless, others have demonstrated that such patients tolerate large volumes of crystalloid well (Virgilio et al,

1979) and it appears that the excess fluid is rapidly mobilized once the stress response abates. Volume replacement with predominantly crystalloid solutions is therefore advocated by some authorities for the uncomplicated, previously healthy patient with traumatic or perioperative hypovolaemia.

Colloidal solutions

These produce a greater and more sustained increase in plasma volume, with associated improvements in cardiovascular function and oxygen transport. They also increase colloid osmotic pressure (Rackow et al, 1983). When capillary permeability is increased, however, these substances may leak across the basement membrane and increase interstitial oncotic pressure, thereby enhancing oedema formation (Holcroft and Trunkey, 1974; Weaver et al, 1978) and slowing its resolution. Furthermore, colloidal solutions may inhibit a saline diuresis (Weaver et al, 1978). Nevertheless, when capillary permeability is increased, all intravenous fluid replacement is hazardous and the use of colloids is probably preferable to administering large volumes of crystalloid, certainly in patients with shock and those at risk of developing ARDS.

1 *Natural colloids.* Because freeze-dried plasma is derived from multiple donors it is a potent source of infection, particularly hepatitis, and is consequently no longer used.

Plasma protein fraction (PPF), which is free of hepatitis antigen and isotonic with plasma, is now widely available, although expensive. In normal subjects, it will expand the circulating volume by an amount roughly equivalent to the volume infused. It has a half-life in the circulation of 15–17 days, although in those with increased capillary permeability this is considerably reduced. As well as its use as a volume expander, it is an excellent source of protein. It has the same sodium content as plasma and this may be a disadvantage in those patients at risk of developing hypernatraemia. Although anaphylactoid reactions are rare, they do occur in less than 1% of cases. PPF should not generally be used for routine volume replacement, particularly if losses are continuing, since other cheaper solutions are equally effective in the short term. In those patients who are seriously hypoalbuminaemic but have sodium retention and/or are at risk from fluid overload, concentrated, salt-poor albumin solutions may be used.

2 *Dextrans.* These are polymolecular polysaccharides contained in either 5% dextrose or normal saline. Low molecular weight dextran (mol. wt 40 000) has a powerful osmotic effect so that fluid moves from the extravascular to the intravascular compartment, thereby expanding the circulating volume by approximately twice the volume infused. Although viscosity is reduced, this may be counterbalanced by a decrease in the flexibility of the red cells. Dextran 40 is rapidly excreted by the kidneys and its effect is, therefore, relatively short-lived. It can form a complex with fibrinogen, thereby inducing a coagulopathy. It also coats the red cell membrane so that blood must be taken for cross-matching before administering dextran. Dextran 70 (mol. wt 70 000) is also hyperoncotic, although less so than dextran 40, and also interferes with cross-matching. It has a longer half-life, however, and is probably the most suitable dextran for routine use. There is a small risk of allergic reactions to all the dextrans (0.07–1.1%) and normally a dose of

$1.5\,g\,kg^{-1}$ body weight should not be exceeded because of the risk of renal damage.

3 *Gelatins*. Haemaccel is a gelatin solution with an average mol. wt of 35 000 which is iso-osmotic with plasma. It appears that large volumes of haemaccel can be administered with impunity since coagulation defects do not occur and it does not impair renal function. It is also very cheap. However, because it readily crosses the glomerular basement membrane, its half-life in the circulation is only 2–3 hours and it can promote a diuresis. The incidence of allergic reactions is probably greater than with the dextrans (0.5–10%).

4 *Hydroxyethyl starches (HES)*. These are rather more expensive than the gelatins but cheaper than PPF. The commonly used HES has a mean mol. wt of approximately 450 000 and a half-life of six hours. Volume expansion is equivalent to, or slightly greater than, the volume infused. The reported incidence of allergic reactions is approximately 0.1%. HES has recently been introduced in the UK.

Oxygen-carrying blood substitutes

The ideal solution for volume replacement in shock would have an oncotic pressure similar to plasma with a long half-life, no adverse side effects, zero incidence of allergic reactions, no requirement for cross-matching and a long shelf-life at room temperature. It would also carry oxygen. Some progress has been made towards attaining the latter objective with the development of fluorocarbon emulsions (Fluosol-DA); these contain HES, electrolytes and an emulsifying agent. Although they are excellent as volume expanders, they have a linear oxygen dissociation curve and only contribute significantly to oxygen delivery when alveolar oxygen tension is relatively high (Tremper et al, 1982). Furthermore, a number of adverse reactions to Fluosol-DA have been reported, possibly related to complement activation initiated by the detergent used to maintain emulsion stability (Tremper et al, 1982). Haemoglobin solutions also have potential as oxygen-delivering resuscitation fluids, but their application is at present limited by a short intravascular retention time and a high affinity for oxygen (DeVenuto, 1982).

Myocardial contractility and inotropic agents

As discussed above, myocardial contractility may be impaired either as the primary abnormality (cardiogenic shock) or as a secondary phenomenon in severe hypovolaemic or septic shock. Before instituting specific measures to stimulate the myocardium, however, it is important to identify, and if possible correct, any of the various associated abnormalities which can impair cardiac performance.

These include hypoxia, severe acidosis, hypocalcaemia and the effects of some drugs (e.g. β-blockers, antidysrhythmics and sedatives). Severe metabolic acidosis may depress myocardial contractility, and can also limit the response to vasopressor agents. On the other hand, therapy with sodium bicarbonate has a number of disadvantages including sodium overload, the subsequent development of a marked alkalosis (see above) and a disadvantageous left-shift of the oxyhaemoglobin dissociation curve. Acidosis should, therefore, only be corrected when it is severe (often arbitrarily taken as pH <7.2) and thought to be impairing cardiovascular performance. Sodium bicarbonate 8.4% should then be administered in small (50 ml) aliquots guided by frequent acid–base measurements, until pH is returned to a safe level. Overcorrection must be avoided.

If the 'best' pre-load and attention to associated factors does not produce an adequate improvement in cardiac output, then a myocardial stimulant may be employed. It must be remembered, however, that all such agents increase myocardial oxygen consumption, particularly if a tachycardia develops, and that this can lead to an imbalance between myocardial oxygen supply and demand with the development and extension of ischaemic area (Lesch, 1976). Thus, a vicious circle may develop in which worsening ischaemia leads to further deterioration in myocardial function and increasing requirement for inotropic support. For this reason, such agents should be used with extreme caution, particularly in cardiogenic shock following myocardial infarction when infarct size may actually be increased.

In patients with septic shock and a high cardiac output, the use of inotropic agents to increase myocardial contractility is often unnecessary and illogical. Nevertheless, when severe hypotension jeopardizes perfusion of vital organs, despite adequate volume replacement, then inotropic agents may be used in an attempt to increase blood pressure and/or redistribute blood flow (e.g. the use of dopamine to increase renal perfusion—see below). Since peripheral resistance is usually low in these patients, some advocate the use of a vasoconstrictor such as adrenaline, or even noradrenaline, to restore perfusion pressures in those with profound, resistant hypotension. This can be combined with a low dose of dopamine in the hope that this will preserve renal blood flow.

Conversely, some authorities have recommended β-blockade in the management of maldistributive septic shock. It is suggested that this can reduce β-induced splanchnic vasodilatation, as well as peripheral arteriovenous and pulmonary shunting. It is also possible that β-blockade inhibits renin release, thereby reducing the risk of acute renal failure. However, such treatment may cause relative bradycardia, a reduction in cardiac output, myocardial depression and prevent the development of a tachycardia in response to hypovolaemia. Consequently, β-blockade is rarely used in the management of septic shock.

The rational selection of an appropriate inotrope depends on a thorough understanding of the cardiovascular effects of the available drugs, combined with an accurate assessment of the individual's haemodynamic disturbance (Herbert and Tinker, 1980). The patient's response must then be closely monitored so that if necessary the inotrope regimen can be altered appropriately. All inotropic agents should be administered via a large central vein.

The most popular of the currently available inotropes are discussed below.

Adrenaline

Stimulates both α- and β-receptors, but at low doses β effects seem to predominate. This produces a tachycardia with an increase in cardiac index and a fall in peripheral resistance, whilst at higher doses, α-mediated vasoconstriction develops. If the latter produces useful increases in cardiac output and perfusion pressure, urine output may nevertheless increase and renal failure may be avoided. However, as the dose is further increased, cardiac output may actually fall, associated with signs of marked vasoconstriction, tachycardia and the development of a metabolic acidosis. Under these circumstances, the reduction in renal blood flow usually causes oliguria and may precipitate acute renal failure, while prolonged administration at high dosage may cause peripheral gangrene. Despite these disadvantages, adrenaline remains an extremely useful inotrope. It is very potent and may prove successful when other agents have failed, particularly in cardiac surgery patients. This may be because it stimulates myocardial α-receptors. Its use in those with severe hypotension associated with a low systemic resistance has already been mentioned. In order to avoid oliguria, renal failure and metabolic acidosis, the minimum effective dose should be used and its administration should be discontinued as soon as possible. It is possible that the addition of 'low dose' dopamine to the regimen may help to preserve renal function (see below).

Noradrenaline

This is predominantly an α-agonist and is therefore rarely used at present. Nevertheless, it may be of value in severe hypotension associated with low peripheral resistance. Some consider noradrenaline to be a useful inotrope in those unresponsive to other measures when combined with an α-blocker such as phentolamine.

Isoprenaline

This β-stimulant has both inotropic and chronotropic effects, as well as reducing peripheral resistance by dilating skin and muscle blood vessels (Holloway et al, 1975). This latter effect means that much of the increased flow is diverted away from vital organs such as the kidneys and may account for the oliguria which can be associated with its use. Most of the increase in cardiac output produced by isoprenaline is due to the tachycardia (Holloway et al, 1975) and this, or the development of dysrhythmias, seriously limits its value. Therefore, there are now few indications for isoprenaline in the critically ill adult.

Salbutamol

This is predominantly a β_2-stimulant and therefore dilates vessels in skeletal muscle and splanchnic beds. It can cause a marked tachycardia, may precipitate dysrhythmias and has only minimal effects on stroke volume. In general, its cardiac effects are less violent than those of isoprenaline and it may therefore occasionally prove useful in post cardiac surgery patients who are bradycardic.

Dopamine

Compared with isoprenaline, this agent causes less tachycardia, is less dysrhythmogenic and has a relatively greater effect on stroke volume

(Holloway et al, 1975). When used in low doses, peripheral resistance falls, largely due to dilatation of splanchnic and renal vasculature. Renal and hepatic blood flow increase (Schmid et al, 1979), urine output and renal function are improved (Davis et al, 1982), and it is possible that failure of these vital organs is thereby prevented. However, dopamine releases noradrenaline and at higher doses vasoconstriction occurs causing an increased after-load and raising ventricular filling pressures. This is particularly dangerous in those in cardiac failure in whom LAP is already dangerously high (Leier et al, 1978). This peripheral vasoconstriction can be avoided by combining high-dose dopamine with a vasodilator such as sodium nitroprusside (see below).

Dobutamine

This is closely related to dopamine and similarly causes less tachycardia and dysrhythmias than does isoprenaline. When compared with dopamine, however, the relative effects of the two agents on heart rate and rhythm are a matter of dispute. Dobutamine has no specific effect on the renal vasculature, although urine output often increases as cardiac output and blood pressure improve. The advantage of dobutamine lies in its ability to reduce systemic resistance, as well as improving cardiac performance, thereby decreasing both after-load and ventricular filling pressures (Leier et al, 1978). Furthermore, it has been claimed that dobutamine produces a greater improvement in cardiac output for a given increase in myocardial oxygen requirements than does dopamine (Leier et al, 1978). For these reasons, dobutamine is probably the agent of choice in those with cardiogenic shock and cardiac failure.

A disadvantage of all these agents when used in patients with respiratory failure is that they increase venous admixture, dopamine possibly being the worst offender in this respect (Regnier et al, 1979). This may be due simply to passive opening of pulmonary vessels by the increased flow and pressure, or to a specific reversal of the hypoxic vasoconstrictor response (Marin et al, 1979).

In most critically ill patients (e.g. those with septic shock with a low peripheral resistance), dopamine is probably the inotrope of choice (Regnier et al, 1979), particularly in view of its effects on renal and hepatic blood flow. Dobutamine may be used as an alternative in patients with cardiac disease, and in septic patients with fluid overload or myocardial failure (Jardin et al, 1981) in whom the vasoconstriction produced by higher doses of dopamine might cause potentially dangerous increases in pre-load and after-load. Dobutamine can be combined with dopamine if large doses of this agent are required. There is now little place for the use of isoprenaline, but adrenaline, because of its potency, remains a useful agent in those patients unresponsive to all other measures, particularly after cardiac surgery. In order to avoid renal failure and the development of an acidosis, its dose must be kept to a minimum and it should be discontinued as soon as possible.

Opiate antagonists

Administration of the specific opiate antagonist, naloxone, can improve cardiovascular function in experimental shock of various aetiologies (Evans et al, 1984), although its value in clinical practice remains unproven. The beneficial haemodynamic effects of naloxone are thought to be due to antagonism of the endogenous opioid systems known to be activated in shock (as discussed at the beginning of this chapter) and a resultant increase in sympathomedullary activity (Hinds, 1985). The clinical use of naloxone is, however, seriously limited by reversal of analgesia and arousal. Furthermore, it has yet to be determined whether this agent has any advantages over currently available inotropes. Perhaps of more interest to the clinician is the finding that some of the newer opiate agonist/antagonist analgesic agents, such as nalbuphine, can also improve cardiovascular performance in experimental shock (Hunt et al, 1984).

Vasodilator therapy, after-load and pre-load reduction
(Cohn and Franciosa, 1977)

In selected cases, after-load reduction may be used to increase stroke volume and decrease myocardial oxygen requirements by reducing systolic wall tension. Vasodilatation also decreases heart size and diastolic ventricular wall tension so that coronary blood flow is improved. The relative magnitude of the falls in pre-load and after-load depends on the pre-existing haemodynamic disturbance, concurrent volume replacement and the agent selected (see below).

Vasodilator therapy is most beneficial in patients with cardiac failure. In this situation, the ventricular function curve is flat, and falls in pre-load have only a limited effect on stroke volume. This form of treatment may therefore sometimes be useful in cardiogenic shock and in the management of patients with pulmonary oedema associated with low cardiac output, mitral regurgitation or an acute ventricular septal defect. Furthermore, because of their ability to improve the myocardial oxygen supply/demand ratio, vasodilators can be used to control angina and decrease ischaemia following myocardial infarction. They may also be valuable in shocked patients who remain vasoconstricted and oliguric despite restoration of an adequate blood pressure, and to control hypertension, e.g. in post cardiac surgery patients.

Such therapy is potentially dangerous and vasodilatation should be achieved cautiously, guided by continuous haemodynamic monitoring. The latter will often include pulmonary artery catheterization or direct measurement of LAP. The circulating volume must be adequate before treatment is started and, except in those with cardiac failure, falls in pre-load should be prevented in order to avoid serious reductions in cardiac output and blood pressure. If diastolic pressure is allowed to fall, coronary blood flow may be jeopardized and, particularly if a reflex tachycardia develops in response to the hypotension, myocardial ischaemia may be precipitated. Provided myocardial performance is not impaired, it is therefore sometimes appropriate to control the tachycardia with a β-blocker. It is also important to appreciate that currently available vasodilators reverse hypoxic pulmonary vasoconstriction and increase shunt (D'Oliveira et al, 1981). Finally, the distribution of the increased blood flow which may follow vasodilator therapy is uncertain but much may in fact be diverted to the splanchnic bed.

Vasodilatation can be achieved using ganglion blockers, α-blockers or drugs acting directly on the vessel wall. The selection of an appropriate agent in an individual patient depends on a careful assessment of the haemodynamic disturbance and on whether the effect required is predominantly a reduction in pre-load, after-load or both.

Ganglion blockers

In the past, continuous infusions of trimetaphan were used to reduce after-load and control blood pressure, particularly after cardiac surgery. This agent rapidly produces vasodilatation and its effects are promptly reversed once the infusion is discontinued. The major disadvantage of trimetaphan is the development of tachyphylaxis. Pentolinium is now rarely used.

α-Adrenergic blockers

These predominantly dilate arterioles and therefore mainly influence after-load. Phenoxybenzamine is unsuitable for use in the critically ill because of its slow onset of action (1–2 hours to maximum effect) and prolonged duration of effect (2–3 days). Phentolamine is very potent with a rapid onset and short duration of action (15–20 minutes). It can be used to control blood pressure acutely in hypertensive crises but can produce a marked tachycardia and is too expensive to administer as a continuous infusion.

Direct-acting vasodilators

This is the group of agents most commonly used to achieve vasodilatation in the critically ill.

Hydralazine predominantly affects arterial resistance vessels. It therefore reduces after-load and blood pressure while cardiac output and heart rate increase. Hydralazine can be administered orally to those with chronic cardiac failure, but in intensive care practice it is usually given as an intravenous bolus (10–20 mg) to control acute increases in blood pressure, particularly after cardiac surgery.

Sodium nitroprusside (SNP) dilates both arterioles and venous capacitance vessels, as well as the pulmonary vasculature. This agent therefore reduces the after-load and pre-load of both ventricles and can improve cardiac output and the myocardial oxygen supply/demand ratio. Some authorities have suggested, however, that SNP can exacerbate myocardial ischaemia by producing a 'steal' phenomenon in the coronary circulation (Chiariello et al, 1976).

The effects of SNP are rapid in onset and spontaneously reversible within a few minutes of discontinuing the infusion. Moreover, in contrast to trimetaphan, tachyphylaxis is not a problem.

An overdose of SNP can cause cyanide poisoning with histotoxic hypoxia caused by inhibition of cytochrome oxidase, the terminal enzyme of the respiratory chain. This is manifested as a metabolic acidosis and a fall in the arteriovenous oxygen content difference. These effects should not inhibit the clinical use of SNP since they are only seen when a gross overdose has been administered and are easily avoided with care. In the short term (a few hours) infusions should be limited to a total dose of 1.5 mg kg^{-1}. There is at present only limited information concerning the safe dosage for long-term administration (several hours to days, or even weeks), although recently, it has been suggested that maximum infusion rates of approximately $4\,\mu g\,kg^{-1}\,min^{-1}$ (certainly less than $8\,\mu g\,kg^{-1}\,min^{-1}$) and a total dose of $70\,mg$ SNP kg^{-1} over periods of up to two weeks are the maximum allowable without risking toxic effects (Vesey and Cole, 1985). Although thiocyanate (SCN) accumulation is not a concern during hypotensive anaesthesia, high plasma levels may be achieved during long-term administration, with possible toxic consequences. Monitoring of SCN levels is therefore recommended during infusions lasting more than three days, particularly in the presence of renal insufficiency (Vesey and Cole, 1985). SNP is broken down during prolonged exposure to light; this problem can be avoided by making up the solution in relatively small quantities or by protecting it with silver foil.

Both nitroglycerine (NTG, glyceryl trinitrate) and isosorbide dinitrate (ISDN) are predominantly venodilators. They can therefore cause marked reductions in pre-load which may be associated with falls in cardiac output and compensatory vasoconstriction. For the reasons discussed above, they are of most value in those with cardiac failure in whom pre-load reduction may reduce ventricular wall tension and improve coronary perfusion without adversely affecting cardiac performance. Furthermore, these agents may reverse myocardial ischaemia by increasing and redistributing coronary blood flow. They can therefore be used to control angina and limit infarct size. These agents are therefore often used in preference to SNP in patients with cardiac failure and/or myocardial ischaemia (Kaplan and Jones, 1979). Finally, both NTG and ISDN reduce pulmonary vascular resistance, an effect which can occasionally be exploited in patients with a low cardiac output secondary to pulmonary hypertension.

Intra-aortic balloon counterpulsation (IABCP) (Swanton, 1984)

Various techniques for mechanical support of the failing myocardium have been described; of these, IABCP has proved most practical and is now widely used in clinical practice.

A catheter with an inflatable, sausage-shaped balloon is inserted via a femoral artery and passed into the aorta until its tip lies just distal to the left subclavian artery (Fig. 10.5). Early in diastole, the balloon is rapidly inflated so that the pressure in the aortic root rises and coronary blood flow is increased. Rapid deflation of the balloon is timed to occur at the onset of systole (usually triggered by the R wave on the ECG) and this leads to a reduction in after-load. Pre-load may also be reduced, as may pulmonary artery pressure and pulmonary vascular resistance. The reduction in left ventricular work reduces myocardial oxygen requirements and this, combined with the increased coronary blood flow, may result in reversal of ischaemic changes and limitation of infarct size. However, IABCP may not increase coronary blood flow distal to significant stenoses. Improved myocardial performance, together with the reduction in after-load, can lead to an increased cardiac output. Inflation and deflation of the balloon must be precisely timed in order to achieve effective counterpulsation (Fig. 10.6).

Originally, insertion of intra-aortic balloons was a time-consuming procedure and required surgical expertise. The femoral artery was exposed and a dacron side arm attached using an end-to-side anastamosis. The

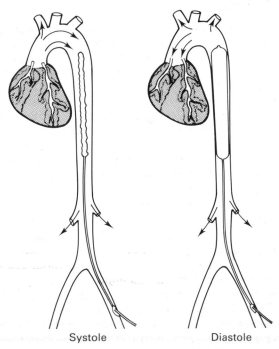

Systole   Diastole

Fig. 10.5 Intra-aortic balloon counterpulsation. Rapid deflation of the balloon occurs at the onset of systole and causes a reduction in after-load. Early in diastole the balloon is rapidly inflated in order to increase the pressure in the aortic root and enhance coronary blood flow.

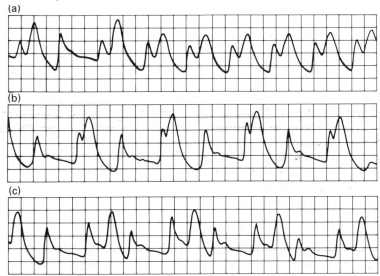

Fig. 10.6 (a) The effect of intra-aortic balloon counterpulsation on the arterial pressure trace. Note: (i) increased diastolic pressure; (ii) slight fall in systolic pressure (due to after-load reduction); (iii) reduced end-diastolic pressure (due to rapid balloon deflation). (b) It is important that the balloon inflates immediately the aortic valve closes (i.e. on the dicrotic notch). In this case the balloon is inflating too early. This will impede left ventricular ejection. (c) In this case balloon inflation is delayed.

catheter was then inserted via this dacron 'chimney'. Surgical closure of the femoral artery and the wound was required when the catheter was removed. Balloons are now available which can be inserted percutaneously using a standard Seldinger technique and this has greatly facilitated the clinical use of IABCP.

The only absolute contraindications to IABCP are aortic aneurysms (or other severe disease of the descending aorta) and marked aortic regurgitation. Relative contraindications include dysrhythmias and extreme tachycardias, both of which limit the ability of the device to trigger balloon deflation accurately.

Complications of IABCP include failure to pass the balloon, aortic dissection, limb ischaemia, thrombosis, embolus and infection. The majority occur at the time of insertion and their incidence seems to be less with the percutaneous technique.

IABCP has proved most useful for weaning patients from cardiopulmonary bypass and for those who develop myocardial ischaemia in the postoperative period. It may also be used to support patients in cardiogenic shock who have surgically correctable lesions, such as ischaemic ventricular septal defects or mitral regurgitation, while they are being prepared for surgery. In patients with severe ischaemia, e.g. those with unstable angina, IABCP may relieve pain and possibly prevent infarction while preparations are made for coronary artery vein grafting or intracoronary thrombolysis. The use of IABCP for the treatment of cardiogenic shock complicating myocardial infarction without a surgically correctable lesion has been less successful, although some feel that this may partly be due to delay in instituting IABCP and extension of the infarct caused by the prior use of inotropes. There is only limited experience with the use of IABCP in myocardial failure complicating septic shock.

HAEMATOLOGICAL PROBLEMS

The most commonly encountered haematological problem in shock is a coagulation defect, usually due to massive blood transfusion and/or consumption coagulopathy (DIC), the latter being particularly common in septicaemia. This can usually be corrected with transfusions of FFP, occasionally combined with platelets, or fresh blood. DIC should be prevented or reversed by aggressive treatment of the underlying condition. Heparinization has been recommended but this is potentially extremely dangerous, particularly in trauma and postoperative cases, and is rarely indicated. Later, coagulation may be impaired secondary to the development of renal and/or hepatic failure.

RENAL FUNCTION

Established acute renal failure still has a high mortality and its prevention is therefore a priority when treating shock. Prevention of acute intrinsic renal failure is best achieved by restoring cardiac output, blood pressure and renal blood flow as rapidly as possible, combined with early and aggressive management of oliguria (see Chapter 15).

ADJUNCTIVE THERAPY IN SHOCK

Steroids

There is evidence from animal studies to suggest that pharmacological doses of steroids can reduce mortality, particularly in septic shock (Hinshaw et al, 1980), possibly by inhibiting complement-induced granulocyte aggregation (Hammerschmidt et al, 1979) and thereby limiting damage to vital organs, particularly the lungs (see Chapter 12). They also inhibit phospholipase A_2 and thereby prevent the liberation of free arachidonic acid from membrane phospholipids (see Fig. 10.3). Other suggested explanations for the beneficial effects of high-dose steroids have included stabilization of lysosomal membranes, a reduction in the affinity of haemoglobin for oxygen and reversal of metabolic derangements.

A variety of cardiovascular responses to steroids has been described, in both experimental and clinical studies, including increases and decreases in cardiac output, as well as vasodilatation and vasoconstriction. These varied cardiovascular effects may be partly influenced by the preceding haemodynamic disturbance, and in one study the overall response to steroids in shock was described as 'normalization' of cardiovascular function (Wilson and Fisher, 1968).

Sharkey et al (1982) showed that the administration of methylprednisolone to animals with high-output normotensive septicaemia improved oxygenation, reduced pulmonary vascular resistance and increased stroke volume.

Nevertheless, the administration of steroids to patients with shock remains controversial (Bihari, 1984; Sibbald, 1984), partly because of deficiencies in the design of many clinical studies. Although Schumer (1976) demonstrated a reduced mortality in patients with septic shock given steroids in a prospective, randomized, double-blind study, this investigation has subsequently been extensively criticized. Sprung et al (1984) undertook a prospective study of high-dose corticosteroids in patients with septic shock which was designed to overcome the limitations of previous studies, but this has done little to resolve the controversy. They administered steroids once, and as a single repeat-dose four hours later only to those who remained shocked. Moreover, a double-blind procedure was not used for all enrolled patients. The analysis of the results of this investigation was complex, but the authors concluded that, although the ultimate mortality was the same in both groups, steroids increased short-term survival and reversal of shock and might be of long-term benefit in certain subgroups.

Because of this conflicting evidence concerning the efficacy of 'pharmacological' doses of steroid in shock, and in view of the risk of complications (hyperglycaemia, secondary infection, gastrointestinal haemorrhage) some consider that, apart from Addisonian crisis, there are few if any indications for steroids in the critically ill (Bihari, 1984). Certainly, if steroids are to be effective it would seem that they must be administered early in the evolution of shock and will only be effective when combined with conventional therapy, in particular appropriate antibiotics (Hinshaw et al, 1980). Our practice is to administer a large bolus dose of methylprednisolone $(30\,mg\,kg^{-1})$ to patients with septic shock as soon as the diagnosis is made and preferably with the first dose of antibiotics. This dose is repeated once, 12 hours later. We do not use steroids in other forms of shock.

Cyclo-oxygenase and lipoxygenase inhibitors

As discussed previously, arachidonic acid metabolites may be important mediators of vascular changes in shock. Prior administration of cyclo-oxygenase inhibitors (such as meclofenamate or indomethacin) can prevent the pulmonary hypertension associated with experimental endotoxin shock, presumably by reducing thromboxane production, although it does not prevent the increase in capillary permeability (Brigham et al, 1982). Furthermore, ibuprofen (another cyclo-oxygenase inhibitor) has been shown to be more effective than naloxone in reversing hypotension in canine endotoxin shock (Toth et al, 1984). Nevertheless, the role of these agents in the management of patients with shock remains to be established.

THERAPEUTIC GOALS IN THE CRITICALLY ILL

It is important to appreciate that in the critically ill patient it may not be sufficient simply to achieve physiological normality. It has been shown that the cardiorespiratory response of those who survive a critical illness involves supranormal values for cardiac index, oxygen delivery and oxygen consumption. In a prospective study, Shoemaker et al (1982) demonstrated that by using the median cardiorespiratory values of survivors as the therapeutic goal, rather than normality, overall mortality was reduced from 48% to 13%. These findings are of obvious relevance to the management of shock and trauma.

FURTHER READING

Bihari DJ & Tinker J (1983) The management of shock. In Tinker J & Rapin M (eds) *Care of the Critically Ill Patient*, pp 188–222. Berlin: Springer-Verlag.
George RJD & Tinker J (1983) The pathophysiology of shock. In Tinker J & Rapin M (eds) *Care of the Critically Ill Patient*, pp 163–187. Berlin: Springer-Verlag.
Messmer K (1983) Plasma substitutes. In Tinker J & Rapin M (eds) *Care of the Critically Ill Patient*, pp 569–575. Berlin: Springer-Verlag.

REFERENCES

Bihari D (1984) The case for steroids. *Intensive Care Medicine* **10:** 113–114.
Brigham KL, Neuman JH, Snapper JR & Ogletree ML (1982) Metabolites of arachidonic acid in the pathophysiology of the pulmonary circulation. In Oates JA (ed.) *The Prostaglandins and The Cardiovascular System*, pp 355–364. New York: Raven Press.
Chiariello M, Gold HK, Leinbach RC, Davis MA & Maroko PR (1976) Comparison between the effects of nitroprusside and nitroglycerin on ischemic injury during acute myocardial infarction. *Circulation* **54:** 766–773.

Cohn JN & Franciosa JA (1977) Vasodilator therapy of cardiac failure (two parts). *New England Journal of Medicine* **297**: 27–31, 254–258.

Collins JA, James PM, Bredenberg CE et al (1978) The relationship between transfusion and hypoxemia in combat casualties. *Annals of Surgery* **188**: 513–519.

Davis RF, Lappas DG, Kirklin JK, Buckley MJ & Lowenstein E (1982) Acute oliguria after cardiopulmonary bypass: renal functional improvement with low-dose dopamine infusion. *Critical Care Medicine* **10**: 852–856.

DeVenuto F (1982) Hemoglobin solutions as oxygen-delivering resuscitation fluids. *Critical Care Medicine* **10**: 238–245.

D'Oliveira M, Sykes MK, Chakrabarti MK, Orchard C & Keslin J (1981) Depression of hypoxic pulmonary vasoconstriction by sodium nitroprusside and nitroglycerine. *British Journal of Anaesthesia* **53**: 11–18.

Editorial (1984) Blood transfusion, haemophilia and AIDS. *Lancet* **i**: 1433–1435.

Emau P, Giri SN & Bruss ML (1984) Role of prostaglandins, histamine and serotonin in the pathophysiology induced by *Pasteurella hemolytica* endotoxin in sheep. *Circulatory Shock* **12**: 47–59.

Evans SF, Varley JG & Hinds CJ (1984) Effects of intravascular volume expansion on the cardiovascular response to naloxone in a canine model of severe endotoxin shock. *British Journal of Pharmacology* **83**: 443–448.

Hagmann W, Denzlinger C & Keppler D (1984) Role of peptide leukotrienes and their hepatobiliary elimination in endotoxin action. *Circulatory Shock* **14**: 223–235.

Hammerschmidt DE, White JG, Craddock PR & Jacob HS (1979) Corticosteroids inhibit complement-induced granulocyte aggregation: a possible mechanism for their efficacy in shock states. *Journal of Clinical Investigation* **63**: 798–803.

Herbert P & Tinker J (1980) Inotropic drugs in acute circulatory failure. *Intensive Care Medicine* **6**: 101–111.

Hewitt PE & Davies SC (1983) The current state of DIC. *Intensive Care Medicine* **9**: 249–252.

Hinds CJ (1985) Opiate antagonists in shock. *British Journal of Hospital Medicine* **34**: 233–234.

Hinshaw LB, Archer LT, Beller-Todd BK et al (1980) Survival of primates in LD$_{100}$ septic shock following steroid/antibiotic therapy. *Journal of Surgical Research* **28**: 151–170.

Holcroft JW & Trunkey DD (1974) Extravascular lung water following hemorrhagic shock in the baboon: comparison between resuscitation with Ringer's lactate and plasmanate. *Annals of Surgery* **180**: 408–417.

Holloway EL, Stinson EB, Derby GC & Harrison DC (1975) Action of drugs in patients early after cardiac surgery 1. Comparison of isoproterenol and dopamine. *American Journal of Cardiology* **35**: 656–659.

Hunt LB, Gurll NJ & Reynolds DG (1984) Dose-dependent effects of nalbuphine in canine hemorrhagic shock. *Circulatory Shock* **13**: 307–318.

Jardin F, Sportiche M, Bazin M, Bourokba A & Margairaz A (1981) Dobutamine: a hemodynamic evaluation in human septic shock. *Critical Care Medicine* **9**: 329–332.

Kaplan JA & Jones EL (1979) Vasodilator therapy during coronary artery surgery. Comparison of nitroglycerin and nitroprusside. *Journal of Thoracic and Cardiovascular Surgery* **77**: 301–308.

Ledingham IMcA, Cowan BN & Burns HJG (1982) Prognosis in severe shock. *British Medical Journal* **284**: 443–444.

Lefer AM & Martin J (1970) Origin of myocardial depressant factor in shock. *American Journal of Physiology* **218**: 1423–1427.

Leier CV, Heban PT, Huss P, Bush CA & Lewis RP (1978) Comparative systemic and regional hemodynamic effects of dopamine and dobutamine in patients with cardiomyopathic heart failure. *Circulation* **58**: 466–475.

Leon C, Rodrigo MJ, Tomasa A et al (1982) Complement activation in septic shock due to gram-negative and gram-positive bacteria. *Critical Care Medicine* **10:** 308–310.

Lesch M (1976) Inotropic agents and infarct size. Theoretical and practical considerations. *American Journal of Cardiology* **37:** 508–513.

Marin JLB, Orchard C, Chakrabarti MK & Sykes MK (1979) Depression of hypoxic pulmonary vasoconstriction in the dog by dopamine and isoprenaline. *British Journal of Anaesthesia* **51:** 303–312.

Messmer K (1975) Hemodilution. *Surgical Clinics of North America* **55:** 659–678.

Puri VK, Weil MH, Michaels S & Carlson RW (1980) Pulmonary edema associated with reduction in plasma oncotic pressure. *Surgery, Gynecology and Obstetrics* **151:** 344–348.

Rackow EC, Falk JL, Fein A et al (1983) Fluid resuscitation in circulatory shock: a comparison of the cardiorespiratory effects of albumin, hetastarch, and saline solutions in patients with hypovolemic and septic shock. *Critical Care Medicine* **11:** 839–850.

Regnier B, Safran D, Carlet J & Teisseire B (1979) Comparative haemodynamic effects of dopamine and dobutamine in septic shock. *Intensive Care Medicine* **5:** 115–120.

Reul GJ, Greenberg SD, Lefrak EA et al (1973) Prevention of post-traumatic pulmonary insufficiency. Fine screen filtration of blood. *Archives of Surgery* **106:** 386–394.

Schmid E, Angehm W, Althaus F, Gattiker R & Rothlin M (1979) The effect of dopamine on hepatic–splanchnic blood flow after open heart surgery. *Intensive Care Medicine* **5:** 183–188.

Schned AR & Silver H (1981) The use of microaggregate filtration in the prevention of febrile transfusion reactions. *Transfusion* **21:** 675–681.

Schumer W (1976) Steroids in the treatment of clinical septic shock. *Annals of Surgery* **184:** 333–341.

Scully MF (1984) Measurement of endotoxaemia by the *Limulus* test. *Intensive Care Medicine* **10:** 1–2.

Scurr JH & Cutting P (1984) Tight jeans as a compression garment after major trauma. *British Medical Journal* **288:** 828.

Sharkey P, Driedger A, Finley R & Sibbald W (1982) Effect of corticosteroids in an animal model of high output systemic sepsis. *Surgical Forum* **33:** 77–79.

Shoemaker WC, Appel PL, Waxman K, Schwartz S & Chang P (1982) Clinical trial of survivors' cardiorespiratory patterns as therapeutic goals in critically ill postoperative patients. *Critical Care Medicine* **10:** 398–403.

Sibbald WJ (1984) The case for steroids: another viewpoint. *Intensive Care Medicine* **10:** 115–117.

Skillman JJ, Restall S & Salzman EW (1975) Randomized trial of albumin vs electrolyte solutions during abdominal aortic operations. *Surgery* **78:** 291–303.

Sprung CL, Caralis PV, Marcial EH et al (1984) The effects of high-dose corticosteroids in patients with septic shock. A prospective, controlled study. *New England Journal of Medicine* **311:** 1137–1143.

Swanton RH (1984) Who requires balloon pumping? *Intensive Care Medicine* **10:** 271–273.

Toth PD, Hamburger SA & Judy WV (1984) The effects of vasoactive mediator antagonists on endotoxic shock in dogs. 1. *Circulatory Shock* **12:** 277–286.

Tremper KK, Friedman AE, Levine EM, Lapin R & Camarillo D (1982) The preoperative treatment of severely anemic patients with a perfluorochemical oxygen-transport fluid, Fluosol-DA. *New England Journal of Medicine* **307:** 277–283.

Vesey CJ & Cole PV (1985) Blood cyanide and thiocyanate concentrations produced by long-term therapy with sodium nitroprusside. *British Journal of Anaesthesia* **57:** 148–155.

Virgilio RW, Rice CL, Smith DE et al (1979) Crystalloid vs colloid resuscitation: is one better? A randomized clinical study. *Surgery* **85**: 129–139.

Weaver DW, Ledgerwood AM, Lucas CE et al (1978) Pulmonary effects of albumin resuscitation for severe hypovolemic shock. *Archives of Surgery* **113**: 387–392.

Wilson RF (1980) The pathophysiology of shock. *Intensive Care Medicine* **6**: 89–100.

Wilson RF & Fisher RR (1968) The hemodynamic effects of massive steroids in clinical shock. *Surgery, Gynecology and Obstetrics* **127**: 769–776.

11
Aspects of Trauma

Trauma, both accidental and non-accidental, is an increasingly common cause of death in young, previously fit adults. Whatever the cause of the injury, the principles of immediate management are always the same. The first priority is to secure the airway and ensure adequate oxygenation and ventilation. Next, external haemorrhage must be arrested and the circulating volume restored. These measures must be undertaken without delay in order to restore oxygen delivery (see Chapter 2) as rapidly as possible and prevent, or minimize, damage to vital organs. The principles of the management of shock are discussed in Chapter 10, and of respiratory support in Chapters 12 and 13; cardiopulmonary resuscitation is described in Chapter 9. Subsequent definitive treatment depends on the nature of the traumatic injury and a number of specific problems are discussed below.

CHEST INJURIES

In Europe and Australasia, most cases of chest trauma are caused by non-penetrating injuries, usually as a result of RTAs. Penetrating injuries caused by knife or gunshot wounds are also seen, but these are much more common in the USA. Occasionally, similar problems are encountered as a result of vigorous closed-chest cardiac massage or intrathoracic surgical procedures.

Resuscitation

As always, the first priority is to establish a clear airway, administer oxygen and ensure adequate ventilation. This is particularly vital in those with chest injuries because, as well as exacerbating hypoxia and hypercarbia, partial airway obstruction produces large fluctuations in intrapleural pressure and increases chest wall instability.

Patients who are comatose, or are confused and require sedation, as well as those with severe faciomaxillary injuries, will require immediate endotracheal intubation or, very occasionally, emergency tracheostomy/cricothyrotomy, in order to secure the airway and protect the lungs from aspiration of blood or gastric contents. The majority of patients will not tolerate the endotracheal tube without sedation and it is then usually safest to institute controlled ventilation. Immediate IPPV will also be required in those with severe respiratory distress, in the presence of massive associated injuries and in patients who are to undergo a general anaesthetic. It is particularly important to ensure adequate oxygenation and ventilation in those with an associated head injury and in such patients IPPV is nearly always required. Before instituting IPPV, it is essential to identify and drain pneumothoraces.

The circulating volume must be replaced as rapidly as possible in order to restore tissue perfusion and avoid further damage to vital organs. Intrathoracic haemorrhage is concealed and therefore easily under-estimated (the entire blood volume can be accommodated within one-half of the thoracic cavity), and many patients with chest trauma will also be bleeding from other associated injuries. Considerable haemorrhage can occur from the lungs and from torn intercostal or internal mammary vessels; this may persist insidiously into the tissues of the chest wall for some time after initial resuscitation and continued transfusion may therefore be required in order to avoid prolonged underperfusion of vital organs. Massive blood loss may follow rupture of major intrathoracic vessels or the heart and this can only be controlled by urgent surgical intervention. Although the extent of the blood loss must never be under-estimated, it is also important to avoid over-transfusion, particularly with crystalloid solutions, since this may exacerbate oedema formation in areas of pulmonary contusion (see below).

Specific injuries

Heart

Penetrating. Surprisingly, a number of patients with penetrating cardiac injuries make a complete recovery, although high-velocity gunshot wounds of the heart are invariably fatal.

In those who remain shocked despite apparently adequate volume replacement, with signs of cardiac tamponade (see Chapter 10), pericardiocentesis must be performed. The pericardial sac can be aspirated using an intravenous cannula or continuously drained using a soft, flexible catheter. Improvement is often dramatic following removal of relatively small amounts of blood. Relief of tamponade may, however, simply encourage further haemorrhage and some patients may be more stable if a degree of cardiac compression is allowed to persist. Emergency thoracotomy is required in the majority of cases. If possible, this should be performed by a competent cardiothoracic surgeon because once the pericardium is opened, haemorrhage can be catastrophic and is most likely to be controlled quickly by those with experience of cardiac surgery. Ideally, the facilities for cardiopulmonary bypass should be available.

Blunt. Myocardial contusion is a common, but often unrecognized, complication of non-penetrating chest injury and may occur in up to 17% of such cases (Macdonald et al, 1981). The diagnosis is suggested by ST segment and T wave changes on the ECG, sinus tachycardia, dysrhythmias and elevated plasma levels of cardiac enzymes, although the latter, with the possible exception of increases in creatine kinase muscle-brain isoenzyme, is a non-specific finding in traumatized patients. Early, and transient, prolongation of the Q–T interval may be a sensitive indicator of myocardial contusion.

Management is as for myocardial infarction. When contusion is severe, myocardial function may be significantly impaired (Torres-Mirabal et al, 1982) in which case insertion of a Swan–Ganz catheter may be indicated to guide volume replacement. Some patients will require inotropic support

(Macdonald et al, 1981). Complications are common and may include sudden unexpected cardiac arrest, as well as supraventricular and ventricular dysrhythmias. The prophylactic use of antidysrhythmics, however, remains controversial.

The heart may rupture either at the time of impact or later as a delayed consequence of myocardial contusions. Intracardiac lesions, such as disruption of a valve or rupture of the interventricular septum, may also occur and are often fatal. These complications are, however, uncommon (Macdonald et al, 1981).

Intrapericardial haemorrhage following blunt injuries originates from torn pericardial and epicardial vessels, or occasionally small myocardial tears. If cardiac tamponade develops it should be relieved by pericardiocentesis. In some cases, bleeding will stop spontaneously while others will require surgical intervention.

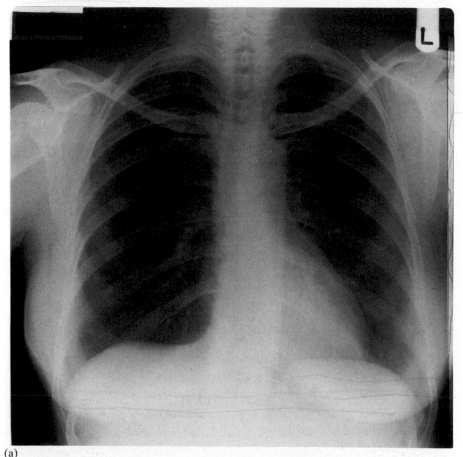

(a)

Fig. 11.1 Traumatic disruption of the aorta. (a) Normal chest x-ray ten days before the accident. (b) Obvious widening of the mediastinum with displacement of right paratracheal stripe. There is a left-sided pleural effusion overlying the apex of the lung in this supine film. (c) Aortagram—complete tear of aorta at the level of isthmus, with an aneurysm extending to the origin of the left subclavian artery.

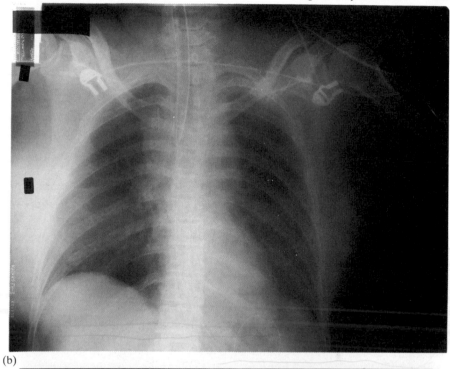

(b)

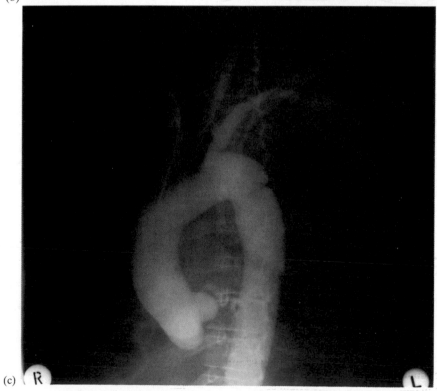

(c)

Pericardium

The pericardium may be torn by a blunt injury, usually in association with rupture of the diaphragm (see below). More often, however, pericardial damage is the result of a penetrating injury. The main danger of a pericardial tear is that the heart will herniate through the defect, severely compromising cardiac function. If this happens, immediate surgery is indicated.

Aorta

The aorta can be disrupted, usually as a result of a rapid deceleration injury, at the junction between the fixed and mobile portions of the aortic arch (i.e. most frequently just distal to the origin of the left subclavian artery). This is usually rapidly fatal in the elderly in whom the aorta is rigid, but young patients may suffer partial rupture and survive for long enough to be investigated and undergo definitive surgery. Disruption of the aorta just above the aortic valve may also occur but is usually fatal.

The diagnosis should be suspected when widening of the superior mediastinum, sometimes in association with some fluid in the pleural cavity, is seen on the chest x-ray of a patient who has suffered an injury compatible with aortic rupture. On examination, there may be a discrepancy between the blood pressure in each arm and femoral pulses may be diminished or absent. However, the significance of mediastinal widening is notoriously difficult to assess in trauma victims and the diagnosis must always be confirmed or excluded by angiography and/or CAT scan (Fig. 11.1).

Lungs and airways

Tears or punctures of lung tissue, often involving small airways, are relatively common following penetrating injuries and chest wall trauma with rib fractures. They are associated with pneumo- or haemopneumothoraces and the presence of surgical emphysema will often alert the clinician to the diagnosis. Rupture of a large bronchus may cause haemoptysis, complete atelectasis of the affected lung and mediastinal emphysema, as well as pneumothorax.

Although, in those breathing spontaneously, a small pneumothorax can be allowed to resolve spontaneously (provided it is not enlarging and not compromising respiratory function), larger collections of air, haemopneumothoraces and those under tension will require insertion of an underwater seal drain. A chest drain should always be inserted when a patient with a pneumothorax requires IPPV. Some authorities recommend prophylactic insertion of chest drains in those with multiple rib fractures who need controlled ventilation, even in the absence of a pneumothorax. This practice is, however, associated with a significant risk of damage to the underlying lung. It is preferable just to be aware of the possibility of this complication and to have the facilities for immediate chest drain insertion available at the bedside.

In order to ensure satisfactory drainage of blood and fluid, the drain should be inserted through the sixth or seventh intercostal space in the midaxillary line. If the pneumothorax fails to re-expand, and the air leak persists, it may be necessary to apply a negative pressure (e.g. $-5\,cm\,H_2O$)

using a high-volume, low-pressure sucker. Patients with a persistent pneumothorax associated with a large air leak may benefit from high-frequency jet ventilation (see Chapter 13) and may require surgical repair or resection of the damaged lung.

Less commonly, the trachea itself may be either partially or totally disrupted. If there is a wide separation of the two ends, the patient usually dies rapidly from asphyxia. Lesser degrees of separation are, however, compatible with survival.

Lung contusion may be diffuse and bilateral, e.g. following a blast injury, or relatively localized, e.g. underlying a limited area of chest wall trauma. Occasionally, an isolated intrapulmonary haematoma is seen. Severe respiratory failure usually ensues in those with extensive contusion, especially when associated with chest wall instability, but oedema formation and chest x-ray changes are often delayed for about 24 hours. As with other causes of non-cardiogenic pulmonary oedema, treatment consists of fluid restriction, diuretics, supplemental oxygen, continuous positive airway pressure (CPAP) and controlled ventilation with positive end expiratory pressure (see Chapter 13). Prophylactic antibiotics should not be used, except possibly in those with pre-existing COAD. Some authorities have suggested that steroids limit the degree of pulmonary abnormality (Trinkle et al, 1975), particularly in those with blast injuries.

Diaphragmatic rupture

This is rare and usually occurs following trauma to the anterior abdominal wall. It may also be associated with acetabular fractures, when the force of the impact is transmitted along the length of the femur and through the abdomen. It is a relatively benign injury and may not be recognized until many years after the accident when, for example, the patient presents with abdominal contents within the left hemithorax. If the right hemidiaphragm is ruptured, the liver usually prevents herniation.

Chest wall

Major chest wall injuries produce instability of the thoracic cage and lung contusion.

If several ribs are fractured in more than one place, or if broken ribs are combined with fracture dislocations of the costochondral junctions or sternum, the negative intrapleural pressure generated on inspiration causes the isolated segment of chest wall to collapse inwards, compromising ventilation. Theoretically, if the area of paradoxical movement, or 'flail segment', was very large, alveolar gas might simply oscillate between the two lungs during the respiratory cycle (pendelluft), causing gross rebreathing. However, it seems that pendelluft is an extremely rare occurrence clinically except, perhaps, when one hemithorax is totally disrupted or open to the atmosphere (Maloney et al, 1961). Nevertheless, these mechanical problems, exacerbated by severe pain, can cause significant hypoventilation, as well as impairing the patient's ability to cough and maintain lung expansion. There is, then, a risk of atelectasis, sputum retention and secondary infection.

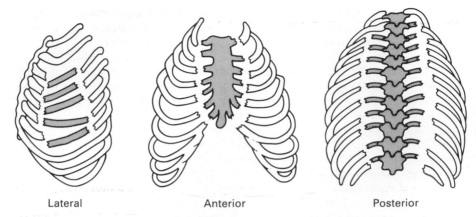

Lateral   Anterior   Posterior

Fig. 11.2 Types of flail chest. A lateral injury is the most common. Anterior injuries are caused by frontal impact and may be associated with damage to the heart. Posterior injuries are unusual and strong muscular support prevents serious paradoxical movement. From Webb (1978), with permission.

Flail segments can be classified according to their anatomical location (Fig. 11.2). An associated fractured clavicle exacerbates chest wall instability, and in this situation ventilation may be further compromised by damage to the phrenic nerve. Sternal fractures can be particularly unstable.

Associated pulmonary contusion (see above) causes hypoxaemia and a progressive fall in lung compliance. The latter exacerbates chest wall instability; as lung compliance falls, increasingly negative intrapleural pressures are generated in order to sustain ventilation and the flail segment becomes progressively more obvious. Indeed, in some cases paradoxical chest wall movement is only noticed when lung mechanics have deteriorated 12–24 hours after the injury.

In the past, instability of the thoracic cage was considered to be the most important abnormality in patients with chest wall injuries. Therefore, treatment consisted of surgical stabilization of the flail segment using strapping, external traction or open reduction and fixation with wires, plates or clamps. These procedures are traumatic, often accompanied by considerable haemorrhage, and relatively ineffective. Moreover, there is a significant risk of serious infection. Finally, those patients with the greatest degree of chest wall instability often also have the most extensive lung contusions; mechanical ventilation is then unavoidable, even if the flail segment is stabilized. Nevertheless, some have continued to advocate surgical stabilization in selected cases in order to reduce the need for, or duration of, mechanical ventilation and to limit the degree of chest wall deformity (Moore, 1975). The majority now rarely resort to these methods except, perhaps, when a thoracotomy has been performed for other indications or to stabilize a particularly mobile sternal fracture.

In 1956, Avery et al described the use of IPPV, with 'alkalotic apnea', in treatment of severe crushing injuries of the chest. They felt that this technique allowed the survival of patients with an apparently hopeless prognosis. Despite this treatment, however, mortality rates were unchanged and the prolonged period of IPPV was associated with a variety of serious complications, including pneumonia, barotrauma and tracheal injury (Shackford et al, 1976). Subsequently, it has been shown that many patients with severe chest injuries can be managed successfully without resorting to prolonged mechanical ventilation. Trinkle and his colleagues (1975) provided analgesia with morphine or intercostal blocks and treated pulmonary contusion with frusemide, methylprednisolone, salt-poor albumin to maintain oncotic pressure, colloids for volume replacement, aggressive physiotherapy and supplemental oxygen. IPPV was only used when the P_aO_2 was less than 8 kPa (60 mmHg) breathing air, or less than 10.6 kPa (80 mmHg) on oxygen, and then only until lung function had improved. With this regimen they claimed a significant reduction in morbidity and mortality when compared with a group of patients treated by early endotracheal intubation and mechanical ventilation. Similarly, Dittman et al (1982) use a thoracic epidural to provide analgesia and recommend elective mechanical ventilation only if the patient is unconscious, if there is severe pulmonary dysfunction (P_aO_2 <8 kPa (60 mmHg) on air, vital capacity <15 ml kg^{-1}) unresponsive to conservative measures and in the presence of serious extrathoracic injuries requiring surgical intervention. Moreover, they suggest that IPPV should be discontinued as soon as the above values have been attained with thoracic epidural analgesia. Others have supported this approach of using mechanical ventilation only in the presence of significant pulmonary dysfunction and weaning the patient once normal gas exchange has been restored (Shackford et al, 1976).

The most appropriate management for a particular patient depends not only on the severity and nature of the chest injury, but is also influenced by the presence of pre-existing obesity or lung disease, the nature of any associated injuries and the patient's age.

Associated injuries to the head, face, abdomen or extremities can significantly complicate the management of chest trauma. In particular, comatose patients should always be intubated and ventilated, while painful laparotomy wounds can further embarrass ventilation. The prognosis following chest wall injury is significantly worse in the obese, the elderly and those with pre-existing COAD, hypertension or myocardial ischaemia. Patients with diseases such as ankylosing spondylitis which interfere with normal chest wall expansion will be particularly seriously compromised by chest wall injuries.

Following initial assessment and treatment, the patient must be closely observed for several days, since deterioration is almost inevitable over the first 24–48 hours. As well as clinical evaluation and blood gas analysis, serial measurements of vital capacity provide a useful means of assessing the patient's progress.

As a guide to the most appropriate management for a particular patient, chest injuries can be categorized into one of three grades of severity:

Grade I (mild). These patients are able to maintain adequate alveolar ventilation and can cough. They may have a small flail segment, but underlying pulmonary damage is minimal and there is no pre-existing lung disease. Associated trauma is limited to moderate peripheral injuries and there is no head or intra-abdominal injury.

168   *Intensive Care*

Grade I injuries can be treated with analgesia, oxygen if required, physiotherapy and early mobilization. Sleep deprivation must be avoided. The success of this regimen depends on the provision of adequate analgesia. In some cases, simple oral anti-inflammatory agents such as aspirin, indomethacin or paracetamol may be sufficient. Others will require narcotics. Intercostal blocks may be useful, but have to be repeated at approximately 12-hourly intervals. This may be facilitated by using a catheter technique. Premixed 50% N_2O in O_2 (Entonox) can be used to provide supplementary analgesia during painful procedures. Although this regimen is often referred to as 'conservative management', this is a misleading term since, to be successful, it requires a particularly active approach to all aspects of patient care and is very demanding of both the patient and staff. If possible, therefore, even patients with grade I injuries should be admitted to the intensive care unit.

Grade II (moderate). Although these patients can ventilate adequately, their ability to cough is seriously impaired. They may have an obvious flail segment and associated lung contusion. As compliance falls and intrapulmonary shunt increases during the first 24–48 hours, these patients can deteriorate sufficiently to be reclassified as grade III. Patients with associated extensive limb injuries, a mild head injury, pre-existing lung disease, obesity or old age are also classified as grade II.

Treatment consists of analgesia, physiotherapy, supplemental oxygen and early mobilization. Some may require endotracheal intubation or tracheostomy to protect their airway and control secretions. Pulmonary contusion should be treated as outlined above with fluid restriction and diuretics. It is especially important to control pain in this category of patient in order to permit coughing and adequate physiotherapy. Thoracic epidurals are particularly effective and can increase FRC, compliance, vital capacity and P_aO_2, as well as decreasing paradoxical movement of the chest wall (Dittmann et al, 1978).

Intercostal blocks are generally less satisfactory, but opiates can be very effective if administered as a continuous intravenous infusion. Some authorities recommend the application of CPAP by face mask (see Chapter 13) for 20–30 minutes each hour in order to increase FRC (Dittman et al, 1982). With this regimen, it may be possible to avoid IPPV, even in those with a large flail segment. However, this may be at the expense of a degree of permanent chest wall deformity and some consider this to be unacceptable, especially in young patients.

Grade III (severe). These patients have severe chest wall instability with extensive pulmonary contusion. They are extremely hypoxaemic, cannot cough and are often unable to sustain adequate alveolar ventilation. They rapidly become exhausted. Patients with associated visceral injuries requiring laparotomy and/or a severe head injury, as well as those with moderate chest injury but who are elderly, obese or who have pre-existing lung disease may be categorized as grade III.

Patients in grade III require controlled ventilation. PEEP can be used to improve oxygenation (see Chapter 13) (Sladen et al, 1973). Although traditionally patients have been prevented from making spontaneous respiratory efforts because of concern that this could perpetuate chest wall instability, some workers recommend the use of IMV with PEEP and have claimed that this can considerably decrease the duration of ventilatory support (Cullen et al, 1975). Patients with severe unilateral pulmonary abnormalities may require independent lung ventilation (see Chapter 13). An alternative is to nurse the patient in the lateral position with the damaged lung uppermost. This diverts pulmonary blood flow away from the damaged lung and limits preferential ventilation of the good lung. In those with a large and persistent air leak, high frequency jet ventilation may prove useful (Chapter 13). Weaning should commence as soon as the lung lesion has resolved and is facilitated by thoracic epidural analgesia.

Although secondary chest infection is common, especially in the presence of lung contusion, antibiotics should be withheld until infection is obvious and preferably until the responsible organism has been identified. Nevertheless, some authorities administer prophylactic antibiotics to those with pre-existing COAD.

Early mobilization is recommended even for these severely injured patients, and it is certainly possible for ventilated patients to stand and sit out of bed.

Prognosis

Reported overall mortality rates for those with chest injuries vary considerably depending on the patient population studied, but death solely attributable to an isolated chest injury is rare. Most often, death is related to associated extrathoracic injuries, particularly head injury, or pre-existing morbidity, such as COAD and old age.

SPINAL INJURIES

Spinal injuries are a feature of modern mechanized societies, the majority of cases being the result of RTAs. Other causes include falls at work or in the home, sports injuries (mainly diving accidents) and battlefield casualties. It is estimated that there are approximately 15–50 new cases of spinal injury per million of the population each year, although this is probably an under-estimate since many immediately fatal cases are unrecognized and many others are inadequately documented.

Initial management

Patients with isolated spinal injury should be resuscitated and, if possible, transferred immediately to a specialized unit (Albin, 1978). Those with serious associated injuries or respiratory failure are usually admitted directly to an intensive care unit. (Chest trauma is common in those with thoraco-lumbar fracture dislocations, and damage to the cervical spine is frequently associated with head injury. A number of patients will have multiple injuries.) High thoracic or cervical lesions may produce immediately life-threatening respiratory failure and cardiovascular disturbances (see below). Some patients may therefore require emergency endotracheal intubation and controlled ventilation, as well as measures to restore haemodynamic stability.

Further damage to the spinal cord must be avoided when removing the patient from the site of the accident and during transfer. Patients must therefore be lifted and extricated from wreckage with extreme care; this will usually require several people. They can then be placed on a 'spine board'. Flexion, extension and lateral movements of the spinal column should be prevented by using a cervical collar, or sandbags placed on either side of the head, and by positioning pillows to maintain the natural curvatures of the spine. Slight hyperextension at the site of the fracture is preferred and traction should be applied to the patient's head and legs.

Spinal injury is easily overlooked in the absence of cord damage and in those who are unconscious. If the patient is comatose, a cord lesion should be suspected if deep tendon reflexes are absent and in the presence of urinary retention or priapism. Lesions above T11 produce intercostal paralysis and an abnormal respiratory pattern, while cervical cord damage may be associated with Horner's syndrome. Nevertheless, all comatose patients should be handled as if a cord injury is present until this possibility has been excluded.

On admission to hospital, a full neurological examination should be performed to determine the level and completeness of the lesion. Subsequently, neurological assessment should be repeated at frequent intervals in order to detect extension of the deficit as cord oedema progresses upwards. It is particularly important to recognize increasing paralysis of respiratory muscles so that controlled ventilation can be instituted without delay. Neck movements should only be examined in conscious patients and by an expert.

Investigations

As well as obtaining appropriate plain x-rays of suspected sites of injury, gas myelography is performed in some centres to delineate bone fragments or intervertebral discs impinging on the spinal cord. CAT scans may be obtained in order to demonstrate the nature and extent of the cord lesion. Somatosensory evoked responses (Chapter 14) can be used to assess the completeness of the cord lesion and to document subsequent recovery or deterioration.

Management of the fracture or fracture dislocation

The stability of the spinal column depends on the integrity of the posterior ligamentous complex. This consists of the supra- and interspinous ligaments, the ligamentum flavum and the capsules of the facet joints. If these are disrupted, the spinal injury will be unstable. In general, controversy continues as to whether operative or non-operative management of spinal fractures and fracture/dislocations is to be preferred.

CERVICAL SPINE INJURIES

In the absence of facet joint dislocation, these can be managed with a cervical collar or skull traction to maintain the position and immobilize the site of injury. If one, or both, posterior facet joints are dislocated, early reduction is indicated. This can be achieved either by manipulation under a relaxant general anaesthetic, guided by an image intensifier, or by graded traction using skull tongs. Some centres perform open reduction in all cases, whereas others only resort to this method when more conservative measures have failed. Subsequently, the position must be maintained with traction. Patients can be nursed in a Stryker frame, although this is unsuitable for those with limb fractures requiring traction and the prone position is poorly tolerated by those with associated chest injuries. Moreover, it is dangerous when an endotracheal or tracheostomy tube is in place. In most situations, therefore, the Egerton Stoke Mandeville tilting and turning bed is more satisfactory.

Specific types of injury

The atlas may be fractured where the arch meets the lateral masses. Displacement occurs if the transverse ligament is torn (Fig. 11.3). Such an injury is usually caused by a vertical force, such as a fall on the head. Neurological damage is generally minimal and the injury can be treated with a cervical collar worn for three months.

The odontoid process may be fractured, usually through the base, most often as a result of an RTA or a severe fall (Fig. 11.4). Cord damage is usually

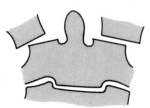

Fig. 11.3 Displaced lateral masses of the atlas. From Johnson (1978), with permission.

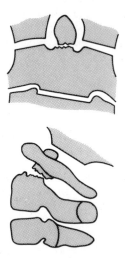

Fig. 11.4 Fractured odontoid process. (a) Antero-posterior view through the mouth of basal fracture. (b) Lateral view in extension. From Johnson (1978), with permission.

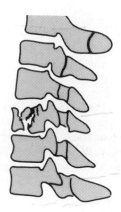

Fig. 11.5 Burst fracture C5. From Johnson (1978), with permission.

mild or absent but skull traction is generally indicated and surgery may be necessary if the fracture fails to unite.

Posterior dislocation of the axis may occur without a fracture. This causes few neurological signs and is treated with traction followed, if necessary, by fusion.

Burst fractures (Fig. 11.5) are very painful but stable. Unless there is marked bony displacement, cord damage is unusual, but they require support in a collar until fusion is seen radiologically.

Lateral x-rays of the cervical spine may appear normal in patients with hyperextension injury, although instability is demonstrable if films are obtained with the neck extended. In some cases, a small fragment of bone may be avulsed from the lower anterior edge of a vertebral body (Fig. 11.6). Because the posterior ligaments remain intact, these injuries are stable in the neutral position and can be treated with a cervical collar. The degree of neurological damage is variable.

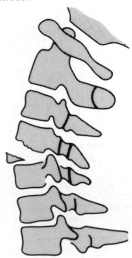

Fig. 11.6 Hyperextension injury of C4/C5: avulsion of fragment from C4. From Johnson (1978), with permission.

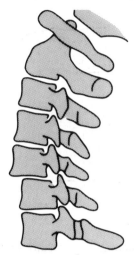

Fig. 11.7 Anterior dislocation: uni-facet dislocation of C5 on C6. From Johnson (1978), with permission.

Anterior dislocations (Fig. 11.7) disrupt the posterior ligaments and are therefore unstable unless the facet joints lock. Tetraplegia may occur as a result of this type of injury, but often neurological damage is minimal. Treatment consists of immediate reduction, e.g. using graded skull traction under x-ray control, followed by fusion approximately three weeks later.

The great majority of serious neck injuries involve fracture/dislocations (Fig. 11.8), most often at C5/6 or C6/7. These injuries are very unstable and are associated with the highest incidence of severe neurological damage. The safest treatment is probably continuous skull traction under x-ray control, although some surgeons will manipulate the injury under general anaesthesia. Traction for four to six weeks may be followed by operative fusion in the absence of satisfactory callus formation.

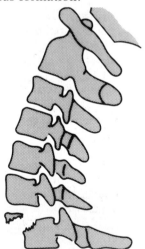

Fig. 11.8 Fracture-dislocation of C6/C7: avulsion of fragment of C7. From Johnson (1978), with permission.

THORACIC SPINE INJURIES

Anterior wedge fractures often occur in association with osteoporosis or malignant deposits. They are stable and should be treated symptomatically. On the other hand, fracture dislocations in this region are irreducible and almost invariably cause paraplegia.

THORACO-LUMBAR INJURIES

Anterior wedge and burst fractures are stable and require only symptomatic treatment. The integrity of the posterior ligaments in this region can be assessed by palpating the midline. If there is a palpable gap between the spinous processes, into which the finger sinks, then the fracture is unstable. These injuries can be treated by postural reduction with the patient extended over a foam bolster positioned at the level of the injury. Some cases will require open reduction and fixation.

Treatment of the spinal cord injury

Although spinal cord trauma produces a variable degree of irreversible neuronal destruction and haemorrhage, there is evidence that the ultimate neurological deficit is exacerbated by ischaemia which may persist for up to 24 hours after injury. This is associated with impaired blood flow, particularly in the grey matter, which may extend beyond the limits of the site of injury (Sandler and Tator, 1976), as well as oedema formation (cf. head injuries, Chapter 14).

A number of measures aimed at preventing or minimizing this secondary cord damage have been evaluated but in general the results have been either inconclusive or discouraging (Albin, 1978).

Thus, although some workers have shown that in animal models of cord injury, local hypothermia can be beneficial if applied within four hours of the injury, others have been unable to confirm these findings and clinically the results have been inconsistent. Possibly, this is because it has proved difficult to achieve adequate cooling of the substance of the spinal cord within less than four hours from the time of injury (Albin, 1978). Hyperbaric oxygen therapy has been suggested as a means of reversing tissue hypoxia in marginally ischaemic areas of the cord, and has been shown to produce improvement in animal models, but its value in human spinal cord injury is uncertain. Similarly, the results obtained with steroids, osmotic diuretics and agents intended to reverse local, noradrenaline-mediated vasoconstriction, such as reserpine and metirosine (α-methyl-L-tyrosine) have been inconsistent (Albin, 1978). At one time, laminectomy was advocated as a means of decompressing the cord, but this has fallen into disrepute.

Nevertheless, it is generally accepted that early immobilization and reduction of fracture dislocations, together with prompt resuscitation to restore oxygen delivery, can minimize neurological damage.

Cardiovascular support

There is some experimental evidence to suggest that spinal cord injury can produce immediate hypertension and bradycardia lasting for approximately

3–4 minutes (Rawe and Perot, 1979). This may be associated with a transient rise in intracranial pressure and an increase in pulmonary artery pressure (Albin et al, 1979). These changes can be compared with those described in neurogenic pulmonary oedema (see Chapter 14, p. 287).

Subsequently, spinal shock supervenes, vasomotor tone is lost and both resistance and capacitance vessels dilate. Since the sympathetic innervation of the heart arises from spinal segments T1–T5 it is interrupted by lesions above this level, while parasympathetic fibres remain intact. Patients with high thoracic or cervical injuries are therefore hypotensive (systolic blood pressure, commonly 80–90 mmHg (10.6–12 kPa), sometimes as low as 40 mmHg (5.3 kPa)) but without an associated tachycardia. Furthermore, vagal stimulation, for example in response to hypoxia or endotracheal suction, is unopposed and can produce a profound bradycardia, or even asystole (Welply et al, 1975). This can be prevented by administering atropine regularly or, in resistant cases, by oral sustained release isoprenaline. Hypoxaemic episodes must be avoided.

Despite the hypotension and relative hypovolaemia, which may or may not be combined with significant blood loss from associated injuries, the circulating volume must be replaced extremely cautiously. Because the CVP is an unreliable guide to volume requirements and cardiovascular function in these patients, pulmonary artery catheterization may be required in the more difficult cases; patients with high spinal injuries are unable to respond to a volume challenge by increasing heart rate and contractility (Troll and Dohrmann, 1975), and there is therefore a considerable risk of overtransfusion. In some cases, an inotropic agent will be required in order to improve myocardial performance and restore the systemic blood pressure to an acceptable level. Furthermore, these patients are particularly prone to pulmonary oedema, possibly because pulmonary capillaries are disrupted during the initial hypertensive episode.

Following the period of spinal shock, reflex activity gradually returns and there is some recovery of sympathetic tone. Nevertheless, although the tendency to bradycardia diminishes, a degree of postural hypotension generally persists.

Respiratory system

Lesions above T11 interrupt the innervation of respiratory muscles. Intercostal paralysis may be partial or complete, and may be asymmetrical. Diaphragmatic breathing in the presence of intercostal paralysis produces a paradoxical pattern of respiration with abdominal distension and indrawing of the affected segments of the chest wall during inspiration. Lesions at or above C4 deprive the diaphragm of its major segmental nerve supply and ventilation is grossly impaired. Immediate intubation and ventilation may be life-saving in such cases.

Associated chest injuries are common, particularly in those with thoraco-lumbar injuries, and can further impair respiratory function. These abnormalities may be exacerbated by aspiration (the patient is usually nursed supine and often has an impaired ability to cough, a reduced conscious level and paralytic ileus) and pulmonary oedema (see above).

It is recommended that controlled ventilation be instituted early on the basis of a clinical assessment, assisted by blood gas analysis, in order to avoid a progressive deterioration in respiratory function. Because of the sympathetic denervation, many of these patients are unable to compensate for the increased mean intrathoracic pressure during positive pressure ventilation and become markedly hypotensive. Cautious volume replacement, with or without inotropic support, may then be required to restore perfusion of vital organs.

The treatment of these respiratory abnormalities is complicated by the positioning and immobilization required to treat the spinal injury, which hampers effective physiotherapy. Moreover, vital capacity is reduced (Ohry et al, 1975) and the ability to cough impaired. Diaphragmatic breathing in the presence of intercostal paralysis is, however, most efficient in the supine position. Intensive physiotherapy is essential.

Urinary tract

Initially, patients admitted to the intensive care unit will require urethral or suprapubic catheterization with continuous drainage. Later, a regimen of intermittent catheterization may be instituted to encourage the return of reflex bladder function.

Gastrointestinal tract, fluid and electrolyte balance, nutrition

In the acute phase, it can be difficult to exclude significant intra-abdominal trauma since patients with spinal injury are unable to appreciate abdominal pain and up to 20% develop a neurogenic paralytic ileus. Peritoneal lavage is a useful diagnostic technique, but interpretation may be complicated by blood leaking into the abdominal cavity from a paravertebral haematoma.

Some patients develop discoordinated bowel activity with progressive abdominal distension and vomiting, despite the presence of bowel sounds. This is associated with an increased risk of aspiration, fluid and electrolyte disturbances and impaired ventilation.

Usually, these abnormalities resolve within 4–7 days and it is then possible to establish enteral nutrition. Occasionally, parenteral nutrition is indicated.

The rectum must be emptied on about the fourth day after injury and this should be followed by regular evacuation on three days of the week. This is achieved with oral aperients, rectal suppositories and, if necessary, manual evacuation. Provided this regimen is started soon after the injury, so that overdistension of the bowel is avoided, a pattern of reflex evacuation can be established and faecal incontinence is prevented.

Body temperature

The ability to adjust skin blood flow and sweating is lost below the level of a complete spinal cord lesion. This is a particular problem for tetraplegics who are therefore prone to hypothermia and require air conditioning during hot weather.

Finally, prophylactic measures to minimize the risk of gastrointestinal haemorrhage and thromboembolic complications are essential (see Chapter

8), as are first-class nursing care and physiotherapy to prevent pressure sores and fixed deformities.

Anaesthetic considerations

Endotracheal intubation is difficult and hazardous in those with unstable cervical spines. In such cases, the head and neck should be immobilized with traction, sandbags or by an assistant prior to intubation. The usual flexion–extension manoeuvres must be avoided. Because of the dangers of vagal stimulation, the patient must be preoxygenated and given atropine (Welply et al, 1975). Suxamethonium can precipitate hyperkalaemia between three days and six months after the injury (Snow et al, 1973) and should therefore be avoided. In the acute situation, however, patients are at risk of aspiration and some recommend rapid sequence induction with suxamethonium and the application of cricoid pressure. Many authorities recommend awake intubation, if necessary using a fibre-optic bronchoscope or laryngoscope, as the safest technique, while emergency cricothyrotomy or tracheostomy is occasionally necessary. Adequate monitoring of cardiovascular and respiratory function is essential throughout.

Prognosis

The outlook for patients with spinal injury has markedly improved since the First World War, when approximately 90% of all cases died within one year, and currently the mortality is only 2–3% in the first 12 months. Furthermore, although the life expectancy of a tetraplegic is undoubtedly reduced, on average by about 15 years, paraplegics can generally anticipate a normal lifespan. However, these figures only apply to young patients. The prognosis is considerably worse in the elderly and very few patients over the age of 60 years will survive for more than a year (Hardy, 1976). Nevertheless, since the majority of spinally injured patients are less than 25 years old, they represent a considerable long-term financial commitment; for example, the average cost over the lifetime of a paraplegic in the USA is estimated at US$500 000. Effective preventive measures are therefore of the utmost importance and must include improvements in safety standards on the roads, at work and in the home. Approximately 80% of patients with incomplete lesions achieve some form of useful recovery, whereas only 10–15% of those with complete lesions recover any neurological function. Of all cases, 74% eventually become independent, either in or out of a wheelchair, 20% remain partly dependent and only 6% are totally dependent.

FAT EMBOLISM SYNDROME (FES)

This syndrome was first described by Zenker in 1862 in a patient who had suffered a crushing thoraco-abdominal injury. Classically, it presents as a triad of respiratory insufficiency, cerebral dysfunction and petechial haemorrhages, although partial syndromes are relatively common (Sevitt, 1973). FES is usually associated with long bone or pelvic fractures, but may occasionally follow minor cracks (e.g. of the ribs or patella) or extensive crush injuries involving adipose tissue. The syndrome may also be encountered after surgical manipulation and stabilization of fractures; a particularly severe or fulminating form may occur after a Thompson's arthroplasty for repair of a subcapital fracture of the femoral neck (Sevitt, 1973).

Pathophysiology

Fractures are almost invariably associated with the presence of fat emboli in the lungs (Editorial, 1972) and the degree of embolization is generally related to the number and severity of the fractures (Sevitt, 1973). Moreover, subclinical hypoxaemia can be detected in up to 50% of patients with long bone fractures, although a number of factors other than fat embolism, such as the effects of a general anaesthetic, may partly account for this finding (Sevitt, 1973). The majority of cases, however, are asymptomatic, and clinically obvious fat embolism occurs in only 1–5% of those with fractures (Sevitt, 1973). It is not understood why most cases are subclinical whereas others, with similar or even less severe injuries, develop FES.

The source of the emboli is still disputed, although there is considerable evidence in favour of the classical view that they originate from ruptured fat cells at the site of injury, usually within the bone marrow, and gain access to the circulation via torn veins (Gossling and Donohue, 1979). This hypothesis is supported by studies demonstrating bone marrow emboli, associated with fat emboli, in the lungs of patients dying within 24 hours of an injury (Sevitt, 1973). Furthermore, in experimental studies the chemical composition of the emboli resembles that of bone marrow and depot marrow fat more closely than that of circulating plasma lipids (Hallgren et al, 1966). An alternative, but much less likely, explanation is that circulating lipomicrons coalesce to form large globules, possibly initiated by intravascular platelet aggregation. The relevance of the observed increase in plasma levels of free fatty acids (FFAs) in trauma victims, which is associated with elevated circulating catecholamine levels, is unclear (Gossling and Donohue, 1979).

The mechanism of organ damage in FES is complex. Embolization almost certainly produces mechanical obstruction of the pulmonary circulation and in the most severe cases fat globules, which are fluid and deformable, are probably forced through the pulmonary capillaries to embolize systemically. Moreover, as the obstruction to the pulmonary circulation becomes progressively more severe, arteriovenous anastomoses may open, exacerbating both pulmonary shunting and systemic embolization. This theory is supported by studies demonstrating that when there is evidence of systemic involvement, pulmonary emboli are invariably present (Sevitt, 1973). Although the concept of mechanical obstruction can account for the presence of haemorrhagic and ischaemic infarcts in the organs of patients dying with FES, it does not explain the inflammatory changes and increased capillary permeability seen in the lungs. It is possible that neutral triglycerides accumulate in the capillaries where they are converted to highly irritant FFAs and it is these which cause the inflammatory response. However, it is still unclear why these changes should be confined to the pulmonary circulation. Further organ damage may be caused by a low-grade DIC associated with impairment of the fibrinolytic system. Findings indicative of altered coagulability in FES may include a fall in haematocrit, thrombocytopenia, increased platelet adhesiveness, red cell aggregation and elevated FDPs (Gossling and Donohue, 1979). Finally, the release of vasoactive substances may contribute to the altered capillary permeability (see Chapter 10), while lung function may be further impaired as a result of inactivation of surfactant by FFAs.

Pathologically, the lung damage in FES is indistinguishable from that seen in ARDS (see Chapter 13). The physiological changes have been described as an initial increase in V_D/V_T ratio caused by embolization, with V/Q mismatch and hypoxaemia (Bruecke et al, 1971). Later, the dead space returns to normal as an interstitial pneumonitis develops. Cerebral changes may be due to embolization, hypoxaemia or both.

Diagnosis

The onset of the symptoms of FES is usually delayed for up to 48 hours after the injury. Generally, the earliest signs are dyspnoea and tachypnoea; hypoxaemia, most often with a low P_aco_2, develops later. Tachycardia, hypotension and pyrexia are common. These signs are followed by diffuse shadowing seen on the chest x-ray. The syndrome may remain mild and resolve or progress to severe respiratory failure with hypoxaemia persisting for up to 14 days. Secondary pulmonary infection is then common. Many fatal cases are fulminating and follow the early onset of coma. Some patients may have associated cerebral involvement manifested as confusion, restlessness and drowsiness following an initial lucid interval. This may progress to convulsions and deep coma. Some cases present with cerebral involvement without respiratory failure. A petechial rash develops in approximately 50% of patients and appears particularly over the anterior axillary fold, the root of the neck and the conjunctivae. This rash is pathognomonic of FES and may be due to capillary occlusion by fat globules or thrombocytopenia, but the explanation for its predilection for these particular areas is not clear. Patients with FES may also have retinal exudates and haemorrhages, and occasionally fat droplets can be seen traversing the retinal vessels. Fat globules may also be detected in urine and sputum but these are not specific for FES. Similarly, thrombocytopenia, elevated FDP levels, hypocalcaemia and a fall in haematocrit may all be demonstrated but are non-specific. Mild jaundice and renal impairment are common. The ECG may show ischaemic ST segment changes and right ventricular strain (Editorial, 1972).

Management

Prompt immobilization of the fracture site may minimize further embolization (Gossling and Donohue, 1979) and even if this is not possible initially, surgical stabilization may be required later if embolic episodes persist. However, such surgical intervention may itself be associated with further deterioration. It is therefore often difficult to select the most appropriate course of action for an individual patient.

A variety of specific agents have been used in an attempt to reduce the severity of organ damage in FES, but none is of proven clinical efficacy (Editorial, 1972; Gossling and Donohue, 1979). For example, it has been suggested that heparin might enhance clearing of fat globules by stimulating lipase activity and that this might be beneficial despite the inevitable increase in circulating FFAs. Moreover, heparin can decrease serotonin release from platelets and inhibit DIC. There is no evidence, however, that heparin administration is of value in FES and its use increases the risk of bleeding into the lungs and from associated injuries. Similarly, the results of administering large doses of alcohol intravenously in order to inhibit serum lipase activity and minimize FFA production have been unimpressive. Dextran 40 has been used to improve tissue perfusion and inhibit platelet aggregation but this has the disadvantage that it may leak across the damaged capillary membrane and exacerbate oedema formation. It is unlikely that clofibrate is of any value.

Anecdotal experience has supported the use of pharmacological doses of steroids in the FES (Fischer et al, 1971) and, as in other circumstances, such treatment is likely to be most effective when given early. Recent evidence has suggested that high-dose methylprednisolone can effectively prevent the FES when administered prophylactically to patients with isolated long bone fractures (Schonfeld et al, 1983), possibly by preventing complement induced leukoaggregation.

In the absence of specific therapy of proven efficacy, treatment of FES is supportive. Respiratory failure is managed according to the principles outlined for ARDS in Chapter 13. Those who are deeply comatose may require treatment aimed at reducing and controlling intracranial pressure. Plasma ionized calcium levels very occasionally fall sufficiently to cause tetany, in which case calcium should be given intravenously. Platelets should be administered only when indicated for the treatment of severe thrombocytopenia.

Prognosis

The mortality of classical FES may approach 10–15%, but a proportion of these deaths are attributable to associated injuries. In a recent series, there were no deaths in a group of 54 patients with FES who did not have associated life-threatening diseases (Guenter and Braun, 1981). The condition is self-limiting and the majority of survivors will make a full recovery.

NEAR DROWNING

In Great Britain, between 1000 and 1500 people die each year as a result of accidental drowning. The incidence is higher in North America and Australia because of the large number of domestic swimming pools and the popularity of water sports. Almost half of those who drown are less than 20 years old, the highest incidence being in the second decade, and approximately 75% of the victims are male (Modell et al, 1976). Blood alcohol levels are often high. About one-third are competent swimmers and a number of these drown during an attempt at prolonged underwater swimming. In this situation, the swimmer hyperventilates prior to diving in order to lower the arterial carbon dioxide tension and extend the length of time he or she can remain under water. Unfortunately, the victim may then lose consciousness due to severe hypoxia before the arterial carbon dioxide tension has reached a level which will stimulate respiration. Subsequently, P_aCO_2 rises sufficiently to generate an inspiratory effort and pulmonary aspiration occurs.

Pathophysiology

It has been suggested that approximately 10–20% of those who drown die without aspirating, presumably as a result of asphyxia due to severe glottic spasm and that this accounts for the so-called 'dry drownings' found at post mortem. This probably occurs most often following submersion in an irritant liquid such as sea water containing particles of sand or heavily chlorinated swimming pool water. Others (Golden and Rivers, 1975) consider this an unlikely explanation since glottic spasm is unlikely to be maintained in the presence of severe hypoxia. Nevertheless, in one series, about 12% of near-drowned patients had apparently not aspirated (Modell et al, 1976); provided they are promptly resuscitated, such cases may not require any further treatment. In contrast, those who have inhaled water often develop respiratory failure and occasionally have significant abnormalities of fluid and electrolyte balance. Cerebral damage and renal dysfunction may complicate the most serious cases. Delayed deaths following near drowning are usually associated with unrecognized pulmonary insufficiency, secondary chest infection, hypoxic cerebral damage or raised intracranial pressure.

Respiratory abnormalities

Aspiration of large volumes of fresh water alters the alveolar surface tension (Giammona and Modell, 1967) and, even though the water is rapidly absorbed into the circulation, this produces hypoxaemia due to V/Q mismatch and alveolar collapse (Modell et al, 1968). Salt water, on the other hand, remains within the alveoli and draws fluid into the lungs from the intravascular space. Although the total amount of surfactant is reduced, that which remains continues to function normally (Giammona and Modell, 1967). This produces predominantly a large fixed right-to-left shunt. In both instances, a severe permeability pulmonary oedema can develop and lung compliance is reduced. In clinical practice, hypoxaemia is common (Modell et al, 1976) but these experimental differences between the pulmonary damage produced by fresh and salt water are rarely obvious, probably because most victims aspirate only small volumes of fluid. A metabolic acidosis is found in a significant proportion of patients and may be severe in some cases (Modell et al, 1976). Development of non-cardiogenic pulmonary oedema may be delayed for up to 72 hours.

Overexpansion of the lungs with areas resembling acute emphysema can frequently be demonstrated at post mortem in those who have drowned, and are probably the result of violent fluctuations in intrathoracic pressure occurring during the period of airway obstruction. In many, there is also evidence of aspiration of particulate matter, such as gastric contents, mud or sand. In those who die later, there may be bronchopneumonia, sometimes with multiple abscess formation, but in those who survive, recovery of lung function is usually complete.

Cardiovascular abnormalities

The most frequent cardiovascular abnormality is bradycardia, often associated with intense vasoconstriction. This response can be elicited by submerging the face in water at less than 20°C, when it is known as the 'diving reflex'. The vasoconstriction may divert blood flow to the brain and myocardium and, together with the protective effect of hypothermia, may account for survival following prolonged submersion in cold water (a 5-year-old Norwegian boy has survived without neurological sequelae following 40 minutes' submersion in iced water (Siebke et al, 1975)). Bradycardia and vasoconstriction can also occur as a response to hypoxaemia and acidosis, while catecholamine release and hypothermia may further contribute to the increased vascular tone.

Theoretically, salt water drowning will cause hypovolaemia, while aspiration of fresh water increases the circulating volume (see above). In clinical practice, however, victims of near drowning rarely inhale sufficient volumes to cause significant changes in blood volume (Modell et al, 1976). Nevertheless, hypovolaemia may be present because of fluid shifts and loss of circulating volume as, for example, pulmonary oedema.

A wide variety of ECG changes have been described in association with near drowning. These have included absent P waves, ST segment elevation, increased P–R interval, AV dissociation and ventricular tachycardia/fibrillation. Generally, these are secondary changes and should revert to normal following correction of hypoxaemia, acidosis, hypothermia and hypovolaemia.

Electrolyte disturbances

Although plasma levels of sodium and chloride may be elevated following experimental salt water drowning (sea water contains 509 mmol l^{-1} of sodium), and low plasma sodium levels have been demonstrated in animal studies of fresh water aspiration, serious electrolyte disturbances are unusual clinically and it is doubtful that they play a significant role in determining survival (Modell et al, 1976). Occasionally, hyperkalaemia occurs in association with metabolic acidosis or acute renal failure, and rarely complicates haemolysis caused by absorption of very large volumes of fresh water. Magnesium levels may be elevated following sea-water drowning.

Body temperature

Hypothermia is a common complication of near drowning and may protect vital organs from hypoxic/ischaemic damage. However, as body temperature falls below 30°C, ventricular fibrillation becomes increasingly likely and at less than 28°C, established ventricular fibrillation is usually resistant to cardioversion. Rapid rewarming may then be necessary (see below).

Renal dysfunction

This is unusual but may occur in association with hypoxia, metabolic acidosis or hypothermia. Established acute renal failure is even more unusual and usually follows an extended period of hypotension.

Neurological damage

Ischaemic cerebral damage can follow prolonged asphyxia, hypoxaemia or cardiac arrest, while some patients develop cerebral oedema and intracranial hypertension.

Management

[handwritten: ABC 1st]

Once the victim has been removed from the water, the first priority is to establish a clear airway followed, if necessary, by mouth-to-mouth resuscitation and external cardiac massage. If it is impossible to reach dry land immediately, expired air ventilation should be attempted in the water since a few breaths may be sufficient to restart spontaneous respiration and cardiac activity. Time should not be wasted in attempting to remove water from the patient's lungs, since the amount recovered, if any, is usually too small to be significant. It is, however, essential to prevent further heat loss by wrapping the victim in blankets or warm clothing.

As discussed above, hypoxaemia is common following immersion and, because the signs of arterial desaturation are unreliable, all patients should receive supplemental oxygen as soon as this is available. Similarly, once experienced personnel arrive at the scene, comatose patients, and those requiring continued artificial ventilation, must be intubated and an intravenous infusion should be established. An ECG will allow the detection and treatment of dysrhythmias. *[handwritten: ABC]*

On admission to hospital it is important to determine the circumstances of the accident (duration of immersion, salt or fresh water, warm or cold, history of alcohol or drug ingestion) as well as the efficacy of any attempts at resuscitation. The patient should be fully examined, including a search for associated injuries. All patients should be admitted to an intensive care unit for observation because of the risk of delayed respiratory failure. *[handwritten: History]*

The principles of treatment for acute respiratory failure are discussed in Chapter 12. Administration of steroids is no longer recommended in near drowning (Modell et al, 1976) since they do not appear to limit the pulmonary abnormality (Calderwood et al, 1975) and may impair lung healing. Although the use of prophylactic antibiotics is advocated by some authorities (Golden and Rivers, 1975), it is generally considered preferable to perform frequent bacteriological investigations and treat only established infections (Modell et al, 1976). Some patients develop irritative bronchospasm requiring bronchodilator therapy. *[handwritten: Rx Resp]*

Cardiovascular support will involve the restoration of sinus rhythm, correction of acidosis and hypoxaemia, volume replacement and, occasionally, inotropic support. In complicated cases, insertion of a Swan–Ganz catheter may provide useful information, particularly in those with pulmonary oedema. The principles of cardiovascular support have been discussed in the preceding chapter. *[handwritten: CVS BP CO]*

The value of aggressive measures aimed at minimizing ischaemic cerebral damage and controlling intracranial hypertension in comatose victims of near drowning is uncertain (see Chapter 14). The management of hypothermia is discussed below.

Associated injuries may significantly complicate the management of near drowning. In particular, cervical spine and head injuries are frequently associated with diving accidents and are easily missed in comatose patients.

Prognosis

In a large retrospective study of near-drowning victims it was found that 87% survived with apparently normal brain function, 2% survived with impaired brain function and 11% died. Approximately 90% of those who are alert, or whose conscious level is merely blunted on admission, should make a complete recovery (Modell et al, 1980). The outlook is less good for those who are comatose and depends on the extent of irreversible cerebral damage.

ACCIDENTAL HYPOTHERMIA

Accidental hypothermia may follow exposure to low environmental temperatures or immersion in cold water and is frequently associated with impaired temperature regulation. Factors predisposing to exposure hypothermia include inadequate or wet clothing, strong winds, contact with snow and strenuous exercise. Paradoxically, it is more common in relatively temperate regions where the dangers of, for example, hill walking in winter are often under-estimated and preventive measures are consequently inadequate. The incidence of immersion hypothermia is rising, probably because of the widespread use of life jackets which support the victim's head above water and prevent drowning (Golden and Rivers, 1975), as well as the increasing popularity of water sports. The rate of heat loss in water is approximately 25 times greater than that in air at the same temperature and this is accelerated by the increase in cutaneous blood flow which accompanies exertion, e.g. swimming, as well as a redistribution of the warmed water layer surrounding the body. Subcutaneous fat provides insulation and obese subjects can generally survive longer periods of immersion; even non-waterproof conventional clothing is protective.

Diseases in which the metabolic rate is reduced, e.g. myxoedema, hypopituitarism and malnutrition, limit the ability to maintain body temperature by increasing heat production. Similarly, patients with spinal cord lesions are unable to produce thermal energy by increasing muscular activity, and this is exacerbated by an inability to adjust skin blood flow (see p. 176). Hypothalamic lesions can impair thermoregulation and patients in coma, e.g. due to a cerebrovascular accident, alcohol abuse or self-poisoning, are frequently hypothermic. Furthermore, alcohol and many sedative drugs, especially the barbiturates, increase heat loss by producing cutaneous vasodilatation. The elderly are particularly vulnerable to cold because of inactivity, impaired shivering, low metabolic rate, malnutrition, reduced subcutaneous fat, decreased vasoconstriction in response to cold, and poor social conditions (Editorial, 1977).

Clinical manifestations and pathophysiology

The clinical manifestations of hypothermia at a particular body temperature are variable and probably depend on the rate of cooling and the duration of hypothermia. Nevertheless, if the core temperature is greater than 33°C, physiological changes are generally minimal and thermoregulatory mechanisms remain intact. At temperatures between 33 and 30°C there is progressive physiological dysfunction, while cooling to below 30°C produces severe cardiorespiratory and neurological abnormalities with failure of thermoregulation. Body temperatures of less than 27–28°C can mimic death, and extreme hypothermia (less than 24–26°C) is usually incompatible with life, although some remarkable cases of survival under these circumstances have been reported (see p. 182).

Metabolic responses

Initially, metabolic rate increases and the victim shivers in an attempt to maintain body temperature. If this is unsuccessful, thermoregulation eventually fails and oxygen consumption falls (e.g. oxygen consumption may be reduced to about $80 \, \text{ml} \, \text{min}^{-1} \, \text{m}^{-2}$ at a core temperature of 32°C) (Harari et al, 1975). As would be expected, the reduction in metabolic rate is greater in those with myxoedema coma.

Neurological manifestations

The severity of the neurological disturbance depends on the rate of cooling. In general, cerebral metabolism is depressed and this minimizes cerebral damage during episodes of ischaemia or hypoxia. At core temperatures below 33°C, the patient is dysarthric and cerebration is slowed. Conscious level falls progressively until at 30°C the victim is usually stuporose and hypertonic, with infrequent voluntary movements. Tendon reflexes are slowed with prolonged contraction and relaxation phases. At core temperatures below 27°C, patients are usually comatose and hypertonic with absent tendon and plantar reflexes. The pupils do not react to light and voluntary movements are absent.

Cardiovascular changes

At first, cardiac output rises to satisfy the increased metabolic demands, but subsequently the cardiovascular system is depressed in proportion to the fall in body temperature. Progressive bradycardia, probably due to a direct effect of cold on the sinus node (30–40 beats min^{-1} at 28–29°C, 10 beats min^{-1} at 25–26°C), produces a dramatic fall in cardiac output, despite a normal or increased stroke volume. Initially, blood pressure is maintained by vasoconstriction and an increase in viscosity, but hypotension usually supervenes at temperatures below 30°C. Moreover, many hypothermic patients are hypovolaemic (Harari et al, 1975) and vasodilatation induced by rewarming can precipitate serious hypotension. Blood pressure may also fall when the increase in viscosity is reversed by intravenous fluid administration. There is some evidence that myocardial performance can be impaired following prolonged exposure to cold (Harari et al, 1975).

Although sinus rhythm is maintained during moderate hypothermia, atrial flutter or fibrillation, sometimes with ventricular premature contractions, often supervenes in the more serious cases. With more profound falls in body temperature, an idioventricular rhythm is common and atrial activity may

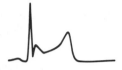

Fig. 11.9 The ECG in accidental hypothermia. Lead V5 showing 'J' wave and ST segment changes.

completely disappear. There is a risk of ventricular fibrillation when core temperature falls below 30°C and this may be precipitated by hypoxia, hypotension or stimulating procedures such as endotracheal intubation. At core temperatures of less than 28°C, there is a pronounced tendency to develop ventricular fibrillation.

The ECG in hypothermia shows evidence of reduced conductivity with prolongation of the PR and QT intervals, as well as widening of the QRS complex. The ST segment is generally depressed or concave, but is sometimes elevated. Classically, a 'J' wave is seen at the junction of the QRS and ST segments (Fig. 11.9) and this finding is almost constant at temperatures below 31°C.

Respiratory changes

Hypothermia reduces the ventilatory response to hypoxaemia and hypercarbia, and tidal volume and respiratory rate fall progressively. This reduction in minute volume is, however, accompanied by a fall in both oxygen consumption and carbon dioxide production. The arterial carbon dioxide tension (corrected to body temperature) may therefore be low, normal or high (McNicol and Smith, 1964) depending on the balance between the reduction in alveolar ventilation and the fall in carbon dioxide production. On the other hand, hypothermic patients are consistently hypoxaemic (when P_aO_2 is corrected to body temperature) with an increased $P_{A-a}O_2$, largely due to ventilation perfusion mismatch (McNicol and Smith, 1964). Although the consequences of a reduction in arterial oxygen tension are minimized by the fall in oxygen consumption, and are generally well tolerated, a metabolic acidosis is common. Moreover, significant tissue hypoxia can develop when the metabolic rate rises during rapid rewarming or shivering, and restoration of blood flow to previously ischaemic areas washes accumulated acid into the general circulation. This metabolic acidosis is exacerbated by impaired hepatic clearance of lactic acid and a reduction in the capacity of the kidneys to excrete hydrogen ions.

Bronchopneumonia is a relatively common complication of hypothermia; both its incidence and severity are related to the duration and the degree of hypothermia.

Renal dysfunction

Hypothermia is associated with diuresis and haemoconcentration, despite a reduction in renal blood flow. This polyuria may be related to a central shift of the blood volume, as well as impaired tubular function due to inhibition of enzyme systems and a reduced responsiveness to ADH. Hypothermic patients therefore produce dilute, eventually almost iso-osmotic urine, with a reduced creatinine clearance, an elevated blood urea and increased sodium excretion. Potassium is retained but this seldom causes significant alterations in plasma levels.

A few patients develop established acute renal failure and require dialysis. This is unlikely to be the result of hypothermia alone and is probably related to associated abnormalities such as hypoxia, hypotension and hypovolaemia.

Other abnormalities

Serum amylase levels are often raised in hypothermia, and this probably reflects a mild acute pancreatitis. Occasionally, this pancreatitis contributes to the development, sometimes delayed, of diabetic ketoacidosis (MacClean et al, 1973).

Initially, glucose is released from liver glycogen and its utilization is increased. Later, glucose uptake decreases, possibly because of insulin resistance or inactivation of hexokinase, and hyperglycaemia is exacerbated by elevated cortisol levels.

Thrombocytopenia and various coagulation abnormalities have been described but these are of doubtful clinical significance.

Management

Monitoring

The diagnosis can be established using a low-reading rectal thermometer. Subsequently, body temperature can be monitored using a rectal probe. This must be inserted at least 10 cm beyond the anal sphincter and will record a temperature 0.25–0.5°C below that of blood. An oesophageal probe may more closely reflect the temperature of the blood and the myocardium. Blood pressure, CVP, the electrocardiogram and urine output should also be monitored in all cases. Insertion of a Swan–Ganz catheter is not recommended since the CVP is usually an accurate reflection of left ventricular filling pressure and passage of the catheter may precipitate ventricular fibrillation. Urea and electrolytes and blood sugar concentrations should be measured frequently.

Determination of blood gas tensions is complicated by the influence of alterations in body temperature on the position of the dissociation curves. Measurements are made at 37°C (see Chapter 4) and if corrected, for example, to a body temperature of 25°C, a P_aO_2 of 13.3 kPa (100 mmHg) and a P_aCO_2 of 5.3 kPa (40 mmHg) become, respectively, 6.7 and 3 kPa (50 and 22.5 mmHg). Changes in temperature also affect pH measurements; a fall of 1°C increases pH by 0.0147 units.

Supportive treatment

Patients who are profoundly hypothermic may survive despite apparently being dead on admission. Moreover, survival has been reported even following prolonged cardiac arrest or ventricular fibrillation. Attempts at resuscitation should therefore continue until rewarming has been achieved or until it is clear that the situation is hopeless. In all cases, underlying diseases must also be treated.

Hypoxaemia must be corrected by securing the airway and administering oxygen; this is particularly important during rewarming when oxygen requirements increase. A few patients will require controlled ventilation. In order to avoid extreme hypocarbia, which can exacerbate peripheral vasoconstriction and may precipitate ventricular fibrillation, the minute volume must be adjusted to match the reduced carbon dioxide production.

Intravenous fluid replacement should be started with 5% or 10% dextrose, combined with sodium bicarbonate as required to correct significant metabolic acidosis. Expansion of the circulating volume is essential during rewarming and this can be achieved using a colloidal solution such as PPF. Subsequent intravenous fluid administration should be guided by frequent estimation of urea, electrolytes and blood sugar levels, and haematocrit.

Occasionally, hypothermic patients develop cardiac failure during rewarming, with an elevated CVP, persistent hypotension, oliguria and acidosis. This may require the administration of an inotropic agent, although there is a considerable risk of inducing dysrhythmias. The heart rate normally increases progressively as body temperature rises and definitive treatment of the bradycardia is not indicated. Intracardiac pacing is generally ineffective and can be harmful. Patients in ventricular fibrillation will require direct current defibrillation. Although successful defibrillation has been reported at temperatures as low as 24°C (Siebke et al, 1975), in general restoration of an effective cardiac rhythm is unlikely until core temperature has reached 28–30°C.

Steroids are of no value in hypothermia, and antimicrobial therapy should be reserved for those with established infection.

Rewarming

The risk of complications such as myocardial failure, bronchopneumonia and neurological dysfunction increases the longer hypothermia persists. Furthermore, spontaneous rewarming takes place more slowly following prolonged hypothermia.

Spontaneous rewarming is the rule in patients whose body temperature is greater than 33°C, and may be possible in a few with core temperatures as low as 26–27°C. Passive rewarming is also preferred by some for elderly patients with prolonged hypothermia and underlying disease, e.g. myxoedema. The patient should be moved to a warm room (25–30°C) and insulated using, for example, a reflective 'space blanket'. It is also important to insulate the patient's head since scalp vessels do not constrict in response to cold and considerable heat can be lost from this region. Reported rewarming rates range from 0.1–3.7°C h^{-1}.

In other patients, particularly those with impaired thermoregulation and an inability to shiver, active measures are required to restore body temperature. This can be achieved with surface heat using hot water bottles, heat cradles, heated mattresses or electric blankets. This method is usually suitable for young patients with moderate hypothermia (28–33°C) of short duration, and for elderly patients who fail to respond to passive rewarming. Warming rates vary between 1 and 4°C h^{-1}. Surface rewarming can, however, produce abrupt vasodilatation and hypotension ('rewarming shock'), while reperfusion of cold ischaemic regions can cause a fall in central body temperature of as much as 3–4°C ('after drop'), as well as exacerbating metabolic acidosis. Moreover, this technique is relatively inefficient and may cause skin burns. Hot baths (at 40–45°C), with the limbs out of the water to avoid after-drop and minimize hypotension, are suitable for fit young adults, particularly following a short period of immersion in cold water, but should not be used in the elderly. Warming rates range from 5–7°C h^{-1}. With this method, active rewarming should be discontinued when the core temperature reaches 33°C.

Theoretically, central rewarming, which warms the 'core' before the 'shell', should avoid some of the dangers of surface heating, as well as ensuring that the myocardium warms early and is able to respond to the increasing metabolic demands. Moreover, it is the only practicable method in those with cardiac arrest.

Central rewarming at a rate of up to 15°C h^{-1} can be achieved using extracorporeal circulation via a femoral artery and vein. This method is relatively complex and its use should be restricted to those with severe hypothermia (<28°C) complicated by myocardial failure or cardiac arrest. Some use veno-venous dialysis to actively warm those whose core temperature is below 31°C and who are not warming steadily (>1°C h^{-1}) with non-invasive methods. Peritoneal lavage with warm fluid is less efficient but may be useful in self-poisoning since it can also hasten drug elimination. Intravenous administration of warm fluids and controlled ventilation with warmed humidified gases are inadequate when used alone but are useful adjuncts to other measures. Indeed, the optimal approach in an individual patient is often to use a carefully selected combination of the available techniques.

Prognosis

The overall mortality of accidental hypothermia may approach 60%, being as high as 75% in patients with an underlying primary disease and as low as 6% in those with hypothermia alone (Weyman et al, 1974). Hypothermia associated with poisoning has the best prognosis.

BURNS (Demling, 1985)

The majority of burn injuries occur in the home and frequently involve children of between one and five years old who are scalded by hot liquids or whose clothing is ignited. Amongst teenagers and adults, men of between 17 and 30 years old are the most frequent victims, usually as a result of accidents with inflammable liquids. Bedding and house fires most frequently affect the elderly and infirm, while about 25% of burns admissions are due to industrial accidents. Major structural fires account for only a small proportion of those admitted to hospital with thermal injury. Although improved fire-fighting techniques and emergency medical services, as well as the increased use of smoke detectors, may have made some contribution to a reduction in burn-related deaths, in general preventive measures have had only limited success. In contrast, there have been major advances in the resuscitation and subsequent care of burns victims which have been responsible for an improved overall survival rate and reduced hospital stay among those admitted to specialized burn centres (Feller et al, 1980). Therefore, high-risk patients must always be admitted to such units following initial resuscitation.

Assessment

The severity of a thermal injury depends on the area damaged and the depth of the burn. The percentage surface area burned can be estimated using the 'rule of nine' (Fig. 11.10), modified in children to take into account the

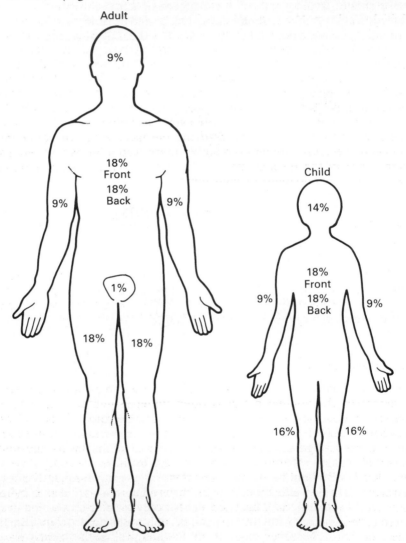

Fig. 11.10 The 'rule of nine' for estimating the percentage surface area burned in an adult and a child.

greater proportion of the body represented by the head and neck and the lesser contribution of the legs. In those with extensive burns, it may be easier to assess the area of undamaged skin and subtract this from one hundred.

The depth of the burn can be classified as erythema only, partial thickness or full thickness. Erythematous changes, without blistering, will usually resolve spontaneously within a few days and should not be included in the calculation of the surface area burned. In areas of partial thickness involvement, some viable deep epithelial elements remain from which regeneration of skin is possible. This occurs beneath the eschar of dead dermis within 1–4 weeks. Because nerve endings are exposed and remain intact, partial thickness burns are extremely painful. In contrast, epithelial structures and nerve endings are virtually completely destroyed following a full thickness burn. Healing can therefore only occur by ingrowth of skin from surrounding structures or by contraction, and pain sensation is absent. Full thickness burns may also involve underlying structures. Finally, it is important to identify associated trauma to other organs and vital structures.

Patients with burns involving more than 15% of their body surface area (BSA), as well as those with pulmonary or electrical injuries, must be referred to a specialist unit. Children with a burn of more than 6% of their BSA have a small, but definite risk of dying and should always be admitted to hospital for observation. Burns involving the face, hands or perineum in a child need specialist care and should be referred to a burns unit, even when less than 6% of the BSA is affected. In some cases, the distribution of the burn suggests the possibility of child abuse.

Management

Analgesia

Initially, this is best achieved by administering small incremental doses of an opiate intravenously (e.g. 2 mg increments of papaveretum up to a total of 15 mg over ten minutes). Subsequently, a continuous intravenous infusion of papaveretum can be given at a rate of 2–5 mg h^{-1}.

Volume replacement

Because fluid losses are not obvious, and the patient may at first appear well, the extent of the volume deficit is often under-estimated. Thermal injury increases microvascular permeability, in part because of the release of vasoactive substances (Harms et al, 1981), and plasma is lost both externally (into blisters and as an exudate on the surface of the burn) and into the interstitial space. Moreover, there is intracellular swelling due to a generalized cell membrane defect (Baxter, 1974). Increases in the osmotic pressure within the interstitium of both burned and adjacent non-burned tissue also appear to be important in the genesis of oedema and may be related to the release of osmotically active cellular elements (Demling, 1985). Recent evidence, however, suggests that although there is an early transient generalized increase in microvascular permeability (which is probably caused by histamine), the oedema which occurs in non-burned tissues is due to severe hypoproteinaemia rather than an increased capillary permeability (Demling, 1985). These changes, combined with evaporation of salt and water from the exposed surfaces, cause a considerable reduction in circulating volume and haemoconcentration. Without aggressive volume replacement, hypovolaemic shock supervenes and, if this is allowed to persist, acute renal failure may follow.

Significant reductions in plasma volume follow burns involving more than 15% BSA in adults and more than 10% BSA in children. Although the magnitude of the losses is variable (e.g. partial thickness scalds may be associated with massive reductions in plasma volume while deep flame burns are often charred and relatively dry), the volume of intravenous fluid required can be estimated using one of a number of formulae. For example, the Mount Vernon formula (Muir, 1981) recommends:

$$\text{Volume of plasma to be given in each period} = \% \text{ area burned} \times \frac{\text{weight (kg)}}{2}$$

Provided the patient's condition remains satisfactory, the calculated volume of plasma is infused in successive periods of 4, 4, 4, 6, 6 and 12 hours. However, it is emphasized that frequent clinical assessment of the adequacy of volume replacement is essential and that the rate of transfusion should be adjusted as indicated. This should be guided by the urine output, which must be maintained at more than $0.6 \, \text{ml} \, \text{kg}^{-1} \, \text{h}^{-1}$, and the PCV. The latter is influenced by red cell destruction, as well as plasma losses, and in the presence of significant haemolysis the PCV should be maintained at 10% below the expected value. When there is obvious haemoglobinuria, a value 20% below normal is ideal. Later, concentrated red cells should be given to restore the red cell mass. Some consider that the CVP is an unreliable guide to volume requirements in burns victims and, in view of the high risk of infection and often limited availability of suitable access sites, avoid cannulating central veins. Others recommend CVP monitoring in all serious burns and the use of a thermodilution pulmonary artery catheter in the most difficult cases (Aikawa et al, 1978).

Severely burned patients require replacement of their circulating volume with large quantities of salt-containing solutions, but the type of fluid used for resuscitation is less important than the volume given and the experience of those responsible for its administration. Some authorities suggest that crystalloids alone should be administered during the first 24 hours because accumulated extravascular water can then be mobilized relatively easily (see pp. 144–146). Subsequently, colloids and blood are given as required to maintain the circulating volume and the PCV respectively. However, for reasons discussed in the preceding chapter, some use colloids even during the early phase of resuscitation while others add colloid to a background crystalloid regimen in order to maintain intravascular volume and the plasma albumin concentration. Some, however, have cautioned against the addition of colloids to crystalloid fluids for resuscitation (Goodwin et al, 1983). These authors found that, although the volumes of fluid required for successful resuscitation were reduced and the cardiac indices were higher in the early phase, the use of colloids promoted accumulation of lung water when oedema fluid was mobilized from the burn wound. Some patients will require intravenous sodium bicarbonate to correct a severe metabolic acidosis.

Despite this aggressive approach to the restoration and maintenance of an adequate circulating volume, acute renal failure or transient episodes of renal impairment may complicate thermal injury. These may follow periods of hypoperfusion and hypoxia, and can be exacerbated by haemoglobinuria or myoglobinuria in those with electrical or crush injuries. Established acute renal failure is associated with a particularly high mortality in burns victims and must be avoided at all costs.

Congestive cardiac failure may occur during the acute phase, or a few days after the injury when oedema fluid is mobilized. Myocardial infarction is a rare complication.

Respiratory care

Inhalation injury may occur in as many as 20% of patients admitted to burn centres. It should be suspected in any patient with facial burns, especially in the presence of stridor, erythema of the nasopharyngeal mucosa, singed nasal vibrissae and in those who are expectorating soot. Such an injury is most likely following facial flame burns or when the victim has been confined within a small, smoke-filled room. Elevated carboxyhaemoglobin (COHb) levels on admission also suggest that there has been significant respiratory involvement provided allowance is made for the time interval between smoke inhalation and admission (Clark et al, 1981). Moreover, COHb levels greater than 15% are associated with a high incidence of potentially lethal cyanide poisoning and could be used to identify those who might benefit from administration of a specific antidote (Clark et al, 1981). The chest x-ray and blood gas analysis may be within normal limits initially, but should be repeated at intervals in order to detect subsequent deterioration. In some centres, indirect laryngoscopy or fibre-optic bronchoscopy is performed early in order to confirm the diagnosis, define the extent and severity of the airway burn and to perform tracheobronchial toilet.

Patients with inhalation burns may develop pharyngeal and laryngeal oedema, with upper airways obstruction, due to thermal and/or chemical damage. Pulmonary parenchymal damage can cause acute hypoxaemic respiratory failure. All those with suspected airway burns must therefore be closely observed for the signs of impending airway obstruction and/or respiratory failure. Early intubation is preferable to a late tracheostomy under unfavourable circumstances. Indeed, tracheostomy should be avoided if possible because it is associated with an increased risk of pulmonary infection in burns injury (Eckhauser et al, 1974).

Few gases, except superheated steam, have sufficient thermal capacity to carry heat beyond the trachea. Pulmonary parenchymal damage is therefore usually chemical and due to water-soluble gaseous products of combustion such as ammonia, chlorine and sulphur dioxide. These react with the water in mucous membranes to produce strong acids and alkalis which can induce bronchospasm, ulceration of the mucous membranes and oedema. Lipid-soluble compounds such as phosgene, nitrous oxide, hydrogen chloride and aldehydes can reach the distal airways on carbon particles that adhere to the mucosa. These damage the cell membrane directly and impair ciliary clearance. Moreover, the inflammation is aggravated by activation of alveolar macrophages (Loke et al, 1984). Early increases in extravascular lung water are rare and may result from the direct chemical toxicity of inhaled gases in the most severe cases of inhalation injury. Delayed increases in lung water occur more frequently and are related to systemic or pulmonary sepsis (Tranbaugh et al, 1983). Presentation is frequently delayed, but early diagnosis may be possible using fibre-optic bronchoscopy, ^{133}Xe lung scans, ventilation/perfusion scans and lung function testing. Subsequently, secondary infection frequently supervenes, often with the organism colonizing the burn wound, and healing is by fibrosis.

Management is supportive, as for other causes of ARDS (see Chapter 13). Some recommend administration of steroids but these have been shown to be ineffective (Levine et al, 1978) and may increase the risk of infection as well as impairing lung healing (Wynne et al, 1979). There is little evidence to support the use of prophylactic antibiotics.

Pulmonary embolism is an unusual complication of thermal injury, but some centres use prophylactic subcutaneous heparin.

Control of infection

A number of immunological abnormalities have been identified in burns victims (Alexander, 1979), including impaired phagocytic function, decreased neutrophil chemotaxis and disturbances of the lymphocyte system. The importance of the observed reduction in fibronectin levels is disputed. It is perhaps not surprising, therefore, that the commonest cause of death following thermal injury is sepsis and multiple organ failure. Most often, this is related to infection of the burn wound or the lungs, but in some cases urinary tract infections or contamination of intravascular catheters are incriminated. As with other infections occurring in the critically ill, the most common pathogens causing burn wound sepsis have altered from the gram-positive cocci (e.g. the β-haemolytic streptococcus) to gram-negative rods, such as *Pseudomonas aeruginosa* and fungi. Methicillin-resistant strains of *Staphylococcus aureus* have, however, been responsible for a number of epidemics of infection in burns units.

The burn wound usually becomes colonized within a few days of admission, as a result either of autogenous infection (usually gram-negative organisms from the patient's own gastrointestinal tract) or of cross-contamination from another patient. The topical application of antibacterial agents for prophylaxis is controversial but may prevent or delay colonization, as well as reducing the concentration of bacteria. The three most commonly used agents are silver nitrate, silver sulphadiazine and mafenide acetate. Antibiotics should only be used to treat documented infection. This is usually diagnosed clinically, and can be confirmed by positive blood culture and/or wound biopsy. The risk of cross-contamination can be minimized by barrier nursing in a single cubicle with plenum ventilation and filtered air. Antitetanus prophylaxis is standard in most units. At present, the value of polyvalent antipseudomonal vaccine and non-specific potentiation of the immune response is being evaluated.

Surgery

Urgent surgical intervention may be required for patients with circumferential burns of the trunk, which can impair respiration, or the limbs, which can constrict blood vessels and cause ischaemic damage. Decompression is achieved by incising the skin and, sometimes, the deep fascia.

Elective surgery is performed to repair areas of full thickness skin loss, and to prevent infection, by excision of eschar and grafting. This is usually first undertaken 2–4 days after burning and can be associated with considerable blood loss.

Nutritional support

Immediately following thermal injury, the metabolic rate is reduced, but later patients become hypercatabolic with marked increases in oxygen consumption and cardiac output. In those with burns involving 60% or more BSA, the severity of this catabolic response can be reduced by nursing in a warm environment (at or above 30°C) (Wilmore et al, 1975) or by using infrared heaters controlled by the patient. Enteral nutrition via a fine-bore nasogastric tube may be adequate, but many patients will require parenteral feeding to supplement their oral intake. The risk of infection is, however, high in those receiving intravenous feeding. Early institution of oral feeding, in combination with antacid prophylaxis, may help to reduce the risk of Curling's ulcer (see Chapter 8).

Prognosis

The mortality of thermal injury is related to the depth of the burn, the percentage of BSA involved and the age of the patient. Survival rates have improved significantly over the last decade or so. For example, in 1964, 50% of patients between 10 and 30 years old with second- and third-degree burns involving 50% of their BSA would have died. Currently, mortality rates of less than 10% are being reported for such cases. Similarly, until recently the mortality rate of 70–80% burns approached 90%, whereas now survival rates of about 50% are being achieved.

FURTHER READING

Stoddart JC (1984) *Trauma and the Anaesthetist*. London: Baillière Tindall.

REFERENCES

Aikawa N, Martyn JAJ & Burke JF (1978) Pulmonary artery catheterization and thermodilution cardiac output determination in the management of critically burned patients. *American Journal of Surgery* **135:** 811–817.
Albin MS (1978) Resuscitation of the spinal cord. *Critical Care Medicine* **6:** 270–276.
Albin MS, Bunegin L, Helsel P, Babinski M & Marlin AE (1979) Intracranial pressure and cardiovascular responses to experimental cervical cord transection. *Critical Care Medicine* **7:** 127.
Alexander JW (1979) Immunological responses in the burned patient. *Journal of Trauma* **19:** 887–889.
Avery EE, Mörch ET & Benson DW (1956) Critically crushed chests: a new method of treatment with continuous mechanical hyperventilation to produce alkalotic apnea and internal pneumatic stabilization. *Journal of Thoracic Surgery* **32:** 291–311.

Baxter CR (1974) Fluid volume and electrolyte changes in the early postburn period. *Clinics in Plastic Surgery* **1**: 693–709.

Bruecke P, Burke JF, Lam K, Shannon DC & Kazemi H (1971) The pathophysiology of pulmonary fat embolism. *Journal of Thoracic and Cardiovascular Surgery* **61**: 949–955.

Calderwood HW, Modell JH & Ruiz BC (1975) The ineffectiveness of steroid therapy for treatment of fresh-water near-drowning. *Anesthesiology* **43**: 642–650.

Clark CJ, Campbell D & Reid WH (1981) Blood carboxyhaemoglobin and cyanide levels in five survivors. *Lancet* **i**: 1332–1335.

Cullen P, Modell JH, Kirby RR, Klein EF & Long W (1975) Treatment of flail chest. Use of intermittent mandatory ventilation and positive end-expiratory pressure. *Archives of Surgery* **110**: 1099–1103.

Demling RH (1985) Burns. *New England Journal of Medicine* **313**: 1389–1398.

Dittman M, Keller R & Wolff G (1978) A rationale for epidural analgesia in the treatment of multiple rib fractures. *Intensive Care Medicine* **4**: 193–197.

Dittman M, Steenblock U, Kränzlin M & Wolff G (1982) Epidural analgesia or mechanical ventilation for multiple rib fractures? *Intensive Care Medicine* **8**: 89–92.

Eckhauser FE, Billote J, Burke JF & Quinby WC (1974) Tracheostomy complicating massive burn injury. A plea for conservatism. *American Journal of Surgery* **127**: 418–423.

Editorial (1972) Fat embolism. *Lancet* **i**: 672–673.

Editorial (1977) The old in the cold. *British Medical Journal* **i**: 336.

Feller I, Tholen D & Cornell RG (1980) Improvement in burn care, 1965 to 1979. *Journal of the American Medical Association* **244**: 2074–2078.

Fischer JE, Turner RH, Herndon JH & Riseborough EJ (1971) Massive steroid therapy in severe fat embolism. *Surgery, Gynecology and Obstetrics* **132**: 667–672.

Giamonna ST & Modell JH (1967) Drowning by total immersion. Effects on pulmonary surfactant of distilled water, isotonic saline, and sea water. *American Journal of Diseases of Children* **114**: 612–616.

Golden FStC & Rivers JF (1975) The immersion incident. *Anaesthesia* **30**: 364–373.

Goodwin CW, Dorethy J, Lam V & Pruitt BA Jr (1983) Randomized trial of efficacy of crystalloid and colloid resuscitation on hemodynamic response and lung water following thermal injury. *Annals of Surgery* **197**: 520–531.

Gossling HR & Donohue TA (1979) The fat embolism syndrome. *Journal of the American Medical Association* **241**: 2740–2742.

Guenter CA & Braun TE (1981) Fat embolism syndrome. Changing prognosis. *Chest* **79**: 143–145.

Hallgren B, Kerstell J, Rudenstam CM & Svanborg A (1966) A method for the chemical analysis of pulmonary fat emboli. *Acta Chirurgica Scandinavica* **132**: 613–617.

Harari A, Regnier B, Rapin M, Lemaire F & LeGall JR (1975) Haemodynamic study of prolonged deep accidental hypothermia. *Intensive Care Medicine* **1**: 65–70.

Hardy AG (1976) Survival periods in traumatic tetraplegia. *Paraplegia* **14**: 41–46.

Harms BA, Bodai BI, Smith M et al (1981) Prostaglandin release and altered microvascular integrity after burn injury. *Journal of Surgical Research* **31**: 274–280.

Johnson PG (1978) Spinal injuries. In Hanson G (ed.) *The Medical Management of the Critically Ill*. London: Academic Press

Levine BA, Petroff PA, Slade CL & Pruitt BA Jr (1978) Prospective trials of dexamethasone and aerosolized gentamicin in the treatment of inhalation injury in the burned patient. *Journal of Trauma* **18**: 188–193.

Loke J, Paul E, Virgulto JA & Smith GJW (1984) Rabbit lung after acute smoke inhalation. *Archives of Surgery* **119**: 956–959.

MacClean D, Murison J & Griffiths PD (1973) Acute pancreatitis and diabetic ketoacidosis in accidental hypothermia and hypothermic myxoedema. *British Medical Journal* **4**: 757–761.

MacDonald RC, O'Neill D, Hanning CD & Ledingham IMcA (1981) Myocardial contusion in blunt chest trauma: a ten-year review. *Intensive Care Medicine* **7**: 265–268.

Maloney JV, Schmutzer KJ & Raschke E (1961) Paradoxical respiration and 'pendelluft'. *Journal of Thoracic and Cardiovascular Surgery* **41**: 291–298.

McNicol MW & Smith R (1964) Accidental hypothermia. *British Medical Journal* **i**: 19–21.

Modell JH, Moya F, Williams HD & Weibley TC (1968) Changes in blood gases and A-aDO2 during near-drowning. *Anesthesiology* **29**: 456–465.

Modell JH, Graves SA & Ketover A (1976) Clinical course of 91 consecutive near-drowning victims. *Chest* **70**: 231–238.

Modell JH, Graves SA & Kuck EJ (1980) Near drowning: correlation of level of consciousness and survival. *Canadian Society of Anaesthetists' Journal* **27**: 211–215.

Moore BP (1975) Operative stabilization of nonpenetrating chest injuries. *Journal of Thoracic and Cardiovascular Surgery* **70**: 619–630.

Muir I (1981) The use of the Mount Vernon Formula in the treatment of burn shock. *Intensive Care Medicine* **7**: 49–53.

Ohry A, Molho M & Rozin R (1975) Alterations of pulmonary function in spinal cord injured patients. *Paraplegia* **13**: 101–108.

Rawe SE & Perot PL (1979) Pressor response resulting from experimental contusion injury to the spinal cord. *Journal of Neurosurgery* **50**: 58–63.

Sandler AN & Tator CH (1976) Effect of acute spinal cord compression injury on regional spinal cord blood flow in primates. *Journal of Neurosurgery* **45**: 660–676.

Schonfeld SA, Ploysongsang Y, Dilisio R et al (1983) Fat embolism prophylaxis with corticosteroids: a prospective study in high-risk patients. *Annals of Internal Medicine* **99**: 433–443.

Sevitt S (1973) The significance of fat embolism. *British Journal of Hospital Medicine* **9**: 784–788.

Shackford SR, Smith DE, Zarins CK, Rice CL & Virgilio RW (1976) The management of flail chest. A comparison of ventilatory and nonventilatory treatment. *American Journal of Surgery* **132**: 759–762.

Siebke H, Breivik H, Rod T & Lind B (1975) Survival after 40 minutes' submersion without cerebral sequelae. *Lancet* **i**: 1275–1277.

Sladen A, Aldredge CF & Albarran R (1973) PEEP vs ZEEP in the treatment of flail chest injuries. *Critical Care Medicine* **1**: 187–191.

Snow JC, Kripke BJ, Sessions GP & Finc AJ (1973) Cardiovascular collapse following succinylcholine in a paraplegic patient. *Paraplegia* **11**: 199–204.

Torres-Mirabel P, Gruenberg JC, Talbert JG & Brown RS (1982) Ventricular function in myocardial contusion: a preliminary study. *Critical Care Medicine* **10**: 19–24.

Tranbaugh, RF, Elings VB, Christensen JM & Lewis FR (1983) Effect of inhalation injury on lung water accumulation. *Journal of Trauma* **23**: 597–604.

Trinkle JK, Richardson JD, Franz JL et al (1975) Management of flail chest without mechanical ventilation. *Annals of Thoracic Surgery* **19**: 355–363.

Troll GF & Dohrmann GJ (1975) Anaesthesia of the spinal cord injured patient: cardiovascular problems and their management. *Paraplegia* **13**: 162–171.

Webb AK (1978) Flail chest: management and complications. *British Journal of Hospital Medicine* **20**: 406–412.

Welply NC, Mathias CJ & Frankel HL (1975) Circulatory reflexes in tetraplegics during artificial ventilation and general anaesthesia. *Paraplegia* **13**: 172–182.

Weyman AE, Greenbaum DM & Grace WJ (1974) Accidental hypothermia in an alcoholic population. *American Journal of Medicine* **56**: 13–21.

Wilmore DW, Mason AD Jr, Johnson DW & Pruitt BA Jr (1975) Effect of ambient temperature on heat production and heat loss in burn patients. *Journal of Applied Physiology* **38**: 593–597.

Wynne JW, Reynolds JC, Hood CI, Auerbach D & Ondrasick J (1979) Steroid therapy for pneumonitis induced in rabbits by aspiration of foodstuff. *Anesthesiology* **51**: 11–19.

12
Respiratory Failure

DEFINITION

Respiratory failure occurs when pulmonary gas exchange is sufficiently impaired to cause hypoxaemia with or without hypercarbia.

TYPES AND MECHANISMS OF RESPIRATORY FAILURE

Acute hypoxaemic (Type I) respiratory failure (ARF)

This is caused by diseases which interfere with gas exchange by damaging lung tissue. In this situation, hypoxaemia is due to right-to-left shunts, ventilation/perfusion (V/Q) mismatch or, most often, a combination of these two. As discussed in Chapter 2, barriers to diffusion are almost never an important cause of hypoxaemia. An increase in right-to-left shunt occurs when alveoli are completely collapsed, become totally consolidated or are filled with oedema fluid. V/Q inequalities result from pulmonary parenchymal disease which causes regional variations in compliance, an increased scatter of time constants (see Chapter 2) and/or abnormalities of perfusion. Furthermore, functional residual capacity (FRC) is reduced so that tidal exchange takes place below closing volume (i.e. airway closure occurs throughout the respiratory cycle), and this is associated with an increase in the number of relatively underventilated lung units.

Initially, there is usually an increase in total ventilation which compensates for the increased dead space and maintains $P_a co_2$ at normal levels. Indeed, relative hyperventilation, possibly in response to severe hypoxaemia and/or stimulation of 'J' receptors within the lungs, may cause a reduction in $P_a co_2$. The degree of hypoxaemia is limited by constriction of vessels supplying those alveoli with a low Po_2—'hypoxic pulmonary vasoconstriction'—although the intensity of this response is very variable and appears to be genetically determined.

As well as the impairment of gas exchanging properties, the lungs deteriorate mechanically with a reduction in compliance (associated with the fall in FRC—see Chapter 2) and/or an increase in resistance so that the work and oxygen cost of breathing is increased. Under these circumstances, patients find it easier to breathe rapidly with low tidal volumes. Finally, these patients are often pyrexial, with a raised metabolic rate, and this further increases both oxygen consumption and the volume of carbon dioxide which has to be excreted. Thus, patients with ARF are classically hypoxic, hypocarbic and tachypnoeic, with small tidal volumes. In contrast to the normal pattern of ventilation, there is little moment-to-moment variation in either respiratory rate or tidal volume.

198

Ventilatory (Type II) respiratory failure

Ventilatory failure occurs when alveolar ventilation is insufficient to excrete the volume of carbon dioxide being produced by tissue metabolism. Carbon dioxide is therefore retained, producing an increase in both arterial and alveolar P_{CO_2}. Due to the operation of the alveolar gas equation (see Chapter 2), this inevitably leads to a fall in alveolar oxygen tension and hypoxaemia, even in a patient with normal lungs. Inadequate alveolar ventilation may be due to reduced ventilatory effort, inability to overcome an increased resistance to ventilation, failure to compensate for an increase in dead space and/or carbon dioxide production, or a combination of these factors. The respiratory muscles have a large reserve, however, and considerable impairment of function may be present without ventilatory failure. Patients with pure ventilatory failure are, therefore, hypercarbic and hypoxic, usually with a reduced rate and/or depth of breathing. They may suffer from an extremely distressing sensation of breathlessness, even when ventilation (judged, for example, by blood gas values) is apparently adequate.

Mixed respiratory failure

Often, the two types of respiratory failure are combined to produce a mixed picture. As discussed above, acute diseases of the pulmonary parenchyma initially cause purely hypoxaemic respiratory failure. In some cases, however, exhaustion eventually supervenes; the patient is then unable to overcome the mechanical impairment of lung function and cannot compensate for the increased dead space and carbon dioxide production. At this stage, the arterial carbon dioxide tension begins to rise and mixed respiratory failure develops.

Ventilatory failure is often complicated by the subsequent development of pulmonary abnormalities. This is because these patients are unable to cough adequately, sigh or take deep breaths and are therefore at risk of alveolar collapse, retention of secretions and secondary infection. Moreover, in those with an associated bulbar palsy, aspiration can occur and further damage the lungs.

CAUSES OF RESPIRATORY FAILURE

Respiratory failure is commonly precipitated by surgical operations (particularly upper abdominal or thoracic), acute respiratory tract infections and the administration of depressant drugs. The causes of respiratory failure can best be considered according to anatomical location (Fig. 12.1).

Respiratory centre

Causes of depression of the respiratory centre commonly seen in the intensive care unit include raised intracranial pressure or direct trauma (e.g. head injury), infections (e.g. meningo-encephalitis), vascular lesions and drug overdose (e.g. narcotics, barbiturates). Patients in traumatic coma with intracranial hypertension may also have associated pulmonary oedema, lung

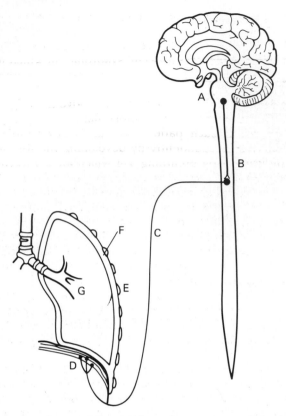

Fig. 12.1 Causes of respiratory failure. (A) respiratory centre; (B) spinal cord; (C) motor nerves; (D) neuromuscular junction; (E) chest wall; (F) pleura; (G) lungs and airways. Pulmonary circulation.

contusion or aspiration pneumonia. Frequently, the laryngeal reflexes are also depressed and in some cases there may be a true bulbar palsy. Both predispose the patient to aspiration pneumonitis. Severe hypoxia and extreme hypercarbia can also reduce the responsiveness of the respiratory centre.

Spinal cord

Very rarely, lesions of the high cervical cord, or brain stem, may interrupt the pathways involved in automatic breathing whilst leaving the conscious pathways intact. Because these unfortunate patients therefore have to remember to breathe, long periods of apnoea occur, even when the subject is awake, and serious CO_2 retention occurs when they fall asleep. The hypercarbia increases cerebral blood flow, causing headaches, nightmares and disturbed sleep patterns. This condition has been called 'Ondine's curse', after a water nymph who, according to German mythology, cursed her husband by abolishing all his automatic functions. When he finally became exhausted and fell asleep, he died.

A similar situation exists with other causes of this 'primary alveolar hypoventilation' in that barely adequate ventilation is maintained by conscious effort but serious CO_2 retention occurs when the patient falls asleep. An example is the 'Pickwickian' syndrome, in which hypoventilation occurs in very obese, somnolent men who are said to resemble the fat boy, Joe, in 'The Pickwick Papers'.

Traumatic damage to the spinal cord at or above the origin of the phrenic nerve (C3, 4, 5) causes severe ventilatory failure since only the accessory muscles are spared. If such patients are artificially ventilated, they may subsequently survive independently by developing the use of the accessory muscles and by using 'frog breathing' (in which air is forced into the lungs using a muscular effort similar to swallowing). Lesions below this level cause less respiratory impairment since diaphragmatic breathing remains intact.

Poliomyelitis has its major impact on the anterior horn cells in the spinal cord and/or the motor nuclei of the cranial nerves, and, in some cases, the respiratory centre itself is damaged. Thus, the patient may suffer from bulbar paralysis, in which case airway protection is vital, or spinal polio, which may cause weakness of the respiratory muscles and ventilatory failure. Sometimes both bulbar and spinal motor nuclei are affected.

If the spasms of tetanus are prolonged and severe, they may interfere with ventilation, but in any case treatment of the most severe cases consists of heavy sedation, paralysis and artificial ventilation (see Chapter 14). There is also some evidence that tetanus causes respiratory depression by a direct effect on the brain stem.

Motor neurone disease is a progressive disorder affecting the cerebral cortex, brain stem and spinal cord and is manifested as muscular atrophy with spasticity and hyperreflexia. It is a disease of middle age which progresses inexorably, and relatively rapidly (2–5 years), until death supervenes from respiratory failure, often associated with aspiration pneumonia. There is no known treatment and mechanical ventilation is inappropriate.

Motor nerves

In Guillain–Barré syndrome, lower motor neurone weakness develops a few days, or even weeks, after a 'flu-like' illness. This initially involves the lower limbs but may later spread to the muscles of the face and trunk. A significant proportion of patients with this syndrome will then develop ventilatory failure and require artificial ventilation (see Chapter 13).

Neuromuscular junction

Although myasthenia gravis may affect any voluntary muscle, ventilatory failure is unusual except during acute exacerbations ('myasthenic crisis'), overdosage with anticholinesterases ('cholinergic crisis') or postoperatively (often following thymectomy) (see Chapter 14).

Botulism is an extremely rare form of food poisoning in which botulinus toxin prevents release of acetylcholine from motor nerve endings, causing flaccid paralysis and ventilatory failure.

Organophosphorus compounds have been developed as chemical weapons and are used as insecticides. They are long-acting anticholinesterases and produce respiratory depression, bronchospasm, salivation, bradycardia, hypertension and convulsions (see Chapter 17).

Failure to reverse the effects of neuromuscular blocking agents used during anaesthesia is a not infrequent cause of admission to intensive care units for artificial ventilation.

Chest wall

If a segment of chest wall becomes unstable due, for example, to multiple rib fractures, particularly when associated with lung contusion, it may be impossible to sustain adequate ventilation (see Chapter 11). Similarly, if the thorax is deformed (e.g. kyphoscoliosis), lung expansion will be impaired. These patients may eventually develop ventilatory failure and are prone to recurrent chest infections. On the other hand, ventilatory failure is unusual when chest movement is restricted but the thorax is uniform (e.g. ankylosing spondylitis). Rarely, patients with myopathies or myositis may develop respiratory failure. Artificial ventilation may be required and can allow time for the diagnosis to be established, for example by muscle biopsy.

Pleura

Pneumothorax, haemothorax, pleural effusion and empyema may all cause, or exacerbate, respiratory failure.

Lungs and airways

As discussed above, diseases affecting primarily the lungs and airways initially cause hypoxaemic respiratory failure but may later progress to the mixed type. Causes of ARF include pneumonia, asthma, left ventricular failure and ARDS (see below). Examples of chronic type I respiratory failure include emphysema and fibrosing lung disease. The commonest cause of mixed respiratory failure is COAD. Upper airway obstruction is usually well tolerated initially but can rapidly progress to frank respiratory failure.

Pulmonary circulation

As well as mechanically obstructing the circulation, acute pulmonary embolism can cause V/Q inequalities, possibly via reflex mechanisms, with hypoxaemia and tachypnoea. Recurrent pulmonary emboli eventually produce chronic pulmonary hypertension and respiratory failure.

PRINCIPLES OF MANAGEMENT

Clearly, the specific treatment of respiratory failure will vary according to the underlying cause, but the same general principles apply in all cases.

Oxygen therapy

Oxygen toxicity (Deneke and Fanburg, 1982)

Since all patients with respiratory failure are hypoxaemic, the administration of oxygen is fundamental. However, although oxygen is present in the air we breathe, and is essential to life, the possibility that prolonged administration of high concentrations of this gas may have toxic effects has been recognized for many years. As long ago as 1775, Joseph Priestley introduced the concept of oxygen toxicity and a century later hyperbaric oxygen was shown to cause convulsions in birds. In 1899, Lorrain-Smith demonstrated that mice and other small animals developed pulmonary complications when exposed to high partial pressures of oxygen. It was not until the 1920s, however, that the therapeutic use of oxygen became common practice and the possibility of oxygen toxicity began to concern clinicians. Even now, the relevance of oxygen-induced lung damage in clinical practice remains controversial.

Experimental work (Kapanci et al, 1969) has shown that mammalian lungs continuously exposed to high concentrations of oxygen develop pulmonary capillary endothelial cell swelling with the formation of interstitial oedema and hyaline membranes. Type I alveolar lining cells are also injured during this early phase of oxygen-induced lung damage. Later, this 'exudative phase' progresses to a 'proliferative phase' with hyperplasia of type II alveolar lining cells (granular pneumocytes), septal thickening, capillary hyperplasia and infiltration with fibroblasts. There may also be damage to the bronchial epithelium and interference with ciliary activity. Survival time can be significantly prolonged if exposure is intermittent or if 100% oxygen is administered at a pressure of about 27 kPa (200 mmHg) (Wright et al, 1966). Neither the presence or absence of nitrogen from the respired gases (Wright et al, 1966) nor artificial ventilation appear to be important factors in the development of pulmonary oxygen toxicity in animals (deLemos et al, 1969). If the animal recovers, the lungs show focal scarring and septal fibrosis with dilatation and proliferation of pulmonary capillaries.

The evidence that high concentrations of oxygen cause lung damage in humans is less conclusive. Nevertheless, volunteers exposed to high concentrations of oxygen for more than 24 hours develop substernal pain with a reduction in vital capacity and pulmonary diffusing capacity (Comroe et al, 1945; Caldwell et al, 1966). Small changes in pressure–volume curves have also been noted in those breathing 100% oxygen for only three hours, but these were not seen when nitrogen was added to the respired gas, nor when atelectasis was prevented during an 11-hour exposure to oxygen at 202 kPa (Burger and Mead, 1969).

It is more difficult to prove that oxygen damages the lungs of patients who receive high concentrations in order to correct hypoxaemia. Such patients obviously already have underlying lung disease, the histological appearances of which are often non-specific. Moreover, there are no pathognomonic chest x-ray or pathological appearances of oxygen-induced lung damage (Winter and Smith, 1972). Finally, there are obvious difficulties in devising a study with a suitable control group. Despite these problems, two prospective, controlled studies have been performed. In one (Singer et al, 1970), post cardiac surgery patients were ventilated with either 100% oxygen or less than

50% oxygen for approximately 24 hours. There were no differences in intrapulmonary shunt, effective compliance, V_D/V_T ratio, or clinical course between the two groups. The other study (Barber et al, 1970), performed in patients with irreversible brain damage, showed that after 30–40 hours, arterial P_{O_2} was lower while intrapulmonary shunt and the V_D/V_T ratio were greater in those ventilated with 100% oxygen than in the control group. Radiographic appearances and measurement of total lung weight supported these findings, although there were no noteworthy histological differences between the two groups. These investigations suggest that 100% oxygen can cause some deterioration in lung function but only if administered for more than 24 hours. Whether this deterioration is associated with characteristic histological changes is not known, although in a retrospective study it was claimed that the early exudative and late proliferative phases could be distinguished and that these correlated with prolonged administration of high concentrations of oxygen (Nash et al, 1967). However, the changes described were non-specific and similar to those seen in ARDS (see below).

The mechanisms by which oxygen damages the lungs are unclear. However, it is possible that high concentrations of oxygen in the lung lead to the formation of free radicals of oxygen which can cause direct cellular damage (Deneke and Fanburg, 1982). Interestingly, this is also one of the postulated mechanisms of the lung lesion in ARDS and in both instances production of oxygen radicals by activated polymorphonuclear leukocytes may be important. Furthermore, high inspired concentrations of oxygen will displace nitrogen from the lungs, creating a huge partial pressure gradient between alveolus and pulmonary capillary. Virtually all the oxygen will then be absorbed and it is suggested that this can cause 'absorption collapse' of underventilated lung units. The contribution of reduced surfactant production to atelectasis in this situation is uncertain. Such progressive collapse may be minimized in ventilated subjects by the use of large tidal volumes and a PEEP or by the application of CPAP in those breathing spontaneously (see Chapter 13). Finally, inadequate humidification of oxygen will exacerbate pulmonary problems by drying both the bronchial mucosa, which impairs the muco-ciliary transport mechanism, and the secretions.

Other adverse effects of administering high concentrations of oxygen include retrolental fibroplasia and bronchopulmonary dysplasia in neonates, whilst hyperbaric oxygen can precipitate convulsions.

Although it is clear that retrolental fibroplasia is caused by excessively high partial pressures of oxygen in arterial blood, it is not certain whether lung damage is related to the alveolar or arterial partial pressure of oxygen. It is worth noting, however, that it is the normal areas of lung which are exposed to the highest partial pressures of oxygen and therefore it is these areas which may be most damaged by the use of high inspired oxygen concentrations.

In conclusion, it seems reasonable to assume that prolonged administration of oxygen can damage the lungs and the clinician should therefore use the lowest $F_{I}O_2$ compatible with adequate arterial oxygenation. Conventionally, the aim is to achieve more than 90% saturation of haemoglobin with oxygen, although in a few cases lower levels may be accepted in order to avoid using potentially toxic concentrations of oxygen. It must be remembered, however, that the patient is then operating on the steep portion of the oxyhaemoglobin dissociation curve where small falls in P_aO_2 will cause significant reductions in oxygen content. Although there is only limited information on safe levels for oxygen therapy, long-term administration of an $F_IO_2 < 0.5$, or of 100% oxygen for less than 24 hours, is traditionally considered to be acceptable. Nevertheless, dangerous hypoxia should never be tolerated through a fear of oxygen toxicity.

Indications for oxygen therapy

In patients with pure ventilatory failure, the primary abnormality is retention of carbon dioxide; specific treatment is therefore directed towards lowering arterial and alveolar carbon dioxide tension. However, the administration of oxygen remains a useful first step when managing these patients since it effectively reverses the hypoxia which is the inevitable consequence of the elevated alveolar carbon dioxide tension. Oxygen therapy is always indicated in patients with acute hypoxaemic or mixed respiratory failure, although for reasons discussed previously it is most effective when the main abnormality is ventilation/perfusion mismatch and is of less value in the presence of a fixed right-to-left shunt (see Chapter 2). Patients poisoned with carbon monoxide will also benefit from oxygen administration. By increasing the arterial oxygen tension, the dissociation of carboxyhaemoglobin is accelerated and the increase in dissolved oxygen improves tissue oxygenation.

Methods of oxygen administration

In patients being artificially ventilated, the inspired oxygen concentration is easily measured (see Chapter 4) and can be maintained at the desired level by mixing air and oxygen in appropriate proportions. This also applies to spontaneously breathing patients with endotracheal tubes, or a tracheostomy, connected either to a T-piece or a CPAP circuit (see Chapter 13).

In the non-intubated, spontaneously breathing subject, measuring the F_IO_2 is not usually a practical proposition. Fortunately, in the majority of patients, the concentration of oxygen delivered is not crucial and a 'variable performance' device, such as a simple face mask or nasal cannulae (Fig. 12.2a and b) will suffice. With these devices, the patient entrains a variable amount of air to supplement the flow of oxygen during inspiration and it is not possible to predict with any degree of accuracy the concentration of oxygen being delivered to the patient's lungs. Furthermore, the F_IO_2 varies during the respiratory cycle and is dependent on the oxygen flow rate as well as the patient's tidal volume and respiratory rate (Goldstein et al, 1982). Since the peak inspiratory flow rate may be as much as $30 \, l \, min^{-1}$ at this point in the respiratory cycle, considerable entrainment of air will occur. On the other hand, if the patient hypoventilates, the F_IO_2 will rise. With these devices, the F_IO_2 probably varies from about 35% to 55% with oxygen flows of between 6 and $10 \, l \, min^{-1}$ (Labrousse et al, 1983).

Nasal cannulae are often preferred to face masks because they are less claustrophobic and do not interfere with sleep, feeding or speaking. However, they may cause ulceration of the nasal or pharyngeal mucosa and in some cases are associated with abdominal distension caused by the patient swallowing oxygen. Although flow rates of between 0.5 and $15 \, l \, min^{-1}$ of

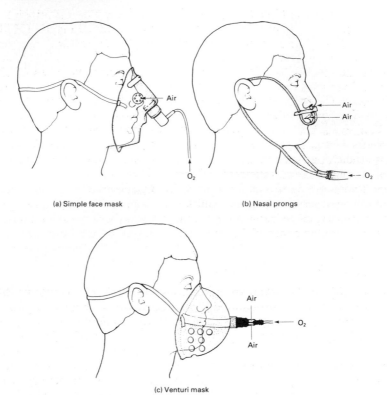

(a) Simple face mask

(b) Nasal prongs

(c) Venturi mask

Fig. 12.2 Methods of administering supplemental oxygen to an unintubated patient:
(a) simple face mask ⎫
(b) nasal cannulae   ⎬ variable performance
⎭
(c) Venturi mask } fixed performance

oxygen can be used through nasal cannulae, high flow rates (more than $2-4 l min^{-1}$) are very uncomfortable and it may be preferable to use them in combination with a face mask. In this way, it is possible to achieve a high F_IO_2 without subjecting the mucosa to such high flows of oxygen. This system has the added advantage that if the face mask is removed, for example, to perform mouth care, the patient continues to receive some supplemental oxygen.

If more accurate administration of oxygen is required, a 'fixed performance' device should be used. There are three ways of delivering a known, constant F_IO_2. Firstly, a gas mixture of the required oxygen concentration can be delivered to the patient via a tight-fitting face mask and a circuit containing a reservoir bag and a one-way valve. The reservoir bag partially collapses during inspiration and supplements the fresh gas flow; during expiration, the bag is refilled. Because there is no entrainment of air, the F_IO_2 is known and remains constant throughout the respiratory cycle. As with the use of tight-fitting face masks for the application of CPAP, these are generally poorly tolerated and can produce pressure necrosis of the facial skin.

The second method involves the application of the Venturi principle (Fig. 12.2c), producing 'high air flow with oxygen enrichment' (HAFOE) (Campbell, 1960a). If oxygen is delivered through an injector at a given flow rate, a fixed amount of air will be entrained and the F_IO_2 can be accurately predicted. Relatively low flows of oxygen entrain large volumes of air and this, combined with the large volume of the mask, ensures that the patient's requirements for fresh gas are satisfied even at peak inspiration. Masks are available which will deliver 24%, 28%, 34% and 60% oxygen. For example, a 24% Ventimask uses an oxygen flow rate of only $2\,l\,min^{-1}$ but produces a total fresh gas flow of $50\,l\,min^{-1}$ downstream of the injector. The design of the mask is crucial, particularly with regard to its volume, and some commercially available devices are unsatisfactory (Campbell, 1982).

Finally, oxygen tents can be used as fixed-performance devices and have proved to be particularly useful in children. They require a high fresh gas flow with a preset F_IO_2. Rebreathing is prevented by allowing gas to escape around the lower, unsealed edges of the tent.

Physiological effects of oxygen therapy

In normal subjects, breathing oxygen causes a reduction in minute ventilation of approximately 10%, probably due to a decrease in chemoreceptor drive. The consequent rise in P_aco_2 is exacerbated by a reduction in the buffering capacity of oxygenated haemoglobin. A redistribution of pulmonary blood flow may occur, causing a rise in V_D/V_T, and absorption collapse (see above) can increase venous admixture. In some cases, reversal of hypoxic pulmonary vasoconstriction may be associated with a fall in pulmonary vascular resistance, while cardiac output may decrease in association with a rise in peripheral resistance. Occasionally, administration of oxygen to those with ARF leads to a transient deterioration in conscious level. This is thought to be due to an acute reduction in cerebral blood flow as reversal of hypoxia leaves the cerebral vasoconstrictor effect of the hypocarbia unopposed.

Monitoring the effects of oxygen therapy

Some clinical improvement may be obvious following the administration of oxygen, e.g. reversal of cyanosis, slowing of the respiratory rate and a reduction in respiratory distress. However, arterial blood gas analysis is essential for proper assessment of the effects of treatment and ideally a baseline sample should first be obtained with the patient breathing air. In most cases, the aim is to achieve a P_aO_2 within normal limits. It is pointless to administer oxygen in concentrations which produce a higher than normal P_aO_2 since, because of the shape of the dissociation curve, oxygen content is not significantly increased. If potentially toxic concentrations of oxygen are required to achieve a normal P_aO_2, lower values may be accepted provided that oxygen content, and by implication oxygen delivery, remains acceptable. In particular, more than 90% saturation of haemoglobin with oxygen is usually considered adequate and this may be achieved at arterial oxygen tensions as low as 8 kPa (60 mmHg). The ultimate goal of oxygen therapy is to ensure adequate tissue oxygenation. Compensatory mechanisms such as polycythaemia, a shift of the dissociation curve, an increase in cardiac output and a redistribution of blood flow may preserve cellular oxygen delivery despite severe arterial hypoxaemia. Clinical assessment of cellular oxygenation is difficult, although a reduction in $P_{\bar{v}}O_2$ or mixed venous oxygen saturation is thought to be a reasonable indication that tissue oxygenation is impaired (see Chapter 2). Other indices such as the development of an acidosis or the lactate/pyruvate ratio are too insensitive to be of value in assessing oxygen therapy. It is also worth re-emphasizing here that when P_{O_2} is low, the patient is operating on the steep part of the oxyhaemoglobin dissociation curve and small increases in P_{O_2} will produce clinically useful improvements in oxygen content. This fact is utilized when administering oxygen to patients who are dependent on a hypoxic drive to respiration in whom too great an increase in P_aO_2 may cause dangerous carbon dioxide retention.

Control of secretions

Many patients with respiratory failure produce large volumes of bronchial secretions and these are often infected. In order to prevent sputum retention, with its attendant dangers of pulmonary collapse and perpetuation of infection, these secretions must be cleared.

Hydration

Patients with severe respiratory failure are often unable to eat or drink and lose large quantities of fluid due to pyrexia, hyperventilation and the excessive work of breathing. Dehydration is therefore frequent, and this may make secretions more tenacious. This can be avoided by humidifying the inspired gases and, more importantly, by achieving adequate systemic hydration with intravenous crystalloid solutions. On the other hand, lung water is frequently increased in patients with respiratory failure, particularly in ARDS and in those receiving artificial ventilation. Under these circumstances, fluid restriction and the use of diuretics may be appropriate.

Mucolytic agents

A number of mucolytic agents have been developed which can reduce sputum viscosity in vitro. For example, various cysteine analogues have been described which reduce the number of cross-linking disulphide bridges of polymeric mucus glycoproteins to produce less viscid thiomonomers. There is, however, no good clinical evidence that these agents are of benefit.

Chest physiotherapy

This usually involves manual hyperinflation, chest compression and endotracheal suction in an attempt to mobilize secretions and expand collapsed lung segments. Chest physiotherapy can, however, be dangerous in hypoxic patients, particularly during endotracheal suction; not only is the oxygen source removed, but oxygen rich gases are aspirated from the lungs and cardiac output can fall. Furthermore, PEEP has to be discontinued. This is associated with an immediate increase in shunt which can take up to an hour to recover following reapplication of PEEP (see Chapter 13). Significant hypoxaemia has been demonstrated during chest physiotherapy in patients maintained on IPPV, particularly those with cardiac pathology, and these authors emphasized the importance of speed when performing endotracheal suction (Gormezano and Branthwaite, 1972). Physiotherapy is probably of no value in those with uncomplicated pulmonary oedema (cardiogenic or associated with ARDS) since fluid simply reaccumulates. These patients are often extremely hypoxic and require PEEP so that physiotherapy is usually best avoided. Later, when secondary infection supervenes, physiotherapy may be reinstituted.

Respiratory stimulants

These may occasionally be used to arouse drowsy patients and to stimulate them to breathe deeply, cough and co-operate with physiotherapy (see below).

Intubation/tracheostomy/bronchoscopy

In some cases, often in an exhausted, confused and uncooperative bronchitic, physiotherapy fails to clear secretions and the patient continues to deteriorate. In the past, a rigid bronchoscopy was sometimes performed to aspirate secretions, but nowadays it is more usual to intubate the patient and perform endobronchial suction via the endotracheal tube. Some of the benefit of this procedure may be due to the fact that it is a strong stimulus to the patient to cough. Clear-cut areas of collapse seen on the chest x-ray, which fail to respond to physiotherapy, may occasionally re-expand if the offending secretions are removed using a fibre-optic bronchoscope. A 'mini tracheostomy', which involves insertion of a small-diameter tube into the trachea through the cricothyroid membrane, provides a route for effective endotracheal suction. This technique is gaining popularity as a means of clearing secretions in those who are unable to cough effectively, and in some cases the need for artificial ventilation can be averted.

Control of infection (see Chapter 6)

When respiratory failure has been precipitated by pulmonary infection, except when this is due to a virus, appropriate antibiotic therapy should be commenced. Ideally, the causative organism should be isolated, and its sensitivity to various antibiotics tested, before treatment is started; in practice, this is often not possible. Many patients have been receiving one or more antibiotics prior to admission to the intensive care unit and in the remainder it is not usually practicable to await the results of bacteriological investigations before starting treatment. The identification of the rarer causes of pneumonia, such as *Mycoplasma*, legionnaires' disease and *Pneumocystis carinii*, can be difficult and time-consuming. It is, however, important to obtain a sputum sample and blood culture prior to initiating or changing antibiotic therapy. A Gram stain of this sputum may give a valuable clue to the aetiology of the pneumonia; later, the results of culture and sensitivities may lead to appropriate modification of the antibiotic regimen. Isolation of an organism from both sputum and blood strongly suggests that this is the pathogen. In the absence of bacteriological information, a reasonable antibiotic regimen should be selected on the basis of the most likely infecting organisms.

Control of bronchospasm

In asthma, reversal of bronchospasm is clearly fundamental but patients with COAD may also have an element of reversible bronchospasm.

β-Stimulants

In the past, isoprenaline was used extensively as a bronchodilator. However, this agent is a non-selective β-stimulant and its use was often complicated by the development of tachycardia and/or dysrhythmias. Selective β_2 agonists, such as salbutamol and terbutaline, are now therefore preferred, although even these can produce β_1 effects in high doses. β-Stimulants can be given orally but are more effective when administered as a nebulized aerosol, e.g. by using a patient-triggered ventilator such as the 'Bird' or by including a nebulizer in the inspiratory limb of the ventilator circuit in those receiving IPPV. Those with severe airway obstruction, however, often fail to respond to inhaled bronchodilators; a continuous intravenous infusion should then be used (Williams and Seaton, 1977). Adrenaline, given intramuscularly, subcutaneously or intravenously, may be effective when other agents have failed.

Theophylline derivatives

The phosphodiesterase inhibitors increase intracellular levels of cyclic AMP but there is some doubt as to whether this mediates their bronchodilator effect. In the UK, aminophylline is the most commonly used member of this group of drugs and can be given intravenously, orally or as a suppository. This agent has a low therapeutic ratio and the dose has to be carefully controlled in order to avoid severe side effects such as tachycardia, dysrhythmias, sweating, tremor, nausea, vomiting, insomnia and seizures. Aminophylline can also exacerbate V/Q mismatch, possibly by reversing hypoxic pulmonary vasoconstriction. Therefore, some recommend measurement of plasma levels (Kordash et al, 1977), which is technically difficult, or the use of nomograms in order to control the dose. The therapeutic range lies between 10 and $20\,\mu g\,ml^{-1}$. Because it may prove difficult to find the optimal dose for an individual patient, aminophylline is usually only used in those unresponsive to other agents.

Steroids

Intravenous steroids (e.g. hydrocortisone 200 mg six-hourly) are often used in combination with β-stimulants or phosphodiesterase inhibitors to relieve severe bronchospasm. Their mechanism of action in this situation is, however, uncertain. As well as their ability to suppress delayed hypersensitivity reactions and the inflammatory response, steroids can increase cyclic AMP levels and restore the responsiveness of the bronchial tree to catecholamines (Shenfield et al, 1975). However, the onset of these effects is slow (3–6 h; maximal effect in 6–8 h) and such large doses of steroids might be deleterious in the presence of infection. In less urgent cases, and in those who are able to take medication by mouth, oral administration of steroids may be preferred. β-Stimulants, steroids and aminophylline can all increase urinary potassium losses.

Volatile anaesthetic agents

Both halothane and ether have bronchodilator properties and may be useful in the occasional patient when conventional treatment has failed (Robertson et al, 1985). Ether is, however, explosive in the presence of oxygen and can damage some ventilators.

Control of lung water

In many patients with respiratory failure, pulmonary capillary permeability is increased and there is an element of pulmonary oedema. This classically occurs in 'shock lung', fat embolism, acid aspiration and other causes of ARDS; it is a less prominent feature of pneumonia. As discussed in Chapter 2, lung water may be further increased if plasma protein levels fall and/or LAP rises. The tendency to develop 'wet lungs' may also be exacerbated by the use of positive pressure ventilation, with or without PEEP, possibly in part because of interference with lymphatic drainage (see Chapter 13). In order to minimize this increase in lung water, some restriction of intravenous fluid therapy is often required, sometimes combined with the administration of a diuretic. Serum proteins, and particularly albumin, should if possible be maintained within normal limits. However, this is often difficult to achieve, even with frequent administration of concentrated albumin solutions and an aggressive approach to nutritional support. This is partly because these patients are often extremely catabolic, but may also be due to persistent leakage of plasma proteins into the interstitial spaces. Similar considerations apply to the controversy surrounding the relative merits of colloids or crystalloids for volume replacement in patients at risk of developing ARDS, or in whom the condition is established (see Chapter 10). Finally, LAP (usually inferred from measurement of PCWP) should be manipulated to produce the optimal cardiac output and oxygen flux without contributing a hydrostatic element to the pulmonary oedema. In general, this means that PCWP should be maintained between 10 and 15 mmHg (1.3 and 2 kPa). Some authorities attempt to take account of oncotic effects and suggest that when the colloid osmotic pressure/pulmonary artery wedge pressure gradient falls to below 7 mmHg (0.9 kPa) there is an increased risk of pulmonary oedema (Puri et al, 1980).

Artificial ventilation (see Chapter 13)

If the patient continues to deteriorate, or fails to respond to the measures outlined above, then artificial ventilation should be considered.

Indications for instituting artificial ventilation

These vary according to the underlying disease process (see below). In hypoxaemic and mixed respiratory failure, the decision is made largely on clinical grounds, aided by blood gas analysis and sometimes simple bedside tests of respiratory function. If the clinical signs of severe respiratory distress (e.g. tachypnoea $> 40\,min^{-1}$, inability to speak, sweating) persist despite maximal treatment and the patient appears exhausted, particularly if this is associated with confusion, restlessness and agitation, artificial ventilation is usually required. Worsening blood gases may confirm that the situation is deteriorating, a rising $P_a co_2$ and/or extreme hypoxaemia ($P_a o_2 < 8\,kPa$) despite oxygen therapy being particularly significant in relation to the need for artificial ventilation. By this stage, bedside tests of respiratory function are rarely helpful.

In contrast, the decision to institute artificial ventilation in patients with ventilatory failure is influenced more by the results of blood gas analysis and bedside tests of respiratory function, in particular the vital capacity, than by clinical assessment. Normally, artificial ventilation should be instituted in a patient with ventilatory failure when the vital capacity has fallen to less than $10–15\,ml\,kg^{-1}$, since this may reduce the incidence of complications such as atelectasis and infection as well as preventing unexpected respiratory arrest. Tidal volume and respiratory rate, on the other hand, are relatively insensitive indicators of the need for artificial ventilation in ventilatory failure because they change only late in the course of the disease. A high $P_a co_2$, particularly if it is rising, is generally an indication for urgent artificial ventilation in these patients.

Treatment as outlined above, particularly the control of lung water, must continue once IPPV has been instituted. Additional measures which may be useful include reduction of oxygen requirements, for example, by heavy sedation, paralysis and cooling, together with maintenance of an adequate cardiac output and haemoglobin level, the ultimate goal being to improve the tissue oxygen supply/demand ratio and prevent organ damage.

Positive end-expiratory pressure (see Chapter 13)

If, despite these measures, it proves impossible to achieve adequate oxygenation of arterial blood without raising the inspired oxygen concentration to potentially dangerous levels (see above), the application of a PEEP should be considered.

Continuous positive airways pressure (see Chapter 13)

Patients with ARF, who are not exhausted and/or hypoventilating, may be allowed to continue to breathe spontaneously whilst a positive pressure is applied to the airway via an endotracheal tube. In those patients in whom retention of secretions is not a problem, CPAP may be applied using a tight-fitting face mask. This technique may become more widely used in the future as a means of avoiding artificial ventilation.

Respiratory failure must not be considered in isolation. Not only do hypoxia and hypercarbia affect the cardiovascular system, but a fall in cardiac output will cause a reduction in $P_{\bar{v}}O_2$ and exacerbate the adverse effects of a given degree of shunt on arterial oxygenation. Many drugs active on the cardiovascular system, such as dopamine and sodium nitroprusside, have been shown to increase venous admixture, probably by reversing hypoxic pulmonary vasoconstriction (see Chapter 10). Myocardial failure often causes pulmonary congestion with increased shunting, and hypotension may lead to an increased dead space, particularly during IPPV. Finally, the increased work and oxygen cost of breathing increases the workload on the myocardium, which may already be compromised.

SOME CAUSES OF RESPIRATORY FAILURE COMMONLY ENCOUNTERED IN THE INTENSIVE CARE UNIT

Postoperative respiratory failure

Surgery and anaesthesia produce alveolar collapse with reductions in FRC, vital capacity and compliance associated with premature airway closure, impaired ability to cough and muscle splinting. Hypoxaemia is invariably present postoperatively and, when this persists for more than a few hours, is probably caused by the reduction in FRC (see Chapter 2). These abnormalities of lung function are particularly severe following upper abdominal surgery (Hewlett and Branthwaite, 1975). There is also depression of macrophage function and ciliary activity, whilst the lower respiratory tract may become colonized with bacteria. It is not surprising that in susceptible patients these changes are often associated with retention of secretions, atelectasis and superimposed infection (either exacerbation of pre-existing bronchitis or secondary pneumonia) or that in some cases they precipitate respiratory failure.

Such postoperative pulmonary complications are much more common in patients with pre-existing respiratory disease, particularly those in whom preoperative assessment of lung function demonstrates significant reductions in maximum breathing capacity and expiratory flow rates or CO_2 retention (Tisi, 1979). Obesity, smoking and prolonged anaesthesia also predispose to postoperative pulmonary complications. Conversely, they are rare in previously fit subjects with normal lung function. It is therefore logical to concentrate preventive measures on those patients known to be most at risk.

In high-risk cases, surgery should be delayed in order to optimize respiratory function and minimize the risk of subsequent serious pulmonary complications (Stein and Cassara, 1970). Thus, patients with bronchiectasis or severe COAD, particularly if associated with cor pulmonale and polycythaemia, will often benefit from a period of intensive physiotherapy, with antibiotic treatment for active infection, prior to surgery. In some cases, bronchodilator therapy may be beneficial. Similarly, those with other forms of chronic respiratory disease will require preoperative treatment of any superimposed respiratory tract infections. Patients must be persuaded to stop smoking, preferably several weeks before surgery.

In the postoperative period, simple but effective preventive measures include chest physiotherapy with deep breathing, coughing, and exercises designed to improve respiratory muscle function. If possible, the patient should be sat up at approximately 45° since in this position diaphragmatic movement is not impeded by the abdominal contents and expansion of basal lung segments is improved. In some centres, the 'incentive spirometer' is used to encourage deep breathing as an alternative to intermittent positive pressure breathing (Van de Water, 1972), whilst the application of CPAP may be a useful means of achieving re-expansion of collapsed lung segments, particularly in those in whom the major abnormality is a reduction in FRC (e.g. the obese patient who has recently undergone upper abdominal surgery).

The provision of adequate analgesia is of paramount importance since pain will seriously inhibit the patient's ability to cough and expand the lungs. Giving intramuscular opiates as and when required is inadequate in the high-risk patient because of wide variations in blood levels (Rigg et al, 1978) and fluctuations in the quality of analgesia.

Recent studies have therefore evaluated continuous intravenous (Church, 1979) or subcutaneous infusions for managing postoperative pain, as well as patient-controlled analgesia systems (Hull and Sibbald, 1981). Unfortunately, both continuous and 'on demand' infusion techniques require relatively expensive pumps with fail-safe mechanisms as well as close monitoring to detect signs of overdosage, although subcutaneous infusions are inherently safer and may be suitable for use on the general ward.

To avoid parenteral administration, oral or sublingual preparations of strong analgesics have been developed—some in long-acting forms. Whilst oral administration and gastrointestinal absorption require a functioning bowel, sublingual administration allows rapid absorption into the systemic circulation. Other innovations have included the introduction of derestricted agonist/antagonist drugs such as buprenorphine (which can be given sublingually), meptazinol and nalbuphine.

The use of regional blockade via extradural or intrathecal routes, using either local anaesthetic agents or opiates, has been extensively investigated. For instance, Bromage and his colleagues (Bromage et al, 1980) used epidural narcotics in 66 patients after surgery under epidural with light general anaesthesia. They found that both narcotics and local anaesthetics administered via the epidural route produced greater improvements in FEV_1 than intravenous morphine. Moreover, epidural narcotics did not cause sympathetic depression or bladder dysfunction. Continuous thoracic epidural infusions of fentanyl, initially at $50 \mu g h^{-1}$ but subsequently at $20 \mu g h^{-1}$, have been shown to produce better analgesia with less sedation than papaveretum postoperatively (Welchew and Thornton, 1982). The analgesia achieved with fentanyl is of shorter duration than that produced by other opiates because of its high lipid solubility. The growing number of fentanyl derivatives (sufentanil, alfentanil) are currently being investigated in various centres.

The complications associated with intraspinal narcotics are legion. The chief side effects include nausea, vomiting, pruritus, urinary retention and delayed respiratory depression. This latter complication is associated with old age, a reduced ventilatory capacity and thoracic extradural puncture (Gustafsson et al, 1982). Correct choice of agent and dosage as well as proper surveillance are essential for the safe use of these techniques, and these constraints preclude their use on general wards.

Despite these measures, some patients will need endotracheal intubation, possibly combined with bronchoscopy, or a mini-tracheostomy to control bronchial secretions, whilst others will deteriorate further and require ventilatory support. Selected cases may therefore benefit from elective, postoperative artificial ventilation.

It is worth considering that in some patients with severe, chronic respiratory disease, e.g. long-standing COAD and hypercarbia, the prognosis of the lung lesion may be considerably worse than that of the disease requiring surgery, even if the operation is not performed.

Acute exacerbations of COAD

Routine treatment consists of controlled oxygen therapy, elimination of bacterial infection with antibiotics, physiotherapy and bronchodilators for reversible airway obstruction. Diuretics may be required in those with pulmonary hypertension and right ventricular failure.

A proportion of these patients have a chronically raised arterial carbon dioxide tension to which they have become accustomed. In these cases, it is hypoxia which stimulates respiration and the administration of high concentrations of oxygen may then attenuate this 'hypoxic drive', decrease alveolar ventilation and precipitate carbon dioxide retention. Because such patients are hypoxic they are operating on the steep portion of their oxygen dissociation curve and small increases in arterial oxygen tension, not sufficient to significantly depress the hypoxic drive, will lead to relatively large increases in arterial oxygen content. This forms the basis for 'controlled oxygen therapy' (Campbell, 1960b) whereby oxygen is administered in low concentrations, just sufficient to produce a useful increase in P_aO_2. This can be achieved using a Ventimask administering 24%, 28% or 34% oxygen, but requires careful monitoring, with frequent blood gas analysis, to obtain the optimal effect.

If the patient continues to deteriorate despite these measures, artificial ventilation should be considered. In general, however, one should be cautious about embarking on artificial ventilation in those with chronic chest disease because in a proportion of cases weaning proves to be impossible. In some patients, artificial ventilation may be avoided by the use of a respiratory stimulant, such as a continuous intravenous infusion of doxapram. This not only stimulates the respiratory centre but also acts as an analeptic, arousing the patient so that he will cough more effectively and co-operate with physiotherapy. Side effects are frequent and include tachycardia, hypertension, tremor and agitation. If this fails, intubation followed by physiotherapy and endotracheal suction may be employed in those patients in whom retention of secretions is the major problem. Such treatment can break the downward spiral of sputum retention, confusion and decreasing level of consciousness.

Selection of those patients who are suitable for artificial ventilation is difficult and is based largely on the severity and nature of the underlying chronic pulmonary disease. The patient's previous exercise tolerance and ability to lead an independent existence are perhaps the most important considerations. Those who were severely incapacitated prior to the present acute episode will be extremely difficult to wean from the ventilator, and even if this is achieved they are unlikely to recover sufficiently to attain a reasonable lifestyle; early relapse is then to be expected. On the other hand, if the patient was leading a full and active life prior to the acute episode, an aggressive approach should be adopted. Other indications that significant hypoxia and hypercarbia have been present for some time (i.e. are a result of severe chronic chest disease) include polycythaemia, a raised bicarbonate concentration and cor pulmonale.

When patients with pure emphysema develop respiratory failure, they do so because of irreversible loss of lung tissue; P_aco_2 is normal, or low, due to compensatory hyperventilation. Such patients will not benefit from artificial ventilation since the process leading to their terminal respiratory failure is irreversible lung destruction and weaning will be impossible. At the other extreme are those who develop respiratory failure mainly due to the accumulation of profuse, infected secretions. Not only are such patients hypoxic but their arterial carbon dioxide tension is raised. Because episodes of acute deterioration are usually due to superadded bacterial infection, they generally benefit from a period of artificial ventilation. The excessive secretions can be removed, the precipitating bacterial infection treated, and lung function improved. Unfortunately, the majority of patients lie somewhere between these two extremes and consequently the decision to institute ventilatory support can be very difficult.

Severe asthma

An asthmatic attack can be considered severe if it is particularly prolonged (i.e. lasting several days) or if it is resistant to therapy. Such episodes are sometimes referred to as 'status asthmaticus', which has been defined as 'an acute asthmatic attack in which the degree of bronchial obstruction is either severe from the beginning or progressively increases in severity and is not relieved by conventional therapy'. Precipitating factors include exposure to high concentrations of allergen and respiratory infection (either bacterial or viral). Alterations in treatment regimens (such as a sudden reduction in the dose of corticosteroids) (James et al, 1977), an overdose of sedatives, desensitization procedures, provocation tests and anaesthesia may all provoke intense bronchospasm. Signs that the attack is particularly severe include extreme dyspnoea (causing an inability to speak, eat, drink or even sleep), use of accessory muscles, mental confusion and exhaustion. Pulsus paradoxus may be difficult to detect and is an unreliable sign, whilst in the most severe cases wheezing may be absent due to the marked reduction in air flow.

The increased airway resistance in asthma is due to oedema of the bronchial mucosa and obstruction by thick, tenacious mucous plugs, as well as an increase in bronchomotor tone. The forced expiratory flow rates and vital capacity are therefore reduced and air trapping causes an increase in FRC and total lung capacity. This helps to maintain the patency of terminal airways but increases both the work of breathing and the risk of pneumothorax. Furthermore, pulmonary vascular resistance is increased, producing right ventricular strain and sometimes a fall in cardiac output. This will be exacerbated if, as is often the case, the patient is hypovolaemic.

A chest x-ray should always be obtained in patients hospitalized with acute severe asthma in order to exclude a pneumothorax. Characteristically, in the absence of pneumothorax, this will show the features of pulmonary hyperinflation with hyperluscent lung fields, horizontal ribs, flat diaphragms and a vertical heart. An ECG may reveal tachycardia, dysrhythmias, ST-T segment changes, P pulmonale in leads II and III and right axis deviation. Initially, the patient is hypoxic due to V/Q mismatch, while relative hyperventilation induces hypocarbia. A normal or high P_aCO_2 is an ominous sign that the patient is tiring. A metabolic acidosis is relatively common and may be due to circulatory failure, a reduction in hepatic metabolism of lactate and an increase in circulating catecholamines.

Patients with acute asthma are managed according to the principles outlined above with oxygen, rehydration, physiotherapy, bronchodilators and antibiotics to control any precipitating bacterial infection. Correction of the metabolic acidosis with sodium bicarbonate will be associated with a transient increase in carbon dioxide production and should, if possible, be avoided. Administration of sedatives, cough suppressants or β-blockers can cause rapid, and sometimes fatal, deterioration.

Improved management of acute asthma has meant that fewer cases require IPPV (0.3% of all admissions for asthma in one series) (Westerman et al, 1979). However, the mortality remains disappointingly high, with many patients dying before they reach hospital and a number of sudden, apparently unpredictable deaths occurring in hospital. In this context, it is important to appreciate that the degree of bronchospasm often worsens appreciably in the early hours ('early morning dips'), possibly because of the reduction in blood cortisol levels at this time (James et al, 1977), or the diurnal variation in catecholamine levels.

Although ventilating severe asthma patients is extremely hazardous, it is equally dangerous to procrastinate when the patient is exhausted. Some characteristic features of those requiring IPPV include youth, a long history of asthma, previous hospital admissions in status and attacks lasting more than 24 hours prior to admission (Westerman et al, 1979). It can be very difficult to assess which patients require ventilation but some generally accepted criteria are extreme exhaustion, increasing mental disturbance and a P_aCO_2 which is >8 kPa and/or rising. Those who suffer respiratory arrest will require immediate intubation and ventilation.

There are a number of important considerations when selecting an appropriate pattern of ventilation for an asthmatic. Because of the severe airway obstruction, a long expiratory phase is required in order to avoid overinflation of the lungs. On the other hand, the time constants of most lung units are markedly increased (see Chapter 2) and inspiration must be prolonged to allow adequate distribution of inspired gases. Thus, a slow respiratory rate, with long inspiratory and expiratory phases, is required. In severe cases, the minute volume is inevitably inadequate and it may be impossible to return the arterial carbon dioxide tension to within normal limits. Although hypercarbia is a strong stimulus for the patient to breathe and 'fight' the ventilator, it has to be tolerated and the patient should be heavily sedated and, if necessary, paralysed.

Apart from increasing the risk of pneumothorax, overinflation of the lungs compresses the heart and attenuates the pulmonary vasculature, further increasing pulmonary vascular resistance. Eventually, the right ventricle fails and cardiac output falls. This may be a terminal event. The risk of this complication can be minimized by ensuring that expiration is completed before the next inspiration begins, either by auscultation or by disconnecting the patient from the ventilator and listening at the endotracheal tube. It may also be helpful to measure the chest circumference in order to detect overinflation.

Similar considerations apply when ventilating those patients with COAD who also have an element of airway obstruction. Moreover, rapidly lowering the arterial carbon dioxide tension towards normal in these patients, some of whom have a compensatory metabolic alkalosis, may cause a marked increase in pH with a reduction in ionized calcium levels, cerebral vasoconstriction and a danger of fitting. There may also be a dramatic fall in cardiac output.

Obstruction by tenacious mucous plugs is an important component of the increased airway resistance in status asthmaticus. Some authorities therefore recommend bronchial lavage in those patients who require IPPV. This is usually performed via a double-lumen tube so that each lung can be lavaged independently, although some centres use rigid or fibre-optic bronchoscopes to isolate smaller lung segments. Nevertheless, these techniques are almost invariably associated with severe hypoxia and hypercarbia and as a consequence are extremely hazardous. An alternative is to instil small quantities of saline into the endotracheal tube at regular intervals, although the efficacy of this technique is questionable.

Weaning and extubation of patients with reversible airway obstruction may precipitate a further episode of severe bronchospasm. A useful technique is to allow the patient to breathe 50% nitrous oxide in oxygen (Entonox) for ten minutes to provide temporary sedation prior to extubation. Alternatively, the patient can be sedated with, for example, a continuous infusion of chlormethiazole during this period.

Upper airway obstruction

There are many causes of upper airway obstruction, including trauma, foreign bodies, burns, tumours, (e.g. lymphoma), haematomas following head and neck surgery (e.g. carotid endarterectomy), acute epiglottitis in children and laryngeal oedema or stenosis following endotracheal intubation/ tracheostomy. Postextubation upper airway obstruction may necessitate reintubation, particularly in children and neonates, and some authorities use dexamethasone in an attempt to reduce mucosal oedema.

Large airway obstruction (mouth down to subsegmental bronchi) presents as dyspnoea with inspiratory stridor and wheezing. Signs that the obstruction is severe include flaring of the alae nasae, retraction of intercostal muscles and a 'tracheal tug' (retraction of the skin and soft tissues in the suprasternal notch).

Patients with upper airway obstruction compensate well in the initial stages by increased respiratory effort and the use of accessory muscles. Tidal volume, respiratory rate and blood gases therefore often remain within normal limits. Once exhaustion develops, however, deterioration occurs alarmingly quickly. Because flow through the obstruction is turbulent, the resistance is dependent on the density of the inspired gas and may be reduced by administering a mixture of helium (which is less dense than air) in oxygen. Often, this simply allows time to prepare for endotracheal intubation and/or tracheostomy. If possible, endotracheal intubation should be attempted in an anaesthetic room, where all the equipment which might be required to secure an airway is available, and with a competent surgeon to hand in case an emergency tracheostomy is required. Gaseous induction of anaesthesia should be followed by laryngoscopy and attempts at intubation with the patient breathing spontaneously.

In some cases a fibre-optic laryngoscope may prove helpful. If all else fails, tracheostomy should be performed, although as discussed previously, this is extremely hazardous under these circumstances and cricothyrotomy may be the preferred technique. In some instances, e.g. severe head and neck trauma, an elective tracheostomy may be performed once the airway has been secured.

Pulmonary oedema is a recognized complication of severe upper airway obstruction (Oswalt et al, 1977) and has been described most often in children with acute epiglottitis. It may be caused by the huge negative intrathoracic pressures generated in order to overcome the resistance to ventilation. A period of IPPV with PEEP is nearly always required in such cases but resolution of the oedema is fairly rapid and weaning can usually commence within 24–48 hours.

Cardiogenic pulmonary oedema

Patients with severe cardiogenic pulmonary oedema unresponsive to normal measures (oxygen, opiates, diuretics, vasodilators and inotropes) often benefit from a period of IPPV. This may be particularly useful in those scheduled for corrective cardiac surgery, e.g. closure of a ventricular septal defect or replacement of a leaking mitral valve. The low cardiac output and hypotension often found in these cases need not necessarily be a deterrent to IPPV, or even IPPV with PEEP (see Chapter 13), since the stiff lungs partially prevent transmission of the positive pressure to the great veins and pulmonary capillaries. In these cases, hypoxaemia is usually very responsive to the application of PEEP and the net effect may be an increase in oxygen delivery. In some cases, a fall in venous return can lead to a beneficial reduction in pre-load and this, combined with reversal of hypoxia, may improve coronary blood flow and myocardial oxygenation. Because the ventricular function curve is flat, the fall in pre-load has little effect on stroke volume and consequently, if myocardial performance improves, cardiac output and blood pressure may actually increase (see also Chapter 13).

Non-cardiogenic pulmonary oedema (adult respiratory distress syndrome, ARDS) (Editorial, 1986)

In 1967, Ashbaugh and his colleagues described a syndrome of acute respiratory distress in adults, characterized by severe dyspnoea, tachypnoea, cyanosis refractory to oxygen therapy, loss of lung compliance and diffuse alveolar infiltrates seen on the chest x-ray (Ashbaugh et al, 1967). They remarked on the similarity between this 'adult respiratory distress syndrome' (ARDS) and that seen in neonates.

ARDS can therefore be defined as diffuse pulmonary infiltrates, refractory hypoxaemia and respiratory distress. A PCWP <16 mmHg

(2.1 kPa) is often included in the definition in an attempt to exclude cardiogenic causes, although even in this situation previously elevated left ventricular filling pressures may have been normalized prior to insertion of the Swan–Ganz catheter, whilst radiological changes take 24–48 hours to resolve. ARDS is a non-specific reaction of the lungs which has been associated with a wide variety of insults, such as shock (especially septic shock, see Chapter 10), fat embolism, massive blood transfusion, trauma, burns, pancreatitis, cardiopulmonary bypass (now very rarely), lung contusion, inhalation of smoke/toxic gases, amniotic fluid embolism and aspiration pneumonia (Fein et al, 1982). Superadded infection is a common feature of ARDS and some would include diffuse pneumonias (e.g. viral, mycoplasma, legionnaires' disease) within the definition of this condition.

Pathophysiology

Although the oedematous pulmonary infiltrates seen in ARDS are distributed diffusely throughout the lung, there are areas of 'spared' normal lung; this causes marked V/Q inequalities. Decreased surfactant may cause atelectasis, and FRC falls, venous admixture increases and lung compliance is reduced. The V_D/V_T ratio rises, particularly in the most severe cases in whom pulmonary vascular resistance is also increased.

The 'non-cardiogenic' pulmonary oedema, which is the main feature of ARDS, is associated with an increased pulmonary capillary permeability. In sheep with respiratory failure induced by *E. coli* endotoxin, lung lymph flow is markedly increased. Although the protein content of this lymph is initially low, suggesting that oedema formation in the early stages is due to elevated microvascular pressures associated with pulmonary hypertension (see below), later the protein content rises, indicating increased pulmonary vascular permeability (Esbenshade et al, 1982). Furthermore, fluid obtained from the airways of patients with ARDS contains a higher concentration of protein, relative to plasma levels, than does that of patients with cardiogenic pulmonary oedema (Snapper, 1981). This increased capillary permeability can be partly explained by the microcirculatory stasis and disseminated intravascular coagulation which can occur in shock, as well as the effects of activated platelets and blood coagulation products (Rinaldo and Rogers, 1982; Zapol et al, 1983). As discussed above, some believe that the debris in stored blood is implicated in the pathogenesis of this condition. Vasoactive substances have already been mentioned as important mediators of platelet aggregation and increased capillary permeability in shock (see Chapter 10) and may also be important in the pathogenesis of ARDS. However, the loss of pulmonary capillary integrity is currently thought to be largely caused by polymorphonuclear leukocytes (PMN) (Heflin and Brigham, 1981) stimulated by activated complement, particularly C5a (Jacob, 1981). Indeed, elevated levels of C5a may be a predictor of ARDS in humans (Hammerschmidt et al, 1980). It is possible that the capillary endothelium is then damaged by toxic oxygen radicals produced by these activated PMN (Babior, 1978). For example, the free radical superoxide O_2^- can participate in a number of chemical reactions yielding hydrogen peroxide (H_2O_2) and hydroxyl radicals (OH^-). These can damage cell membranes and interfere with the function of a number of enzyme systems. This may be valuable when directed against bacteria, but detrimental when capillary endothelium is the target. However, it is worth noting that because the lung is the only organ to be perfused with virtually all of the cardiac output, it is probably uniquely vulnerable to the damaging effects of circulating substances.

Pulmonary vascular resistance (PVR) is often elevated in patients with ARDS (Zapol and Snider, 1977). High right-sided filling pressures are then required in order to maintain cardiac output and the right ventricle dilates, increasing myocardial wall tension and reducing coronary perfusion. In severe cases, the interventricular septum may be distorted so that it impinges on the left ventricular cavity, causing a rise in LAP. LVEDV and stroke index thus remain low, whilst PCWP is paradoxically high (Sibbald and Prewitt, 1983).

There are a number of causes of the pulmonary hypertension in ARDS (Zapol et al, 1983). Initially, mechanical obstruction of the pulmonary circulation may occur as a result of vascular compression by interstitial oedema and subsequently oedema of the vessel wall itself. Later, constriction of the pulmonary vasculature may occur in response to increased autonomic nervous activity as well as circulating substances such as catecholamines, serotonin, $PGF_{2\alpha}$, thromboxane, fibrin/fibrinogen degradation products, complement and activated leukocytes. Those vessels supplying alveoli with low oxygen tensions constrict (the 'hypoxic vasoconstrictor response'), diverting pulmonary blood flow to better oxygenated areas of lung, thus limiting the degree of shunt. This response may be enhanced by local acidosis and hypercarbia, but may in some cases be inhibited by vasodilator products of arachidonic acid metabolism. In some patients with ARDS and pulmonary hypertension, angiography will reveal 'beading' of the arterioles and peripheral 'pruning' of the pulmonary vasculature. This suggests fibrin deposition and is associated with a marked increase in dead space and a poor prognosis despite attempts to reverse the process using heparin and streptokinase. In this situation, subpleural lung segments are infarcted but continue to be ventilated and are therefore liable to rupture. In others, both angiography and PVR are normal and the 'wet lung' usually responds to dehydration and respiratory support.

The hyaline membranes seen microscopically in the lungs of patients with ARDS consist of necrotic type I alveolar cells and coagulated intra-alveolar proteins derived from the pulmonary exudate. Within seven days of the onset of ARDS, activated fibroblasts are seen in the interstitial spaces. Subsequently, interstitial fibrosis progresses with loss of elastic tissue and obliteration of the pulmonary vasculature (Fein et al, 1982). These changes are probably irreversible, although in patients who recover from ARDS, lung function often returns virtually to normal, particularly in young, non-smokers (Lakshminarayan et al, 1976) and residual x-ray changes are usually limited to a few linear scars. A more recent study concluded that spirometry and lung mechanics are restored to normal within six months of extubation but that gas exchange remains impaired. Exercise tolerance may be limited by a reduction in the pulmonary capillary blood volume (Buchser et al, 1985).

Presentation

Clinically, the first sign of the development of ARDS is often an unexplained tachypnoea, followed by increasing hypoxia. Later, the chest x-ray shows

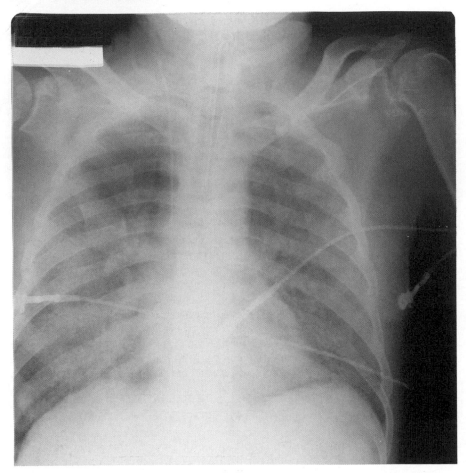

Fig. 12.3 Chest x-ray appearances in adult respiratory distress syndrome. Bilateral diffuse alveolar shadowing without cardiac enlargement.

bilateral, diffuse shadowing with an alveolar pattern and air bronchograms which may then progress to the picture of complete 'white out' (Fig. 12.3).

Management

This is based on treatment of the underlying condition (e.g. eradication of sepsis), and supportive measures such as oxygen, CPAP, and IPPV/IMV with or without PEEP. Oedema formation should be minimized by controlling left-ventricular filling pressure and, if possible, maintaining plasma proteins, particularly albumin, close to the normal range. However, once plasma enters the interstitial space, the transvascular oncotic gradient disappears and the main determinants of interstitial oedema formation become the microvascular hydrostatic pressure and lymphatic drainage. There is therefore considerable controversy concerning the relative merits of colloids or crystalloids for volume replacement in patients likely to develop ARDS, or in whom the condition is established (see Chapter 10). As discussed above, cardiovascular support and reduction of oxygen requirements are also important.

Specific treatment

Prior administration of steroids to sheep given endotoxin prevents the subsequent increase in lung vascular permeability (Brigham et al, 1981) and the early administration of high-dose steroids to patients with septic ARDS may in some cases reduce alveolar-capillary permeability (Sibbald et al, 1981). Pretreatment with cyclo-oxygenase inhibitors (see Chapter 10) can abolish the early pulmonary hypertension associated with endotoxin administration, although it does not prevent the increase in capillary permeability (Snapper, 1981), while the combination of steroids and cyclo-oxygenase inhibitor can virtually abolish the pulmonary response to endotoxin in sheep (Begley et al, 1984). Other suggested approaches based on the presumed importance of arachidonic acid metabolites have included the administration of prostacyclin and vasoactive intestinal peptide (which counteracts some effects of leukotrienes). Free radical scavengers may also prove to be of value.

Nevertheless, the place of these agents in the clinical management of ARDS remains unclear, although it seems certain that to be of benefit, they must be given early. Currently, investigators are searching for markers which will allow early identification of those who are at high risk of developing ARDS. Possibilities include C5a, leukotrienes and oxidant activity in exhaled breath (Baldwin et al, 1986).

Prognosis

Despite the supportive treatment outlined above, the mortality of established severe ARDS remains depressingly high: more than 50% overall. Approximately 40% of uncomplicated cases die but the mortality rises with increasing age and failure of other organs.

FURTHER READING

Pontoppidan H, Geffin B & Lowenstein E (1972) Acute respiratory failure in the adult (first and second of three parts). *New England Journal of Medicine* **287**: 690–698, 743–752.
Sykes MK, McNicol MW & Campbell EJM (1976) *Respiratory Failure*. Oxford: Blackwell Scientific.

REFERENCES

Ashbaugh DG, Bigelow DB, Petty TL & Levine BR (1967) Acute respiratory distress in adults. *Lancet* **ii**: 319–323.
Babior BM (1978) Oxygen-dependent microbial killing by phagocytes (two parts). *New England Journal of Medicine* **298**: 659–668 and 721–725.

Baldwin SR, Simon RH, Grum CM et al (1986) Oxidant activity in expired breath of patients with adult respiratory distress syndrome. *Lancet* **i:** 11–14.

Barber RE, Lee J & Hamilton WK (1970) Oxygen toxicity in man. A prospective study in patients with irreversible brain damage. *New England Journal of Medicine* **283:** 1478–1484.

Begley CJ, Ogletree ML, Meyerick BO & Brigham KL (1984) Modification of pulmonary responses to endotoxaemia in awake sheep by steroidal and non-steroidal anti-inflammatory agents. *American Review of Respiratory Disease* **130:** 1140–1146.

Brigham KL, Bowers RE & McKeen CR (1981) Methylprednisolone prevention of increased lung vascular permeability following endotoxemia in sheep. *Journal of Clinical Investigation* **67:** 1103–1110.

Bromage PR, Camporesi E & Chestnut D (1980) Epidural narcotics for post-operative analgesia. *Anesthesia and Analgesia* **59:** 473–480.

Buchser E, Leuenberger Ph, Chiolero R, Penet U & Freeman J (1985) Reduced pulmonary capillary blood volume as a long-term sequel of ARDS. *Chest* **87:** 608–611.

Burger EJ & Mead J (1969) Static properties of lungs after oxygen exposure. *Journal of Applied Physiology* **27:** 191–197.

Caldwell PRB, Lee WL Jr, Schildkraut HS & Archibald ER (1966) Changes in lung volume, diffusing capacity, and blood gases in men breathing oxygen. *Journal of Applied Physiology* **21:** 1477–1483.

Campbell EJM (1960a) A method of controlled oxygen administration which reduces the risk of carbon-dioxide retention. *Lancet* **ii:** 12–14.

Campbell EJM (1960b) Respiratory failure. The relation between oxygen concentrations of inspired air and arterial blood. *Lancet* **ii:** 10–11.

Campbell EJM (1982) How to use the Venturi mask. *Lancet* **ii:** 1206.

Church JJ (1979) Continuous narcotic infusions for relief of postoperative pain. *British Medical Journal* **i:** 977–979.

Comroe JH, Dripps RD, Dumke PR & Deming M (1945) Oxygen toxicity. The effect of inhalation of high concentrations of oxygen for twenty-four hours on normal men at sea level and at a simulated altitude of 18,000 feet. *Journal of the American Medical Association* **128:** 710–717.

deLemos R, Wolfsdorf J, Nachman R et al (1969) Lung injury from oxygen in lambs: the role of artificial ventilation. *Anesthesiology* **30:** 609–617.

Deneke SM & Fanburg BL (1982) Oxygen toxicity of the lung: an update. *British Journal of Anaesthesia* **54:** 737–749.

Editorial (1986) Adult respiratory distress syndrome. *Lancet* **i:** 301–303.

Esbenshade AM, Newman JH, Lams PH, Jolles H & Brigham KL (1982) Respiratory failure after endotoxin infusion in sheep: lung mechanics and lung fluid balance. *Journal of Applied Physiology* **53:** 967–976.

Fein AM, Goldberg SK, Lippmann ML, Fischer R & Morgan L (1982) Adult respiratory distress syndrome. *British Journal of Anaesthesia* **54:** 723–736.

Goldstein RS, Young J & Rebuck AS (1982) Effect of breathing pattern on oxygen concentration received from standard face masks. *Lancet* **ii:** 1188–1190.

Gormezano J & Branthwaite MA (1972) Effects of physiotherapy during intermittent positive pressure ventilation. Changes in arterial blood gas tensions. *Anaesthesia* **27:** 258–264.

Gustafsson LL, Schildt B & Jacobsen K (1982) Adverse effects of extradural and intrathecal opiates: report of a nationwide survey in Sweden. *British Journal of Anaesthesia* **54:** 479–485.

Hammerschmidt DE, Weaver LJ, Hudson LD, Craddock PR & Jacob HS (1980) Association of complement activation and elevated plasma-C5a with adult respiratory distress syndrome. Pathophysiological relevance and possible prognostic value. *Lancet* **i:** 947–949.

Heflin AC & Brigham KL (1981) Prevention by granulocyte depletion of increased vascular permeability of sheep lung following endotoxaemia. *Journal of Clinical Investigation* **68:** 1253–1260.

Hewlett AM & Branthwaite MA (1975) Post-operative pulmonary function. *British Journal of Anaesthesia* **47:** 102–107.

Hull CJ & Sibbald A (1981) Control of postoperative pain by interactive demand analgesia. *British Journal of Anaesthesia* **53:** 385–391.

Jacob HS (1981) The role of activated complement and granulocytes in shock states and myocardial infarction. *Journal of Laboratory and Clinical Medicine* **98:** 645–653.

James OF, Mills RM & Allen KM (1977) Severe bronchial asthma: factors influencing intensive care management and outcome. *Anaesthesia and Intensive Care* **5:** 11–18.

Kapanci Y, Weibel ER, Kaplan HP & Robinson FR (1969) Pathogenesis and reversibility of the pulmonary lesions of oxygen toxicity in monkeys 11. Ultrastructural and morphometric studies. *Laboratory Investigation* **20:** 101–118.

Kordash TR, Van Dellen RG & McCall JT (1977) Theophylline concentrations in asthmatic patients after administration of aminophylline. *Journal of the American Medical Association* **238:** 139–141.

Labrousse J, Tenaillon A & Chastre J (1983) Equipment for respiratory therapy. In Tinker J & Rapin M (eds) *Care of the Critically Ill Patient*, pp 387–403. Berlin: Springer-Verlag.

Lakshminarayan S, Stanford RE & Petty TL (1976) Prognosis after recovery from adult respiratory distress syndrome. *American Review of Respiratory Disease* **113:** 7–16.

Nash G, Blennerhassett JB & Pontoppidan H (1967) Pulmonary lesions associated with oxygen therapy and artificial ventilation. *New England Journal of Medicine* **276:** 368–374.

Oswalt CE, Gates GA & Holmstrom FMG (1977) Pulmonary edema as a complication of acute airway obstruction. *Journal of the American Medical Association* **238:** 1833–1835.

Puri VK, Weil MH, Michaels S & Carlson RW (1980) Pulmonary edema associated with reduction in plasma oncotic pressure. *Surgery, Gynecology and Obstetrics* **151:** 344–348.

Rigg JRA, Browne RA, Davis C, Khandelwal JK & Goldsmith CH (1978) Variation in the disposition of morphine after IM administration in surgical patients. *British Journal of Anaesthesia* **50:** 1125–1130.

Rinaldo JE & Rogers RM (1982) Adult respiratory-distress syndrome. Changing concepts of lung injury and repair. *New England Journal of Medicine* **306:** 900–909.

Robertson CE, Steedman D, Sinclair CJ, Brown D & Malcolm-Smith N (1985) Use of ether in life-threatening acute severe asthma. *Lancet* **i:** 187–188.

Shenfield GM, Hodson ME, Clarke SW & Paterson JW (1975) Interaction of corticosteroids and catecholamines in the treatment of asthma. *Thorax* **30:** 430–435.

Sibbald WJ, Anderson RR, Reid B, Holliday RL & Driedger AA (1981) Alveolo-capillary permeability in human septic ARDS. Effect of high-dose corticosteroid therapy. *Chest* **79:** 133–142.

Sibbald WJ & Prewitt RM (1983) Right ventricular function. *Critical Care Medicine* **11:** 321–322.

Singer MM, Wright F, Stanley LK, Roe BB & Hamilton WK (1970) Oxygen toxicity in man. A prospective study in patients after open-heart surgery. *New England Journal of Medicine* **283:** 1473–1478.

Snapper JR (1981) Septic pulmonary edema. *Seminars in Respiratory Medicine* **3:** 92–96.

Stein M & Cassara EL (1970) Preoperative pulmonary evaluation and therapy for surgery patients. *Journal of the American Medical Association* **211:** 787–790.

Tisi GM (1979) Pre-operative evaluation of pulmonary function. *American Review of Respiratory Disease* **119:** 293–310.

Van de Water JM, Watring WG, Linten LA, Murphy M & Byron RL (1972) Prevention of postoperative pulmonary complications. *Surgery, Gynecology and Obstetrics* **135:** 229–233.

Welchew EA & Thornton JA (1982) Continuous thoracic epidural fentanyl. *Anaesthesia* **37:** 309–316.

Westerman DE, Benatar SR, Potgieter PD & Ferguson AD (1979) Identification of the high-risk asthmatic patient. Experience with 39 patients undergoing ventilation for status asthmaticus. *American Journal of Medicine* **66:** 565–572.

Williams S & Seaton A (1977) Intravenous or inhaled salbutamol in severe acute asthma? *Thorax* **32:** 555–558.

Winter PM & Smith G (1972) The toxicity of oxygen. *Anesthesiology* **37:** 210–241.

Wright RA, Weiss HS, Hiatt EP & Rustagi JS (1966) Risk of mortality in interrupted exposure to 100% O_2: role of air vs lowered Po_2. *American Journal of Physiology* **210:** 1015–1020.

Zapol WM & Snider MT (1977) Pulmonary hypertension in severe acute respiratory failure. *New England Journal of Medicine* **296:** 476–480.

Zapol WM, Trelstad RL, Snider MT, Pontoppidan H & Lemaire F (1983) Pathophysiological pathways of the adult respiratory distress syndrome. In Tinker J & Rapin M (eds) *Care of the Critically Ill Patient*, pp 341–358. Berlin: Springer-Verlag.

13
Artificial Ventilation

Although orotracheal intubation was first used to facilitate anaesthesia by MacEwen, a Glasgow surgeon, as long ago as 1878, it only became a routine procedure following the work of Magill, Rowbotham and others in the 1920s. Using endotracheal intubation, the anaesthetist was able to control the patient's ventilation, and in the 1940s neuromuscular blockade with IPPV, usually performed manually, became a standard anaesthetic technique. Nevertheless, mechanical ventilation for therapeutic purposes was initially performed using negative pressure devices (Fig. 13.1). Not only were

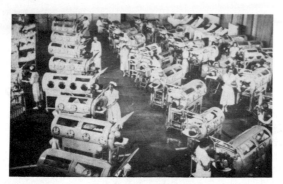

Fig. 13.1 'Tank' ventilators in use during an epidemic of poliomyelitis.

morbidity and mortality high with this technique, but it was much less successful in those with abnormal lungs. Therefore, apart from the treatment of ventilatory failure due to poliomyelitis, it was used infrequently; when polio became a rare disease, the use of artificial ventilation declined further. During the polio epidemic in Copenhagen in 1952, however, the advantages of positive pressure ventilation (see below) had been clearly demonstrated and in 1955 the use of IPPV for the treatment of acute exacerbations of chronic obstructive airway disease was described (Bjorneboe et al, 1955). Subsequently, clinicians increasingly accepted that IPPV could be used to treat patients with a variety of diseases affecting the lung parenchyma, as well as those with neuromuscular problems. This has led to a resurgence in the therapeutic use of artificial ventilation, particularly over the last two decades.

The various techniques of ventilatory support currently available are shown in Table 13.1.

227

Table 13.1 Techniques for respiratory support.

Negative pressure ventilation	Tank ventilators Cuirass ventilators
Intermittent positive pressure ventilation (IPPV)	ZEEP NEEP PEEP (CPPV)
Intermittent mandatory ventilation (IMV)	ZEEP PEEP
Continuous positive airway pressure (CPAP)	Endotracheal tube Mask
High-frequency jet ventilation (HFJV)	

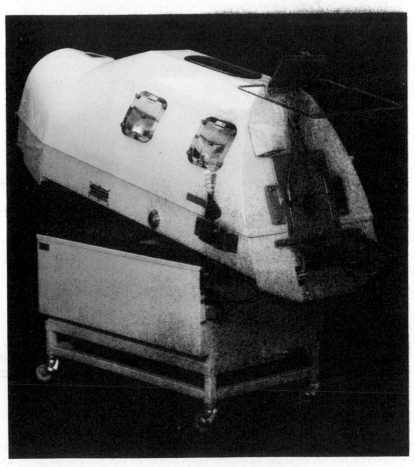

Fig. 13.2 The Cape Warwick portable tank respirator. This has been developed for use in the home; it is quiet, compact and allows the patient to enter and leave the tank unaided.

NEGATIVE PRESSURE VENTILATION

'Tank' ventilators ('iron lungs') (Figs. 13.1 and 13.2)

At one time, these were widely used for the treatment of ventilatory failure complicating polio. They are still occasionally employed for long-term ventilation of patients with chronic respiratory failure due to neuromuscular disease or skeletal deformity since they avoid some of the disadvantages of long-term IPPV. The patient's body is enclosed in an airtight 'tank' within which a negative pressure is created intermittently by a separate pump. During the negative pressure phase, the patient's thorax expands, drawing air into the lungs. Expiration then occurs passively. Although those patients who are conscious can speak and swallow in time with the ventilator, this technique has a number of disadvantages. Firstly, the ventilator itself is, of course, very bulky (although recent designs are more compact (Fig. 13.2)) and access to the patient is restricted, making it difficult to perform nursing and medical procedures. Secondly, the patient's airway is unprotected and there is no route for endotracheal suction. This technique is therefore only suitable for those with competent swallowing, laryngeal and cough reflexes, and even under these circumstances pulmonary aspiration can be a problem. Lastly, because the negative pressure is applied to the whole body, the normal inspiratory pressure gradient is lost, venous return is reduced and cardiac output may fall.

Cuirass ventilators

Cuirass ventilators, which encase only the thorax, were originally most frequently used during the recovery phase of poliomyelitis. However, they proved to be inefficient and difficult to use, a particular problem being the creation of an airtight seal around the lower thorax and abdomen. Nevertheless, such devices can be useful when used to assist ventilation, particularly during sleep, in those with borderline respiratory function. The Tunnicliffe jacket or its alternative, the 'pneumosuit', is a more efficient alternative.

Chest compression

Cuirass-type ventilators which create an intermittent positive pressure have been described. Gas is squeezed out of the lungs during the expiratory phase, while inspiration occurs passively due to the elastic recoil of the chest wall. Tidal exchange is inadequate, however, and progressive alveolar collapse causes rapidly worsening hypoxia. These ventilators are now only of historical interest.

Rocking beds

These can be used for those patients with neuromuscular disease whose respiratory reserve is limited but who only develop significant hypercapnia when they fall asleep. The rocking motion of the bed causes the abdominal contents to push the diaphragm in and out of the thorax, thereby assisting tidal exchange.

POSITIVE PRESSURE VENTILATION

Adequate pulmonary gas exchange can be achieved by intermittently inflating the lungs with a positive pressure applied via either an endotracheal tube or a tracheostomy. As mentioned above, IPPV has a number of important advantages over negative pressure ventilation. In particular, the airway is secured and protected, secretions can be aspirated more easily and IPPV can be used more successfully in those with diseases involving the lung parenchyma. Furthermore, access to and movement of the patient is relatively unrestricted. IPPV has therefore largely superseded the use of negative pressure devices in clinical practice.

In recent years, a number of refinements and modifications of IPPV have been described, including intermittent mandatory ventilation (IMV), mandatory minute volume (MMV) and IPPV with PEEP (sometimes known as continuous positive pressure ventilation, CPPV). These will be discussed later in this chapter.

Classification of positive pressure ventilators

A mechanical ventilator has to perform four operations during each respiratory cycle:
1 inflate the lungs;
2 change from inspiration to expiration;
3 allow expiration to take place;
4 change from expiration to inspiration.
Mechanical ventilators can therefore be classified according to the method used to inflate the lungs (the 'driving mechanism') and the means by which they change from one phase of the respiratory cycle to the other ('cycling') (Table 13.2).

Table 13.2 Classification of mechanical ventilators according to the driving mechanism and mode of cycling.

Driving mechanism	
Pressure generator	
Flow generator	
Mode of cycling	
Expiration to inspiration	*Inspiration to expiration*
Time	Time
Volume	Volume
Pressure	Pressure
Flow	Flow
Patient triggered	Mixed
Mixed	Other
Other	

Pressure preset ventilators

These are designed either to generate a preset pressure or they are cycled from inspiration to expiration when a designated airway pressure is reached.

The magnitude and shape of the inspiratory pressure waveform produced by these ventilators is therefore uninfluenced by changes in lung mechanics, whereas the pattern of flow during inflation depends on the interaction between the generated pressure pattern and the mechanical properties of the lung and chest wall. Thus, if pulmonary compliance falls, or resistance increases, there will be a reduction in the delivered tidal volume, unless the operator increases the inflation pressure. Pressure preset ventilators will, however, compensate for small leaks in the circuit.

Volume preset ventilators

These are designed to deliver a fixed tidal volume regardless of alterations in lung mechanics. The pattern of flow is therefore not affected by changes in lung compliance or airway resistance: if, for example, the lungs become stiffer, there will be a compensatory increase in inflation pressure and the tidal volume will remain unchanged. This type of ventilator does not, however, compensate for leaks in the circuit.

Cycling

The change from inspiration to expiration is usually time cycled, whilst inspiration is nearly always time cycled and/or patient triggered. A few ventilators have been designed which are volume cycled from inspiration to expiration and others are pressure cycled or flow cycled. Most sophisticated, modern electronic ventilators are time-cycled flow generators.

Selecting positive pressure ventilators for use in the intensive care unit

There are now a large number of positive pressure ventilators available, many of which are very sophisticated and, consequently, extremely expensive. Cost is therefore an important consideration when equipping a unit with ventilators and it is often sensible to provide a number of cheap but reliable ventilators, such as the Brompton-Manley, and to purchase only a few sophisticated machines, such as a Servo 900C, for use in complicated cases.

In general, ventilators should be as small, quiet and simple to operate as possible. The more complex the controls, the greater the opportunity for errors. Similarly, there is some advantage in restricting the number of different types of ventilator available on a particular unit since familiarity with the equipment generates confidence and reduces the incidence of mishaps. Suitable alarms are another important aspect of safety. These should be activated in the event of disconnection or obstruction and if the fresh gas supply fails.

The danger of cross infection can be minimized by using autoclavable patient circuits and these are now an essential feature of ventilators intended for use in an intensive care unit. Some ventilators also incorporate heated bacterial filters on both the inspiratory and expiratory limbs of the circuit, although the value of these is uncertain. There must be a safe and efficient means of humidifying inspired gases, and a 'kettle' type humidifier heated to 60°C has the advantage of effectively preventing bacterial contamination of the water reservoir.

It should be possible to adjust the duration of both the inspiratory and expiratory phases, as well as the ratio of one to the other. It should also be possible to apply PEEP (see below), if only by placing the tubing of the expiratory limb under water. Sophisticated ventilators should have facilities for synchronized intermittent mandatory ventilation (SIMV) both with and without PEEP. Other features which are often incorporated, but not of proven benefit, include sigh functions and a selection of inspiratory waveforms.

These criteria are adequately fulfilled by most modern electronic ventilators; indeed, these are often so technologically advanced that they have outstripped our clinical understanding. With the increasing use of SIMV as a routine mode of ventilation, one of the most important considerations when selecting a sophisticated ventilator is the performance of the SIMV/CPAP circuit (Cox and Niblett, 1984).

The rational use of IPPV depends on a clear understanding of its potential beneficial effects, as well as its dangers.

BENEFICIAL EFFECTS OF IPPV

Improved carbon dioxide elimination

Using mechanical ventilation, it is possible to remove the carbon dioxide which accumulates in some patients with respiratory failure and return the $P_a\text{CO}_2$ to within normal limits. Because of the operation of the alveolar air equation (see Chapter 2), the reduction in alveolar $P\text{CO}_2$ inevitably leads to a rise in alveolar $P\text{O}_2$ and improved arterial oxygenation. By adjusting the delivered minute volume, it is possible to compensate for any changes in the patient's dead space and/or carbon dioxide production. Under certain circumstances, improved distribution of inspired gases may lead to a fall in dead space and further benefit may accrue from abolishing the work of breathing, thereby reducing carbon dioxide production.

Improved oxygenation

Percentage venous admixture, whether due to alveolar collapse or ventilation/perfusion mismatch generally falls slightly when IPPV is instituted, but this effect is variable and therefore usually of only marginal benefit. Indeed, prolonged artificial ventilation with small tidal volumes may actually cause an increase in venous admixture and a deterioration in lung function (see below). Far more important is that artificial ventilation removes the work of breathing and relieves the extreme exhaustion which may be present in patients with respiratory failure (see Chapter 12). In those with severe pulmonary parenchymal disease, the lungs may be very stiff, the work of breathing is therefore greatly increased and institution of artificial ventilation may then significantly reduce oxygen consumption (Wilson et al, 1973). This reduction in oxygen requirements allows mixed venous oxygen tension, and consequently $P_a\text{O}_2$, to rise. Finally, because ventilated patients are connected to a leak-free circuit it is possible to administer high concentrations of oxygen, up to 100%, accurately and to apply PEEP. In selected cases, the latter may reduce shunt and increase $P_a\text{O}_2$ (see below).

INDICATIONS FOR ARTIFICIAL VENTILATION

Respiratory failure

Mechanical ventilation is most clearly indicated in the treatment of patients with severe respiratory failure who fail to respond to conventional medical treatment (see Chapter 12).

Prophylactic artificial ventilation

Artificial ventilation may also be used to prevent deterioration to respiratory failure in susceptible patients. For example, prophylactic postoperative IPPV is now a well-established practice in poor-risk patients in whom some degree of respiratory failure might otherwise be anticipated. Ventilatory support may also be used prophylactically in patients with neuromuscular or skeletal abnormalities. In these cases, a fall in vital capacity impairs the patient's ability to cough, sigh and take deep breaths; consequently, retention of secretions and progressive alveolar collapse eventually lead to respiratory failure, often in association with secondary infection. Under certain circumstances, it may be appropriate to prevent this sequence of events by instituting IPPV when the vital capacity has fallen to approximately one-quarter of the predicted value (see p. 304).

However, by no means all patients with respiratory failure and/or a reduced vital capacity will require artificial ventilation and clinical assessment of each individual case is of paramount importance. Factors such as age, general condition, degree of exhaustion and level of consciousness are at least as important as blood gas values (see p. 212).

Raised intracranial pressure and cerebral ischaemia

In patients with intracranial hypertension, e.g. following severe head injury, it is most important to avoid hypercarbia and/or hypoxia, since both will increase intracranial blood volume and exacerbate cerebral oedema. Furthermore, elective hyperventilation, even in those not in respiratory failure, can temporarily decrease cerebral blood flow and, secondarily, intracranial pressure, although the value of such treatment remains uncertain (see Chapter 14). Artificial ventilation may also be indicated in some patients following an episode of cerebral ischaemia (see Chapter 9).

DANGERS OF IPPV

General

Any patient undergoing IPPV is subjected to all the dangers and complications inherent in endotracheal intubation or tracheostomy (see below). Moreover, disconnection from the ventilator is an ever present danger. Mechanical failure is unusual but equally dangerous, and a suitable means of manually ventilating the patient with oxygen, e.g. an Ambu bag, must always be available by the bedside.

Barotrauma

Overdistension of the lungs during IPPV can rupture alveoli and cause air to dissect centrally along the perivascular sheaths. This pulmonary interstitial air is difficult to detect but can sometimes be seen on a good quality chest x-ray as linear or circular perivascular collections or, most specifically, subpleural blebs (Rohfling et al, 1976). In some cases, this progresses to produce pneumothorax (when gas under pressure in the pulmonary ligament penetrates the thin visceral pleura or a subpleural bleb ruptures), pneumomediastinum, pneumoperitoneum, air in the retroperitoneal space and subcutaneous emphysema (Fig. 13.3). Each of these may occur in

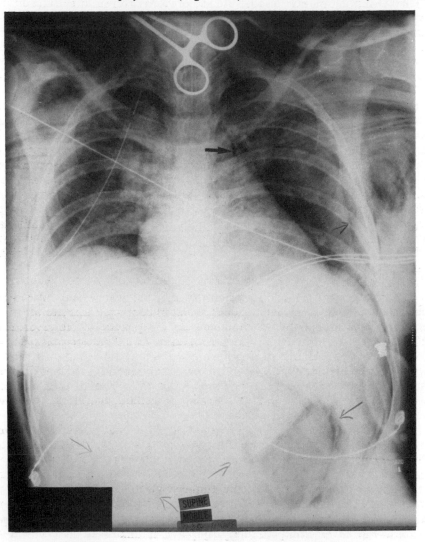

Fig. 13.3 Pulmonary barotrauma. Note subcutaneous air, left pneumothorax, right pleural drain, pneumomediastinum (air outlining aortic arch), and retroperitoneal air outlining left and right kidneys. (Courtesy of Dr K.M. Hillman.)

isolation or in combination with any of the others. Pneumomediastinum, pneumoperitoneum and subcutaneous emphysema can all precede the appearance of a pneumothorax and their presence should alert the clinician to the possibility of this complication. Intra-abdominal air originating in the lungs is probably always associated with pneumomediastinum and this can help distinguish pneumoperitoneum due to barotrauma from a ruptured viscus.

The incidence of barotrauma is greatest in those patients who require high inflation pressures, with or without PEEP, and the risk of pneumothorax is increased in those with destructive lung disease (Fig. 13.4) (e.g. staphylococcal pneumonia, emphysema) (Rohfling et al, 1976), asthma or fractured ribs. Because a life-threatening tension pneumothorax can develop extremely rapidly in patients receiving IPPV, the facilities for chest drain insertion should be immediately available at the bedside of all such high risk cases. Barotrauma may also be the result of endotracheal tube obstruction, intubation of a main bronchus or overvigorous manual ventilation (Rohfling et al, 1976).

Because tension pneumothorax can be rapidly fatal in ventilated patients with respiratory failure (Rohfling et al, 1976), intensive care personnel must always be alert to the possibility of this complication. Suggestive signs include the development, or worsening, of hypoxia, cyanosis, fighting the ventilator, an unexplained increase in inflation pressure, hypotension and tachycardia, sometimes accompanied by a rising CVP. Examination may reveal that one side of the chest is expanding more than the other, that there is mediastinal shift (deviated trachea, displaced apex beat) and that one or other hemithorax is hyperresonant. Although, traditionally, breath sounds are diminished over the pneumothorax, this sign can be extremely misleading in ventilated patients. If there is time, the diagnosis can be confirmed by chest x-ray.

In an extreme emergency, the tension can be relieved by inserting a large-bore intravenous cannula anteriorly through the second intercostal space in the midclavicular line. Indeed, some recommend this site as being the safest for insertion of chest drains by the inexperienced. However, it is preferable to place the drain through the sixth or seventh intercostal space in the midaxillary line. In this position, fluid as well as air can be removed, and it is cosmetically more acceptable. It is important not to insert the drain posteriorly, since it is very uncomfortable and easily kinked in this position. Chest drain insertion can be a very painful procedure; therefore, generous amounts of local anaesthetic should be used.

Pulmonary interstitial air is also important in neonates with respiratory distress syndrome as a harbinger of bronchopulmonary dysplasia, in which individual small areas of emphysema distend and compromise the expansion of remaining areas of lung. In those who survive, the lung remains damaged with interstitial fibrosis, microscopic emphysema and mucosal destruction. However, this gradually recovers over the next few years and pulmonary function is usually clinically normal by the time the child reaches school age. The aetiology of bronchopulmonary dysplasia is unknown, but as well as increased airway pressures, high concentrations of inspired oxygen are thought to contribute to its development.

Bronchiolectasis (a pronounced dilatation of terminal and respiratory

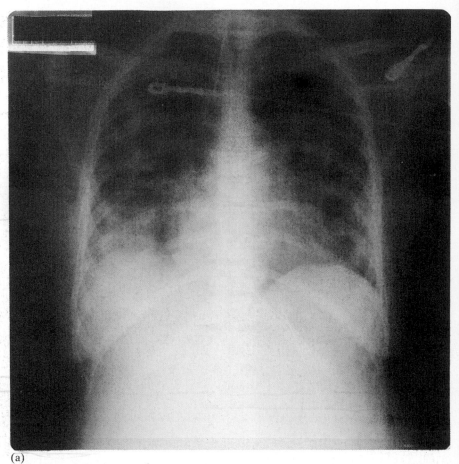

(a)

bronchioles) has been described in the lungs of adults dying following positive pressure ventilation with sustained high levels of PEEP (Slavin et al, 1982). These changes were associated with an increased V_D/V_T ratio, but the authors felt that oxygen toxicity was unlikely to be important in the pathogenesis of the lung lesions. A subsequent study suggests that these changes are reversible in those who survive (Navaratnarajah et al, 1984).

Respiratory

During spontaneous breathing, ventilation is preferentially distributed to the lower lung zones and this is matched by a similar increase in blood flow (see Chapter 2). During IPPV, however, ventilation is more evenly distributed throughout the lungs, leading to an increase in the overall V/Q ratio. This effect is enhanced when high intra-alveolar pressure (high inflation pressures, PEEP) and/or a reduced PAP divert blood flow away from apical lung zones. The net effect of IPPV is therefore normally an increase in V_D/V_T, but this is variable and usually of little clinical significance.

Patients ventilated with small tidal volumes become progressively more hypoxic. This is probably due to collapse of peripheral alveoli and can be

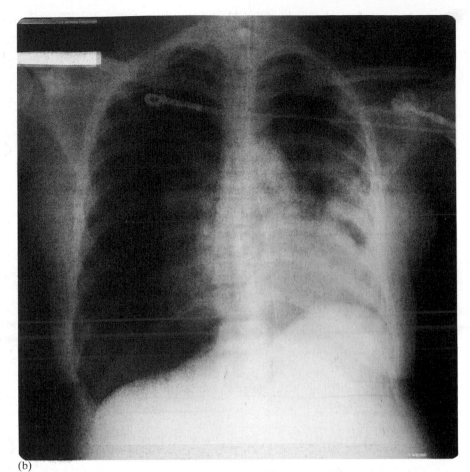

(b)

Fig. 13.4 (a) Bilateral consolidation with multiple cavities. (b) The same patient has developed a right tension pneumothorax (displacing the right hemidiaphragm inferiorly and the mediastinum to the left).

largely prevented by using greater tidal volumes ($10–15\,ml\,kg^{-1}$) and reducing the respiratory rate to avoid hypocarbia. Some ventilators incorporate a 'sigh' mechanism which regularly hyperinflates the lungs in an attempt to re-expand distal lung segments and prevent hypoxia. However, the benefits of 'sigh functions' have not been established; they may damage the lung tissue and in any case are unnecessary if sufficiently large tidal volumes are used.

Nosocomial pulmonary infection is a common and ominous complication of IPPV. This topic is discussed in Chapter 6.

Cardiovascular

The intermittent application of positive pressure to the lungs and thoracic wall reduces pre-load and distends alveoli, thereby 'stretching' the pulmonary capillaries and causing a rise in pulmonary vascular resistance. Both these mechanisms can produce a fall in cardiac output in patients on IPPV. It has been suggested that this may be exacerbated by a reduction in myocardial contractility caused by humoral (Grindlinger et al, 1979) or reflex mechanisms and, possibly, impaired coronary perfusion. Finally, reductions in carbon dioxide tension may also be responsible for a fall in cardiac output (Editorial, 1981).

In normal subjects, the fall in cardiac output is prevented by constriction of capacitance vessels which restores venous return. Hypovolaemia, pre-existing pulmonary hypertension, right ventricular failure and autonomic dysfunction (as may be present in those with Guillain-Barré syndrome, acute spinal cord injury and diabetes) will exacerbate the haemodynamic disturbance. Expansion of the circulating volume, on the other hand, can often restore cardiac output. In some cases, inotropic support is required in addition to volume expansion.

In patients with heart failure, a paradoxical rise in blood pressure and cardiac output may occur in response to both IPPV and IPPV with PEEP. This may be due to reversal of hypoxia and a reduction in oxygen consumption, both of which will reduce the burden on a failing heart. A further possible benefit in those with cardiac failure is that a reduction in pre-load will reduce ventricular wall tension, allowing increased coronary blood flow and improved myocardial function. Moreover, when the ventricular function curve is flat, the fall in pre-load has little effect on stroke volume, whilst stiff lungs limit the transmission of high inflation pressures to the great veins and pulmonary capillaries. One should therefore not hesitate to institute IPPV in patients with cardiogenic pulmonary oedema who have severe respiratory distress and exhaustion (see also Chapter 12).

Gastrointestinal

Initially, many artificially ventilated patients will develop abdominal distension associated with an ileus. The cause is unknown, although the use of non-depolarizing neuromuscular blocking agents may be in part responsible.

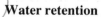

Water retention

IPPV, particularly with PEEP, may cause increased ADH secretion and this, combined with a fall in cardiac output and a reduction in renal cortical blood flow, can cause salt and water retention (Kumar et al, 1974). This excess fluid is distributed throughout the body compartments and, particularly if capillary permeability is increased and/or serum albumin levels are low, interstitial oedema will develop. This fluid retention is often particularly noticeable in the lungs, possibly because IPPV interferes with pulmonary lymphatic drainage, and may cause a deterioration in lung function. It is therefore advisable to restrict the total amount of salt and water administered to ventilated patients; approximately $20\,\mathrm{ml\,kg}^{-1}$ per day of 5% dextrose intravenously is usual in the first instance.

INSTITUTION OF IPPV

If the patient is conscious, the procedure must be fully explained before anaesthesia is induced.

Intubating patients in severe respiratory failure is an extremely dangerous undertaking and should only be performed by experienced staff. The patient is usually hypoxic, and may be hypercarbic, with increased sympathetic activity, and the oxygen mask has to be removed to allow intubation (although nasal cannulae can be left in situ). Under these circumstances, the stimulus of laryngoscopy followed by intubation can precipitate dangerous arrhythmias and even cardiac arrest. If possible, therefore, the ECG should be monitored during the procedure. The patient should be preoxygenated and ventilated with added oxygen, using a face mask and a self-inflating bag, prior to laryngoscopy. In some deeply comatose patients, no sedation will be required although when there is a possibility of intracranial hypertension, an intravenous anaesthetic agent should be administered to prevent surges in intracranial pressure. In the majority of patients, a short-acting intravenous anaesthetic agent followed by muscle relaxation will be necessary. In those at risk of regurgitation and aspiration of stomach contents, preoxygenation should be followed by administration of an intravenous anaesthetic agent and a rapidly acting muscle relaxant (usually suxamethonium). Cricoid pressure should be applied as soon as the patient loses consciousness and should not be released until the endotracheal tube is in place with the cuff inflated. It must be remembered that there is a risk of precipitating dangerous hyperkalaemia when suxamethonium is used in those with burns, renal failure, spinal injury or neuromuscular disease (see Chapter 11). Following endotracheal intubation, it is important to avoid the temptation to hyperventilate the patient, since this can lead to overinflation of the lungs and a fall in cardiac output, particularly in those with airway obstruction (see pp. 217–218).

MANAGEMENT OF PATIENTS ON VENTILATORS

General

Because the upper respiratory tract has been bypassed, the inspired gases must be artificially warmed, humidified and filtered. Patients on ventilators are unable to cough, sigh or take deep breaths and therefore regular physiotherapy, manual hyperinflation of the lungs and endotracheal suction are normally employed. This is of little value, however, in those with pulmonary oedema and, because removal of ventilation, PEEP and oxygen during endotracheal suction can precipitate extreme hypoxia, these techniques are often abandoned in such cases. The use of large tidal volumes, and possibly sigh functions, may help to prevent progressive collapse of alveoli. On the rare occasions when physiotherapy fails to re-expand a clearly defined area of collapsed lung, a fibre-optic bronchoscope may be used to aspirate secretions. (For further discussion of the general aspects of managing these patients, see Chapters 5, 6, 7 and 8).

Settling the patient on the ventilator

It is most important that mechanically ventilated patients do not 'fight the ventilator'. Not only can this increase oxygen consumption and carbon dioxide production, but the rise in mean intrathoracic pressure can reduce cardiac output. It is also distressing for the patient, relatives and staff.

Frequent explanation, reassurance and encouragement are essential for all alert patients. Manual hyperventilation with 100% oxygen will often assist initial synchronization with the ventilator by ensuring adequate oxygenation and a degree of hypocarbia. Most ventilated patients will require sedation. In the majority, the drug of first choice is a parenteral narcotic, which also provides analgesia and some respiratory depression. Many patients will also need an anxiolytic agent and usually a benzodiazepine is administered in combination with the opiate. In most cases—provided large tidal volumes are used, the arterial oxygen tension is within normal limits, there is moderate hypocarbia and sedation/analgesia is adequate—the patient will not fight the ventilator. If, despite these measures, the patient continues to make spontaneous respiratory efforts, synchronization may be achieved by using even larger tidal volumes. This is thought to increase the afferent impulses from stretch receptors in the lungs and inhibit the inspiratory neurones. Undue hypocarbia can be avoided by decreasing the respiratory rate and/or adding an extra dead space.

Causes of persistent failure to synchronize with the ventilator include hypoxia/hypercarbia, obstructed ventilation, severe pulmonary parenchymal disease (e.g. pulmonary oedema), bladder distension, metabolic acidosis and raised intracranial pressure. If specific treatment is not possible, then heavy sedation with opiates and benzodiazepines, and occasionally muscle relaxation, may be required. However, muscle relaxants should only be used as a last resort, or in certain special situations (e.g. in those with severe hypoxia or airway obstruction—see Chapter 12). The administration of muscle relaxants must always be accompanied by sedative/analgesic drugs in order to avoid the intolerable situation of a patient who is aware, and often in pain, but unable to move.

Clearly, bolus administration of these agents produces wide fluctuations in conscious levels, whilst intravenous opiates in particular often produce episodes of hypotension. Moreover, the administration of nitrous oxide in oxygen to critically ill patients has been implicated in the development of megaloblastic bone marrow change (Amos et al, 1982) and can no longer be recommended as a means of providing continuous analgesia and sedation for ventilated patients. More recently, therefore, continuous infusions of intravenous anaesthetic agents (such as etomidate or althesin), or a benzodiazepine (such as midazolam) sometimes combined with opiates, have been used to provide a consistent level of sedation and analgesia. However, neither althesin nor etomidate is currently available for use in this way. Althesin has been withdrawn by the manufacturers because of the relatively high incidence of anaphylactoid reactions to the solubilizing agent used in this preparation (Cremophor EL) (Morgan and Whitwam, 1985), whilst etomidate has been shown to suppress adrenocortical function (Moore et al, 1985). Furthermore, it is questionable whether, except in certain specific situations such as traumatic coma, it is desirable to anaesthetize ventilated patients for long periods. Indeed, there is a trend towards limiting the quantities of sedative and analgesic agents used to the minimum required to keep the patient relaxed, comfortable and pain-free. Under these circumstances, SIMV can be used so that the patient is able to make some spontaneous respiratory efforts (see below).

Selection of pattern of ventilation

The aim is to achieve optimal gas exchange while minimizing adverse effects on the cardiovascular system.

IPPV with negative end-expiratory pressure (NEEP)

In order to minimize the fall in cardiac output which occurs with IPPV, it was suggested that the application of a NEEP might increase venous return and restore cardiac output. Although this is in fact the case, NEEP also causes progressive alveolar collapse and hypoxia so that its use is now rarely, if ever, indicated.

IPPV with zero end-expiratory pressure (ZEEP)

As discussed above, IPPV per se may improve oxygenation by re-expanding collapsed alveoli, improving gas distribution and reducing oxygen require-ments. In order to prevent progressive alveolar collapse, large tidal volumes of $10-15 \, \text{ml kg}^{-1}$ should be used (see above).

The length of the inspiratory phase must be sufficient to allow filling of all distal lung segments. Since an alveolus will be 95% filled in three time constants (i.e. on average within 1.8 seconds in a normal lung), inspiration should last for between 1.5 and 2.0 seconds (see Chapter 2). In order to minimize the fall in cardiac output, the expiratory phase should be at least twice as long as inspiration (I : E ratio of 1 : 2) and both inflation and deflation should be relatively rapid. However, in those with severe lung disease there is an increased 'scatter' of time constants (see Chapter 2), and it may therefore be beneficial to prolong the inspiratory phase. In some cases, markedly extending inspiration so that the I : E ratio is reversed, sometimes to as much as 4 : 1, can improve gas distribution, re-expand collapsed areas of lung and increase P_aO_2 (Cole et al, 1984). The obvious danger of reversing the I : E ratio is cardiovascular depression, and in this respect the same considerations apply as during CPPV (see below).

The influence of the shape of the inspiratory waveform on the efficiency of gas exchange is less certain and probably of little clinical relevance (Fig. 13.5). A decelerating flow pattern is produced when a constant pressure is applied to the airway. This pattern of ventilation probably achieves the optimal distribution and uptake of inspired gas. It is also thought to be the most effective for re-expanding collapsed lung. However, mean intrathoracic pressure is highest with this 'square wave' pattern of positive pressure ventilation and it therefore causes the greatest reduction in cardiac output. In contrast, the pressure wave required to produce a constant flow pattern is associated with a relatively low mean intrathoracic pressure and minimal cardiovascular depression. A rising flow pattern appears to offer little clinical advantage.

Neonates and infants should be ventilated at a higher respiratory rate (25–30 breaths per minute) than older children and adults. They will normally require a minute volume of $100-200 \, \text{ml kg}^{-1}$.

INSPIRATORY WAVE FORM

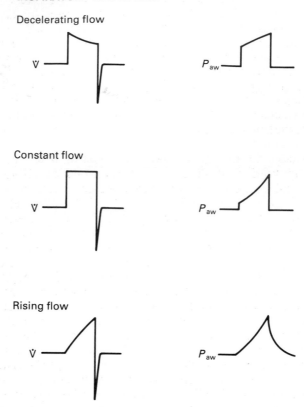

Decelerating flow

Constant flow

Rising flow

Fig. 13.5 Inspiratory waveforms (see text). $\dot{V}$ = flow; P_{aw} = airway pressure.

IPPV with PEEP

This is also frequently referred to as continuous positive pressure ventilation (CPPV). If it proves impossible to achieve adequate oxygenation of arterial blood (more than 90% saturation) without raising the inspired oxygen concentration to potentially dangerous levels (conventionally, $F_IO_2 > 0.5$, see Chapter 12), then the application of PEEP should be considered. PEEP is not, however, a panacea for all patients who are hypoxic and indeed can sometimes be detrimental, not least because the use of high levels is associated with an increased risk of barotrauma. Furthermore, it is not certain that the application of PEEP influences the ultimate outcome of acute respiratory failure (Petty, 1981a). Although some have suggested that the early or prophylactic use of PEEP in those at risk of developing ARDS can decrease the incidence and severity of subsequent pulmonary complications (Weigelt et al, 1979), a more recent controlled study has shown that early application of PEEP has no effect on the incidence of ARDS or other associated complications (Pepe et al, 1984). The rational use of PEEP is based on a knowledge of its physiological effects and of the pathophysiology of the patient's pulmonary disease.

The primary effect of PEEP is to expand underventilated lung units and increase FRC. Provided that shunting is due to alveolar collapse, this will reduce venous admixture and improve arterial oxygenation (Ashbaugh and Petty, 1973). As long as the rise in arterial oxygen content is not offset by a fall in cardiac output (see below), oxygen delivery also improves and there may be an associated increase in oxygen consumption. In general, the worse the shunt the greater the response to PEEP. It seems unlikely that PEEP primarily decreases extravascular lung water (Miller et al, 1981); indeed, it may have the opposite effect by interfering with lymphatic drainage. In some cases, the application of PEEP may be associated with an increased V_D/V_T ratio.

Unfortunately, the inevitable rise in mean intrathoracic pressure which follows the application of PEEP may further reduce pre-load, increase pulmonary vascular resistance and thus reduce cardiac output (Ashbaugh and Petty, 1973; Qvist et al, 1975; Editorial, 1981). This effect may be proportional to lung compliance (i.e. the stiffer the lungs the less the fall in cardiac output), although some studies do not support this contention (Beyer et al, 1982). It has also been suggested that a substance with negative inotropic activity is released when the lungs are stretched (Grindlinger et al, 1979; Editorial, 1981). Moreover, at levels of PEEP > 10 cmH$_2$O (1 kPa), the rise in pulmonary vascular resistance, and thus right ventricular after-load, may be associated with dilatation of the right ventricle. Because lateral expansion is restricted by the pericardium, the interventricular septum is displaced and encroaches on the left ventricular cavity. This is thought to restrict left ventricular filling and reduce stroke volume, despite a slight increase in myocardial contractility (Jardin et al, 1981; Editorial, 1981). The fall in cardiac output can be ameliorated by volume loading (Qvist et al, 1975), although when PEEP is removed relative hypervolaemia may precipitate pulmonary oedema (Qvist et al, 1975; Laaksonen et al, 1977), and in some cases inotropic support may be required. Thus although arterial oxygenation is often improved by the application of PEEP, a simultaneous fall in cardiac output can lead to a reduction in total oxygen delivery. This reduction in cardiac output is associated with a redistribution of blood flow favouring vital organs such as brain, heart and kidneys which may precipitate ischaemia of less important structures such as stomach, pancreas and liver. Although total renal blood flow is preserved, oliguria, with salt and water retention, is often observed and may be due to intrarenal redistribution of blood flow (Beyer et al, 1982) exacerbated by increased circulating ADH levels (Kumar et al, 1974). Nevertheless, if the same oxygen flux can be achieved with a lower cardiac output, PEEP may be beneficial by reducing myocardial work (Ashbaugh and Petty, 1973). Furthermore, some have demonstrated that cardiac index can be paradoxically higher during CPPV than IPPV or even spontaneous respiration (Laaksonen et al, 1977), and it has been suggested that low cardiac output need not be a deterrent to its use (Colgan et al, 1974).

The net effect of PEEP in an individual patient is therefore unpredictable and dependent on a balance of several factors. It is clear, however, that the most beneficial effects are likely to occur in those patients with low FRCs, large shunts, stiff lungs and good cardiovascular function. This is exemplified by the young fit patient with ARDS (see Chapter 12). On the other hand, in those with normal or high FRCs, compliant lungs and only a modest degree of shunting, the improvement in P_aO_2 may be negated by the fall in cardiac output, particularly in those with poor cardiovascular function. Thus, PEEP should not be used in patients with emphysema or asthma and is usually of little benefit in those with fibrotic lung disease or bacterial pneumonia (Ashbaugh and Petty, 1973). Furthermore, in patients with only localized areas of diseased lung (e.g. unilateral aspiration pneumonia), PEEP may adversely affect oxygenation by overexpanding normal lung tissue and diverting blood to underventilated lung units (see below).

Obviously, careful monitoring of the effects of PEEP is essential and it should now be clear that simply measuring P_aO_2 is often not sufficient. It is also important to select the level of PEEP at which oxygen flux is maximal: so-called 'best PEEP'. By measuring P_aO_2, $P_{\bar{v}}O_2$ and cardiac output, the effect of PEEP can be accurately assessed; it is also possible to calculate venous admixture and oxygen delivery. In difficult cases, it is therefore often necessary to insert a Swan–Ganz catheter. A few centres actually measure the changes in FRC in response to PEEP.

If PEEP is removed, P_aO_2 falls almost immediately, whilst following its reapplication P_aO_2 may take up to 60 minutes to return to previous levels (Kumar et al, 1970).

Children under six years old have low FRCs, which are less than their closing volume, and they should therefore always be ventilated with 5 cmH$_2$O (0.5 kPa) PEEP unless this is specifically contraindicated.

Continuous positive airway pressure

CPAP achieves for the spontaneously breathing patient what PEEP does for the ventilated patient. Not only can it improve oxygenation by the same mechanism, but the lungs become less stiff, breathing becomes easier, respiratory rate falls and both vital capacity and inspiratory force have been shown to improve (Feeley et al, 1975; Venus et al, 1979). The cause of the increased compliance can be appreciated by referring to Fig. 2.19 (p. 27), which shows the compliance curve for the lung and chest wall combined. Normally, tidal exchange takes place from the resting expiratory position at which the tendency for the lungs to collapse is exactly counterbalanced by the tendency of the chest wall to expand and the pressure difference is zero. It can be seen that this is also the steepest point on the curve at which relatively small changes in pressure produce a large change in volume, i.e. compliance is greatest and the work of breathing minimal. As lung volume falls, however, the curve becomes flatter, i.e. the lungs become stiffer and the work of breathing increases. The application of positive airway pressure re-expands the lungs and compliance increases. If the lungs are overexpanded, then compliance will again fall.

Because mean intrathoracic pressure is lower with CPAP than with IPPV plus PEEP, haemodynamic depression is minimized (Venus et al, 1979; Simonneau et al, 1982), renal perfusion is maintained and the incidence of barotrauma may be reduced. Furthermore, heavy sedation is unnecessary. A circuit suitable for applying CPAP is shown in Fig. 13.6.

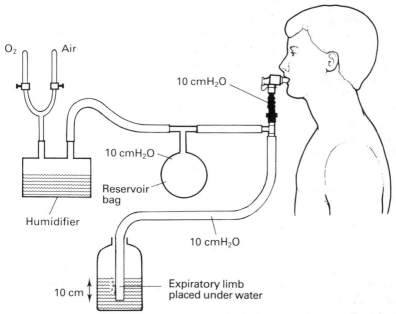

O₂   Air

10 cmH₂O

10 cmH₂O

Reservoir
bag

Humidifier

10 cmH₂O

Expiratory limb
placed under water

10 cm

Figure 13.6 Circuit for applying a continuous positive airway pressure. The fresh gas flow must be sufficient to maintain the reservoir bag distended throughout the respiratory cycle, with continuous bubbling of the underwater seal; i.e. the circuit is pressurized to the required level throughout the respiratory cycle.

CPAP can be used as the primary treatment in patients with acute hypoxaemic respiratory failure who are not exhausted and in whom alveolar ventilation is adequate (Venus et al, 1979). The use of a tight-fitting face mask allows the application of CPAP without the need for endotracheal intubation or tracheostomy (Greenbaum et al, 1976). However, such masks are uncomfortable to wear for prolonged periods and the technique is only suitable for those who are alert, able to clear secretions and protect their airway. Gastric distension, vomiting and aspiration are a potential risk and a nasogastric tube should be inserted in all patients receiving mask CPAP.

CPAP is also useful for weaning patients who have required PEEP while being ventilated since it prevents the alveolar collapse and hypoxia which might otherwise occur (Feeley et al, 1975). In general, therefore, patients who have required CPAP should not be allowed to breathe spontaneously through an endotracheal tube with ZEEP but rather should be extubated directly from 5 cmH₂O (0.5 kPa) of PEEP. Once extubated, patients probably provide their own 'PEEP' using, for example, pursed lip breathing.

Infants are obligate nose breathers and thereby produce their own CPAP. Therefore, when breathing spontaneously through an endotracheal tube, they should always receive CPAP. Positive pressure can also be applied via a 'nasal prong' or, in neonates, using a head box.

Independent lung ventilation (Hillman and Barber, 1980)

Occasionally, a patient with predominantly unilateral lung disease, e.g. following aspiration of gastric contents, will require positive pressure ventilation. Under these circumstances, conventional IPPV may fail to achieve satisfactory gas exchange. The normal 'compliant' lung tends to become overinflated, while the stiff, diseased lung collapses progressively, causing further mechanical deterioration. Furthermore, pulmonary blood flow is diverted away from normal alveoli to underventilated areas of lung and shunt is increased. The application of PEEP in an attempt to re-expand the diseased lung simply exacerbates the situation. Finally, the 'good' lung is exposed to the high concentrations of oxygen required to combat hypoxia and as a result may itself be damaged.

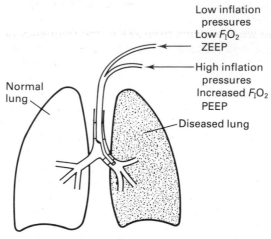

Fig. 13.7 Independent lung ventilation.

In such cases, it is possible to ventilate each lung independently, using separate ventilators, through a double lumen endotracheal tube (Fig. 13.7). The diseased lung can then be ventilated using high inflation pressures, an increased $F_I O_2$ and, if indicated, PEEP or a reversed I : E ratio. The good lung is ventilated conventionally and is therefore protected from the adverse effects of exposure to high airway pressures and potentially toxic concentrations of oxygen. Initially, it was thought that in order to avoid marked reductions in cardiac output, both lungs should inflate and deflate synchronously. It is possible to achieve this by linking two ventilators electronically but it is not, in fact, necessary to do so (Hillman and Barber, 1980). Numerous variations of the technique have been described, including the application of CPAP or high frequency jet ventilation (see below) to the diseased lung.

Assisted mechanical ventilation (AMV)

This technique, in which the patient's own respiratory efforts trigger a positive pressure inflation, has been used in some centres, particularly in North America, as an alternative to controlled mechanical ventilation (CMV). Using AMV, it is not necessary to abolish the patient's respiratory efforts and the use of heavy sedation and paralysis can in some cases be avoided.

Intermittent mandatory ventilation (IMV)

This was originally introduced as a technique for weaning patients from artificial ventilation (Downs et al, 1973) but is increasingly being used as an alternative to conventional IPPV (either CMV or AMV). IMV allows the patient to breathe spontaneously between the 'mandatory' tidal volumes delivered by the ventilator. Most modern ventilators will time the mandatory breath to coincide with the patient's own inspiratory effort (synchronized IMV, SIMV) and IMV can be used with, or without, PEEP/CPAP. Since its introduction, considerable controversy has surrounded the use of this technique both for weaning and as a means of ventilatory support (Petty, 1981b; Downs and Douglas, 1981).

When used to wean patients from IPPV, the frequency of the mandatory breaths is progressively reduced so that spontaneous respiration accounts for an increasing proportion of the total minute volume (see below). As a technique for providing ventilatory support, IMV has a number of potential advantages when compared with CMV (Weisman et al, 1983). Firstly, because it is unnecessary to abolish all respiratory efforts, heavy sedation and muscle relaxation can be avoided. This, combined with the reduction in mean intrathoracic pressure, means there is less cardiovascular depression, and renal function is preserved (Steinhoff et al, 1984). It has also been suggested that the risk of barotrauma is reduced (Mathru et al, 1983). Respiratory alkalosis may be avoided and intrapulmonary gas distribution may be more uniform. Finally, because patients continue to breathe, the strength and co-ordination of respiratory muscles is relatively well maintained. Suggested disadvantages of IMV include increased work of breathing with respiratory muscle fatigue and a risk of carbon dioxide retention. Moreover, the potential advantages of IMV are less clear when compared with AMV rather than CMV.

Mandatory minute volume (MMV) (Hewlett et al, 1977)

This modification of IMV ensures that the patient always receives the preset minute volume despite moment-to-moment variations in the level of spontaneous ventilation. Although MMV is inherently safer, it is in fact used less frequently in clinical practice than SIMV.

High-frequency jet ventilation (HFJV)

Surprisingly, it is possible to achieve adequate oxygenation and carbon dioxide elimination by injecting gas into the trachea at rates of up to several thousand breaths per minute. In clinical practice, ventilation at between 60 and 300 breaths per minute, with tidal volumes of $1-5\,\mathrm{ml\,kg^{-1}}$, is usually employed. Although it is known that adequate oxygenation can be produced by 'apnoeic diffusion', it is unclear how carbon dioxide elimination is achieved with this technique. Some consider that this can be explained by the reduction in dead space which is known to occur as tidal volume falls (see Chapter 2). Others feel that conventional physiology cannot account for the removal of carbon dioxide and attribute the gas exchange produced with this technique to 'augmented' or 'facilitated' diffusion.

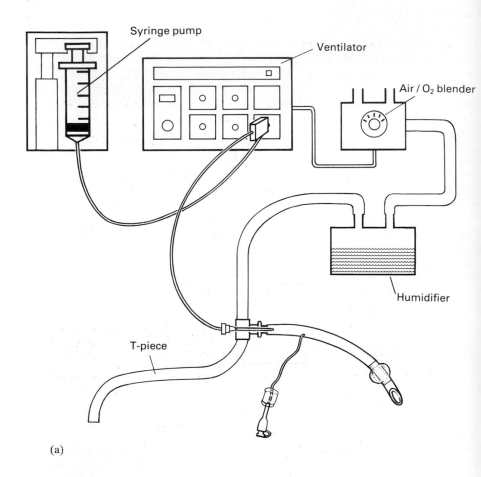

(a)

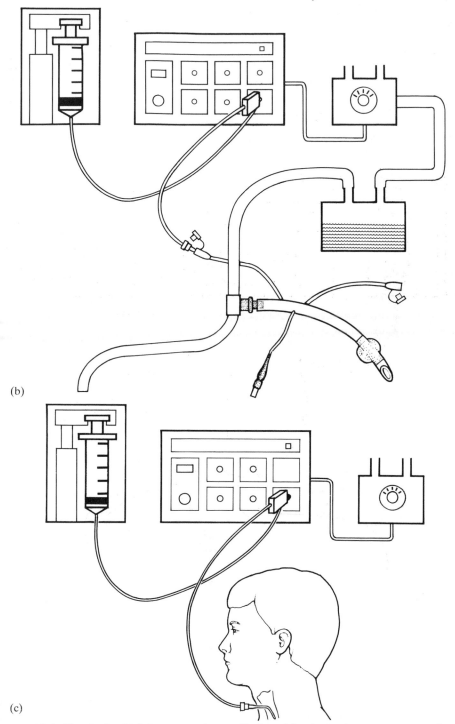

(b)

(c)

Fig. 13.8 Circuits for high frequency jet ventilation: (a) using an intravenous cannula positioned in an endotracheal tube; (b) using a modified endotracheal tube; (c) using a cannula positioned in the trachea via the cricothyroid membrane.

HFJV can be applied via an intravenous cannula positioned centrally in an endotracheal tube or a transtracheal catheter placed within the trachea via the cricothyroid membrane. Alternatively, a modified endotracheal tube with a small additional lumen opening distally can be used. It has been suggested that HFJV via the cricothyroid membrane may be a useful approach in emergencies. However, this could be dangerous in the presence of upper airway obstruction, when overinflation of the lungs may cause serious barotrauma, and correct positioning of the cannula is clearly essential. Aspiration will be prevented as long as 'jetting' continues (Klain et al, 1983), but most clinicians inflate the cuff on the endotracheal tube in order to protect the airway in the event of a technical mishap or disconnection. The main practical difficulty is provision of adequate humidification. Suitable circuits for HFJV are shown in Fig. 13.8.

Potential advantages of HFJV are largely related to the low peak airway pressures; thus, venous return is preserved, changes in pulmonary vascular resistance are minimal and cardiac output is well maintained. Furthermore, the risk of barotrauma is negligible. Another possible advantage is that HFJV appears to suppress the respiratory drive and unobstructed spontaneous respiration can take place via the T-piece circuit. Therefore, many alert patients find this form of artificial ventilation particularly easy to tolerate and weaning from ventilatory support can normally be achieved relatively smoothly. Indeed, in some patients HFJV may facilitate weaning when other methods have failed (Klain et al, 1984).

Clinical experience of HFJV is at present limited. Nevertheless, it is clear that this technique is valuable in the management of patients with large air leaks (e.g. those with bronchopleural fistulae or lung lacerations) who require ventilatory support (Derderian et al, 1982). In such patients, the air leak is markedly reduced on changing from IPPV to HFJV, and indeed in some cases, spontaneous healing of the damaged lung may then occur.

The place of HFJV in the management of patients with ARF is less clear (Schuster et al, 1982). Although it is possible to apply a PEEP to the expiratory limb of the circuit (and also to achieve a small PEEP effect by increasing the respiratory rate to above 200 per minute), the institution of HFJV may be associated with a temporary increase in shunt (Sladen et al, 1984), and this justifies the initial administration of a high $F_I O_2$ (0.8–1.0) until oxygenation can be assessed. In general, however, it appears that at the same $F_I O_2$ and level of PEEP, arterial oxygenation is either unchanged (Schuster et al, 1982) or improved (Vincken and Cosio, 1984) when HFJV is compared with IPPV. HFJV has therefore been recommended for those with stiff lungs who require very high inflation pressures during IPPV, and in those in whom conventional IPPV produces severe cardiovascular depression (Vincken and Cosio, 1984).

Extracorporeal membrane oxygenation (ECMO)

This technique was developed in an attempt to save the lives of some patients who would otherwise inevitably have died from severe, progressive ARF. It was based on the premise that the lungs of such patients would eventually recover, provided death from hypoxia could be avoided. This proved not to be the case since in the majority of cases the lung lesion continued to progress, culminating in irreversible pulmonary fibrosis. Moreover, prolonged respiratory support with ECMO presents formidable logistic difficulties and requires a disproportionate allocation of resources. When a randomized prospective study demonstrated that the mortality of groups of patients with severe ARF was similar whether or not ECMO was employed (Zapol et al, 1979), its use was abandoned.

Low-frequency positive pressure ventilation with extracorporeal carbon dioxide removal (Gattinoni et al, 1980)

Following the disappointing results obtained with ECMO, an alternative approach was developed. This involves the removal of carbon dioxide by passing a relatively low flow of blood over a membrane while oxygenation is achieved via the lungs. The latter are ventilated two or three times per minute and are continuously maintained at a positive pressure with an appropriate fresh gas flow. Initial results are encouraging and are attributed to enhanced resolution of the pulmonary lesion as a result of 'resting' the lungs. It is, however, too early to be certain of the value of this technique.

Weaning (Feeley and Hedley-Whyte, 1975; Browne, 1984)

As discussed above, the use of IPPV can be complicated by alveolar collapse, pulmonary oedema, barotrauma and secondary pneumonia. Moreover, cardiac output and renal blood flow are reduced. It is therefore important to discontinue artificial ventilation, and, if possible, to extubate the patient as soon as possible. On the other hand, premature attempts at weaning may be dangerous and can adversely affect the morale of conscious patients.

Because they perform no work during conventional mechanical ventilation, the respiratory muscles eventually become weak and uncoordinated. Moreover, there is usually some persisting abnormality of lung function. Thus, in patients who have been artificially ventilated for any length of time, spontaneous respiration normally has to resume gradually.

Criteria for weaning patients from artificial ventilation

Clinical. Clinical assessment is of paramount importance when deciding whether a patient can be weaned from the ventilator. The patient's conscious level, psychological state, metabolic function, the effects of drugs, cardiovascular performance and lung mechanics must all be taken into account.

An altered level of consciousness does not necessarily prevent weaning, but patients should not be extubated until they can cough, co-operate with physiotherapy and protect their own airway. However, weaning will often prove difficult in those who are restless, confused and uncooperative. In such cases, it is sometimes preferable to continue artificial ventilation and to institute measures to improve the patient's mental state. Some patients who have undergone a prolonged period of artificial ventilation become psychologically dependent on the ventilator (see Chapter 7); they will require particular care and continual reassurance throughout the weaning period.

Malnourished patients may have difficulty in sustaining adequate alveolar ventilation. For this, and many other reasons (see Chapter 5), malnutrition should if possible be prevented or corrected by providing an adequate protein/energy intake during the patient's hospitalization and by correcting any specific deficiencies, in particular hypophosphataemia (Aubier et al, 1985). On the other hand, some patients with borderline respiratory function may be unable to excrete the large quantities of carbon dioxide produced by the metabolism of high energy glucose feeds (see Chapter 5). Similarly, increased oxygen demands, e.g. in response to fever or shivering, can prevent successful weaning. It is also important to correct any significant abnormalities of acid–base balance. This is because a metabolic alkalosis can blunt the respiratory drive and cause carbon dioxide retention, while patients with a metabolic acidosis will attempt to hyperventilate to produce a compensatory respiratory alkalosis.

The possibility that the residual effects of drugs are impairing respiration must also be considered. Of most importance in this respect are the opiates and the non-depolarizing muscle relaxants; both are a particular problem in the presence of renal failure.

Cardiovascular stability is another important prerequisite for successful weaning. In particular, weaning is unlikely to be accomplished, and may be dangerous, in patients with a low cardiac output; indeed, in some cases failure to wean is associated with an unexpected fall in cardiac output (Beach et al, 1973). This is partly because when cardiac output is low, there is a reduction in pulmonary artery pressure and the number of relatively underperfused alveoli increases. The V_D/V_T ratio therefore rises. Moreover, oxygen delivery is very precarious under these circumstances. Life-threatening dysrhythmias and bleeding likely to require surgical intervention, e.g. after cardiac surgery, are other contraindications to discontinuing ventilation. On the other hand, provided the patient is stable, dependence on inotropic support and/or IABCP is not a contraindication to commencing cautious weaning.

Finally, mechanical factors likely to impair ventilation, such as abdominal distension and pleural effusions should, if possible, be corrected.

Objective. Although many objective criteria for the ability to wean have been suggested (Skillman et al, 1971; Sahn and Lakshminarayan, 1973; Feeley and Hedley-Whyte, 1975), these sometimes prove misleading (Michel et al, 1979). In most cases, a clinical assessment as outlined above, together with blood gas analysis (considered in conjunction with the F_IO_2 and the minute volume) and an assessment of the mechanical state of the patient's lungs, will be sufficient to make the correct decision. Certainly, the quantitative criteria for weaning described below are not absolute and should only be used as guidelines.

The gas exchanging properties of the lungs may be considered adequate for weaning if the P_aO_2 is >10 kPa (80 mmHg) with an F_IO_2 <0.5 (some suggest a P_aO_2 >8 kPa (60 mmHg) with an F_IO_2 of 0.4), if the $P_{A-a}O_2$ is <40–47 kPa (300–350 mmHg) with an $F_IO_2 = 1.0$, if the percentage venous admixture is <15% and if the V_D/V_T ratio is <0.58–0.6 (Skillman et al, 1971; Feeley and Hedley-Whyte, 1975). The patient should not require >15 cmH$_2$O (1.5 kPa) PEEP. The strength of the respiratory muscles in relation to the mechanical properties of the lungs can be assessed by measuring vital capacity (which should be >10–15 ml kg^{-1} to commence weaning) and the maximum inspiratory force (which should be $>-20\,\mathrm{cmH_2O}$ ($-2\,\mathrm{kPa}$)). In one study, all those patients who were able to produce a peak negative pressure of $>-30\,\mathrm{cmH_2O}$ weaned successfully, while a resting minute volume of $<10\,\mathrm{l\,min^{-1}}$ and the ability to double this voluntarily correlated well with weaning (Sahn and Lakshminarayan, 1973). If the cardiac index can be measured, it should be $>2\,\mathrm{l\,min^{-1}\,m^{-2}}$. Finally, the pH should be between 7.3 and 7.5.

Techniques for weaning

Patients who have undergone artificial ventilation for less than 24 hours, e.g. elective IPPV after major surgery, can usually resume spontaneous respiration immediately and no weaning process is required. They should be connected to a T-piece circuit and provided with humidified fresh gas of an appropriate F_IO_2 (Fig. 13.9). This procedure can also be adopted for those who have been ventilated for longer periods but who clearly fulfil the criteria for weaning outlined above. The traditional method of weaning in difficult cases is to allow the patient to breathe entirely spontaneously for a short time, following which he is reconnected to the ventilator. The periods of spontaneous breathing are gradually increased and periods of IPPV are reduced. Initially, it is usually advisable to ventilate the patient throughout

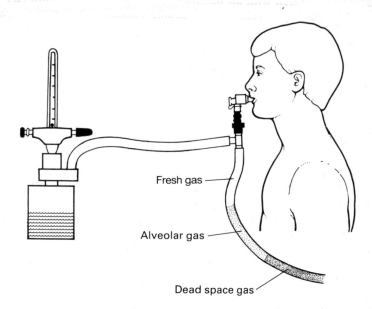

Fresh gas

Alveolar gas

Dead space gas

Fig. 13.9 A T-piece circuit: situation at end-expiration. Expired gases are prevented from entering the inspiratory limb by the flow of fresh gas. During the end-expiratory pause fresh gas enters the expiratory limb, pushing the expired gases distally. At peak-inspiration, when the fresh gas flow may be insufficient, fresh gas can be entrained from the expiratory limb of the T-piece. In order to prevent rebreathing of alveolar gas, the fresh gas flow must exceed 2½ times the patient's minute volume. In order to prevent entrainment of air, the volume of the expiratory limb must be greater than the patient's tidal volume.

the night. This method has several practical disadvantages; during the period of spontaneous respiration, the patient may develop progressive hypoxia and/or hypercarbia as well as increasing sympathetic drive with tachycardia and hypertension. After a predetermined period, or earlier if tachypnoea and exhaustion develop, the patient is reconnected to IPPV. At this time, respiratory drive is high, synchronization with the ventilator is difficult and heavy sedation may be required. It is then necessary to wait until the effects of these drugs have worn off before trying another period of spontaneous respiration. This method is stressful and tiring for both patients and staff. However, some patients do not tolerate IMV and this method of weaning may then prove more successful.

These disadvantages may be overcome by using IMV or MMV. As described above, these techniques provide a smoother, more controlled method of weaning; they may also enable weaning to commence at an earlier stage than is possible using the conventional method. There is no evidence, however, that they enable patients who could not be weaned using conventional methods to resume spontaneous respiration, and in some cases the weaning process may be unnecessarily prolonged. The performance of the IMV circuits on some ventilators is unsatisfactory (Cox and Niblett, 1984) and this may actually hinder weaning in those with borderline respiratory function.

The application of CPAP can prevent the alveolar collapse, hypoxaemia and fall in compliance which may otherwise occur when patients start to breathe spontaneously (Feeley et al, 1975; Feeley and Hedley-Whyte, 1975). It is therefore often used during weaning with IMV and in spontaneously breathing patients prior to extubation, particularly when they were previously receiving CPPV. As mentioned above, it is important to extubate such patients from $5\,cmH_2O$ (0.5 kPa) PEEP rather than following a period of spontaneous ventilation at ZEEP.

Extubation

This should not be considered until the patient can cough, swallow, protect his own airway and is sufficiently alert to be co-operative. Patients who fulfil these criteria can be extubated provided their respiratory function has improved sufficiently to sustain spontaneous ventilation indefinitely. This is often difficult to assess and is usually largely based on the patient's ability to breathe spontaneously via the endotracheal tube over a period of time. In those who have undergone prolonged artificial ventilation, this period may be for 24–48 hours, or even longer, while patients ventilated for less than 12–24 hours can often be extubated within 10–15 minutes. During this 'trial of spontaneous respiration', the patient should be closely observed for any signs of respiratory distress (tachypnoea, use of accessory muscles, 'gasping' respirations, tachycardia, sweating) and the tidal volume and respiratory rate should be recorded frequently. Some suggested quantitative criteria for extubation include a respiratory rate of <35 per minute, a vital capacity of >10–$15\,ml\,kg^{-1}$ and an inspiratory force of $>-25\,cmH_2O$ (-2.5 kPa). The criteria relating to oxygenation are similar to those for weaning mentioned above, except that the patient should not require $>5\,cmH_2O$ (0.5 kPa) CPAP.

ENDOTRACHEAL INTUBATION

Indications

Apart from providing a route for mechanical ventilation and the application of CPAP, endotracheal intubation may be required to secure and maintain a clear airway, protect the lungs and to allow control of bronchial secretions.

Complications

Early

All the common immediate hazards of endotracheal intubation cause difficulty with inflation of one or both lungs. It is therefore essential to ensure that both sides of the chest are expanding equally and adequately at all times and that the inflation pressure is not excessive.

A common mistake is intubation of one or other bronchus, usually the right since this is most directly in line with the trachea, and in one series this occurred in 9% of all endotracheal intubations (Stauffer et al, 1981). As a result, the left lung, and often the right upper lobe, collapse and the patient becomes hypoxic. Therefore, the length of an endotracheal tube must always be checked on the chest x-ray and if the tip is close to or beyond the carina, the tube should be withdrawn. Some authorities recommend that a mark should be made a few centimetres proximal to the cuff and that the tube should be positioned so that this mark lies between the vocal cords.

Accidental intubation of the oesophagus can sometimes be surprisingly difficult to recognize. Hypoxia with gaseous distension of the stomach may then develop rapidly. Endotracheal tubes can migrate out of the trachea so that they come to lie in the pharynx; this process is often accelerated by overinflation of the cuff in an attempt to abolish the leak which inevitably develops when the cuff herniates between the vocal cords. A leak around the tube will also develop if the cuff ruptures; this is usually clearly audible.

Obstruction may be due to inspissated secretions, kinking, biting on the tube, cuff herniation, compression of the tube by an overinflated cuff or the bevel of the tube impinging on the tracheal wall or carina.

All these acute complications are potentially extremely dangerous and must be recognized promptly and dealt with appropriately. If at any time the tube becomes obstructed (indicated by the patient becoming distressed and/or cyanosed with inadequate or absent expansion of one or both sides of the chest, accompanied by a rise in inflation pressures and activation of the ventilator alarm), the following procedure should be adopted:
1 Attempt manual inflation with 100% oxygen.
2 Check and adjust position of tube. If correct,
3 Deflate cuff (relieves obstruction if due to cuff herniation or tube compression).
4 Apply endotracheal suction (may confirm or relieve obstruction).
5 Check that the tube is not kinked in the oropharynx.
6 Change endotracheal tube.
If a significant leak develops which cannot be abolished by reinflating the cuff, either the endotracheal tube has dislodged into the oropharynx or the cuff has ruptured. If the tube has become misplaced, it should be removed and the

patient ventilated using a face mask and Ambu bag prior to reintubation. If the cuff is leaking, the endotracheal tube should be replaced electively.

Late

Prolonged pressure on the structures of the upper respiratory tract, caused either by the tube itself or the cuff, causes mucosal oedema which may then progress to ulceration. This later heals by granulation with the development of fibrotic scar tissue and tracheal narrowing. The points at which excessive pressure may occur are shown in Fig. 13.10. At the level of the glottis, the posterior aspect of the vocal cords, the arytenoid cartilages and the cricoarytenoid joints may be damaged while in some, the lesions extend down into the subglottic space (Stauffer et al, 1981). Damage may also occur at the

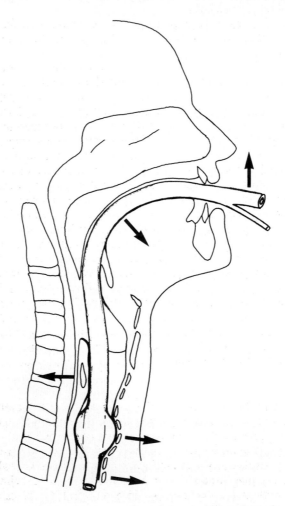

Fig. 13.10 Points at which excessive pressure is exerted by endotracheal tube. From Lindholm & Grenvik (1977), with permission.

level of the cuff, often anteriorly, and this may be extensive with complete loss of mucosa and exposure of underlying tracheal cartilage. Granuloma formation is unusual (Stauffer et al, 1981). The ways in which this damage may be minimized are as follows:

1 *Tube size.* In order to avoid the risk of circular subglottic stenosis, a tube with an external diameter well below the internal diameter of the cricoid ring should be used. This is particularly important in children in whom an uncuffed tube, small enough to allow an audible leak, should be used (see below).

2 *Tube shape.* It is important that the endotracheal tube is made of thermolabile material so that once in place it conforms to the shape of the airway. Conventional red rubber tubes are not thermolabile and have a pronounced curvature. Consequently, undue force is exerted, particularly on the medial aspects of the arytenoid cartilages and on both sides of the midline at the cricoid plate (Fig. 13.10).

3 *Movements of the larynx.* Coughing and straining on the tube is thought to increase the risk of mucosal damage, and the arytenoid cartilages are again particularly vulnerable.

4 *Tube cuff.* High pressures are required to inflate the cuffs of standard red rubber endotracheal tubes and, because their shape does not conform to that of the trachea, this high pressure is concentrated on a small area of the tracheal wall, impairing capillary blood flow in the underlying tracheal mucosa. In addition, prolonged high cuff pressures may lead to distension of the trachea, with eventual erosion of the cartilagenous rings. It has been shown that by using high-volume, preshaped, low-pressure cuffs made of non-irritant material, the severity of the tracheal injury can be minimized (Grillo et al, 1971). It is important that these cuffs are not overinflated since, once a seal has been created, further inflation causes a steep rise in intracuff pressure. Inflation of the cuff beyond this point can be avoided by monitoring the intracuff pressure, or by using a pressure-limiting valve, and this may reduce the incidence of cuff-related complications (Lewis et al, 1978). Nevertheless, severe laryngotracheal injury may still occur (Stauffer et al, 1981) and progressive, but temporary, tracheal dilatation, mainly affecting the muscles of the posterior wall, has been described following the prolonged use of low pressure cuffs (Leverment et al, 1975). This may partly account for the observation that low-pressure cuffs are not an entirely reliable barrier to the aspiration of liquid such as acid gastric secretions. Intermittent deflation of the cuff is no longer practised since it is unnecessary and may precipitate aspiration of pooled infected material from the oropharynx.

Other factors thought to increase the risk of mucosal damage include prolonged intubation, episodes of hypotension during which mucosal blood flow is further compromised, the administration of steroids and tracheitis due to pooling of infected material above the cuff. Despite the relatively high incidence of laryngeal injury detected at autopsy, late laryngeal sequelae of prolonged endotracheal intubation are rare in survivors. Tracheal stenosis is more common and in one series was detected in 19% of cases following endotracheal intubation. The incidence was even higher after tracheostomy (65%) but in most of these patients tracheal narrowing occurred at stomal, rather than cuff, level. However, only one patient with tracheal stenosis had symptoms of upper airway obstruction (Stauffer et al, 1981).

Oral or nasal endotracheal intubation?

Many patients are unable to tolerate oral endotracheal tubes and this applies particularly to those who are fully conscious and require prolonged intubation. In these cases, the nasal route may be preferred since it is more comfortable and secure fixation of the tube is more easily achieved. Furthermore, damage to, or occlusion of, the tube by the teeth is avoided. However, nasal endotracheal intubation has a number of disadvantages, including epistaxis, damage to the nasopharyngeal mucosa (including submucosal insertion of the tube), erosion of the alar cartilages, necrosis of the nasal septum (Stauffer et al, 1981), difficulty with bronchial suction and increased resistance to gas flow. Nasal intubation is contraindicated in those with adjacent facial or skull fractures and may be associated with septicaemia secondary to sinus infection or otitis media (Stauffer et al, 1981). On the other hand, ulceration of the corners of the mouth and superadded fungal infection may complicate the use of oral tubes. Furthermore, laryngeal injury may be more common with oral, as opposed to nasal, intubation (Stauffer et al, 1981). The choice of route in an individual patient often depends largely on the experience and preference of a particular unit, but each undoubtedly has its place.

Endotracheal intubation in paediatric practice

Secure fixation of the endotracheal tube is particularly important in paediatric practice since displacement is a constant danger in these small patients. This is

Table 13.3 Recommended sizes of endotracheal tubes in relation to age.

Age	Tube size in mm (internal diameter)
<2 months	2.5–3.0
3–5 months	3.0–3.5
6–9 months	3.5–4.0
10–12 months	4.0–4.5
2–4 years	4.5–5.0
5 years	5.0–5.5
6–7 years	5.5–6.0
8–9 years	6.0–6.5
10 years	6.5–7.0
11–12 years	7.0–7.5

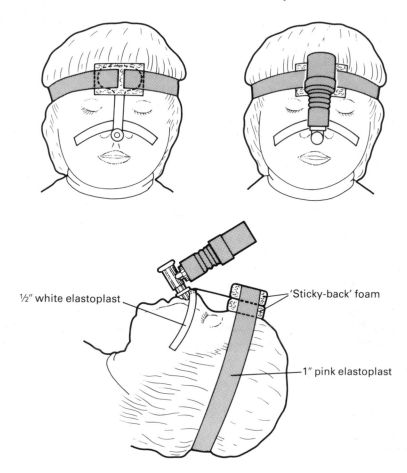

Fig. 13.11 A suitable method for fixation for paediatric endotracheal tubes using a Tunstall connector.

best achieved using the nasal route which has the additional advantages of reducing the risk of kinking in the oropharynx and avoiding the danger of palatal ulceration. Moreover, in neonates, infants and young children, as large a tube can be passed via the nasal route as can be inserted orally. Uncuffed tubes should always be used in prepubertal patients and, because of the risk of stenosis at the level of the cricoid cartilage (which is extremely difficult to treat), there should be as large a leak around the tube as is compatible with efficient positive pressure ventilation. An approximate guide to suitable tube sizes in relation to age is shown in Table 13.3. If long-term ventilation is envisaged, the smaller of the two sizes should be used and, if there is any doubt, one-half size smaller than that. A Tunstall connector is preferred for tube sizes <6.0 mm and a suitable method of fixation is shown in Fig. 13.11.

It is always safest to first control the airway with an oral tube. If this is the correct size, it can then be replaced by a nasal tube of the same size, measured and cut to length under direct vision. The cut end of the tube should be taped to the bed so that its diameter can be easily checked and a tube of the same size should be immediately available.

Care of the intubated child

A daily check should be made for the presence or absence of a leak around the tube. If the leak disappears and the tube was originally a loose fit, it is not necessary to change down to a smaller size. However, if there was any doubt about its size initially, it is prudent to change down one-half size. Otherwise, it is generally recommended that endotracheal tubes be changed weekly unless extubation is imminent.

The risk of obstruction of small diameter endotracheal tubes with encrusted secretions must be minimized by ensuring adequate humidification and by regular tracheobronchial suction. It is important to use suction catheters of the correct size in order to avoid large negative intrathoracic pressures on one hand or inefficient suction on the other. Recommended sizes of suction catheters are shown in Table 13.4.

Table 13.4 Recommended size of suction catheters in relation to internal diameter of endotracheal tube.

Tube size in mm	Suction catheter (French gauge)
2.5	6
3.0–4.5	8
>4.5	10

To reduce the possibility of aspiration of gastric contents, a nasogastric tube should always be passed and left on free drainage. This also helps to avoid gastric distension which may compromise respiration in those breathing spontaneously. Head-up tilt can also be used if the circulation permits. An oropharyngeal pack is irritant and unnecessary unless there is a particular likelihood of regurgitation, or if the leak around the endotracheal is too great to allow effective IPPV.

TRACHEOSTOMY

Indications

There is a small, but significant, mortality (up to 3%) associated with tracheostomy and the morbidity is greater than that of prolonged endotracheal intubation (Stauffer et al, 1981). Although the use of tracheostomy has therefore declined, there are a number of situations in which the technique remains invaluable. Furthermore, the long-term laryngeal dysfunction which may occur following prolonged intubation, although rare, is difficult to treat.

The only indication for immediate tracheostomy is a life-threatening obstruction of the upper respiratory tract which cannot be bypassed with an endotracheal tube. Tracheostomy performed under these circumstances can, however, be extremely hazardous, mainly because of engorgement of the blood vessels in the neck. An emergency tracheostomy may also be necessary to secure the airway in patients with head and neck injuries, including burns to the face and upper airway.

Tracheostomy may be required for the long-term control of excessive bronchial secretions, particularly in those with a reduced conscious level, and/or to maintain an airway and protect the lungs in those with impaired pharyngeal and laryngeal reflexes.

Because endotracheal tubes can now safely remain in place for several weeks (Stauffer et al, 1981), tracheostomy is less often performed simply for prolonged control of the airway. However, when patients are extubated following an extended period of intubation, their vocal cords are oedematous and rigid, impairing their ability to cough. This may influence the decision to perform a tracheostomy, particularly in those who continue to produce excessive secretions and/or are unable to co-operate fully with physiotherapy. The reduction in dead space which occurs when tracheostomy is performed is no longer considered to be significant.

Techniques

It is important to avoid damaging the first tracheal ring, since this renders the larynx unstable. On the other hand, a low tracheostomy increases the risk of erosion of the innominate artery. The trachea should therefore be opened through the second, third and fourth tracheal rings following ligation and division of the thyroid isthmus. Duke's modification of the Bjork flap, in which an inverted U incision is made in the trachea and the flap is sutured to the lower skin edge, remains a popular technique. It has the advantages of supporting the tracheostomy tube, thereby minimizing erosion of the lower border of the trachea, and facilitating reinsertion (Price, 1983). Alternatively, a simple 'window' of tracheal wall can be removed. Both these methods weaken the tracheal wall and some now prefer a vertical slit, the edges of which are held apart with hooks while the tracheostomy tube is inserted, or a T-shaped incision with stay sutures. Certainly in neonates and infants a vertical slit should always be used. In general, however, there are a large number of surgical approaches and there is little information concerning the influence of these various techniques on the incidence of long-term complications.

Although cricothyroidotomy was for many years considered to be associated with an unacceptably high incidence of complications, more recent evidence suggests that this technique may in fact be safer than tracheostomy, particularly in emergencies and in those with a median sternotomy incision (Brantigan and Grow, 1976; Boyd et al, 1979). Bleeding is seldom a problem with this approach since no significant structures overlie the cricothyroid membrane, pneumothorax has not been reported and infection rates may be lower (Brantigan and Grow, 1976). Furthermore, the technique requires minimal expertise, few instruments and can be performed by non-surgical personnel. Misplacement of the tube is unusual. Boyd et al (1979), however, caution against the use of cricothyroidotomy following prolonged endotracheal intubation since, in their experience, severe laryngeal stenosis may ensue under these circumstances. They recommend the use of this technique only in emergencies and in patients with median sternotomy incisions.

In an extreme emergency, a large intravenous cannula can be inserted into the trachea percutaneously via the cricothyroid membrane. Alternatively, the Penlon cricothyrotomy cannula can be used. This technique involves extending the patient's head, making a small skin incision and pushing the cannula blade through the cricothyroid membrane into the trachea. The blade is then retracted and the integral metal dilators advanced and opened, allowing insertion of a tracheostomy tube. Recently, 'mini tracheostomies' have gained some popularity as a means of performing tracheobronchial toilet in the uncooperative or debilitated patient. The cricothyroid membrane is punctured percutaneously with an endotracheal tube and a sharp introducer. The latter is removed and the edges of the endotracheal tube are sutured to the skin.

Tracheostomy tubes

During IPPV, and for protection against aspiration, a cuffed tracheostomy tube is clearly required. As with endotracheal tubes for long-term use, these should be constructed of non-irritant material and have low-pressure, high-volume cuffs. The tip is normally cut square, rather than bevelled, to decrease the risk of obstruction.

When the patient's condition has improved, it is usual to change to an uncuffed tube. Traditionally, these are made of silver which is non-irritant and bactericidal. They have an inner tube which can be removed for cleaning at regular intervals. They can also be modified with a one-way flap valve and a window at the angle of the tube to allow the patient to speak. Alternatively, the patient can simply use a finger to temporarily occlude the tracheostomy. Plastic, uncuffed tubes are now available, some with disposable inner cannulae, both with and without 'windows'. Recently, various tracheal 'buttons' have been introduced which maintain patency of the tracheostomy and provide a route for endotracheal suction.

Once the tracheostomy has been decannulated and covered with a dry dressing, it closes spontaneously. This can occur surprisingly quickly and reinsertion of a tracheostomy tube may prove difficult within as little as 24 hours. Occasionally, a persistent sinus develops.

Complications

Because a tracheostomy tube is merely a short endotracheal tube inserted via the neck, the complications of intubation occurring below the level of the glottis are common to both. There are, however, certain additional complications peculiar to tracheostomy.

Early

The tracheostomy tube is easily misplaced in the pretracheal subcutaneous tissue, particularly during emergency reinsertion in the early postoperative period. This danger is minimized by using a Bjork flap (Price, 1983). The tube may obstruct if tilted, and leaks around the cuff can give rise to surgical emphysema. Pneumothorax, pneumomediastinum and perioperative haemorrhage are other well-recognized complications (Stauffer et al, 1981).

Intermediate

As with endotracheal intubation, ulceration of the trachea may occur at the level of the cuff and, because a tracheostomy tube is prone to tilting, the mucosa may also be damaged by the tip of the tube. Erosion of the tracheal cartilages and neighbouring structures may lead to fatal haemorrhage from the innominate artery, or to a tracheo-oesophageal fistula.

Tracheostomy wounds are usually colonized with resident bacteria which are often resistant to the commonly employed antibiotics. Sometimes, these are responsible for serious infection, particularly of sternotomy wounds in those who have undergone cardiac surgery.

Late

Tracheal stenosis may occur at the level of the stoma, the cuff, or the tip of the tube; sometimes, the tracheal rings collapse at stomal level. The incidence of these complications may be decreased by preserving as much tracheal cartilage as possible at operation, correct positioning of the tube and minimizing movement of the tube relative to the trachea.

These complications are particularly serious in paediatric patients and, if possible, tracheostomy should be avoided. Uncuffed tracheostomy tubes must always be used before puberty.

FURTHER READING

Lindholm CE & Grenvik A (1977) Flexible fibreoptic bronchoscopy and intubation in intensive care. In Ledingham I McA (ed.) *Recent Advances in Intensive Therapy 1*, pp 47–66. Edinburgh: Churchill Livingstone.

Gi RTN & Wilson RS (1983) High-frequency ventilation. In Ledingham IMcA & Hanning CE (eds) *Recent Advances in Critical Care Medicine 2*, pp 1–13. Edinburgh: Churchill Livingstone.

Pontoppidan H, Geffin B & Lowenstein E (1972) Acute respiratory failure in the adult (second and third of three parts). *New England Journal of Medicine* 287: 799–806.

Suter PM (1983) Intermittent and continuous positive pressure ventilation. In Tinker J & Rapin M (eds) pp 371–386. Berlin: Springer-Verlag.

Sykes MK, McNicol MW & Campbell EJM (1976) *Respiratory Failure*, 2nd edn, chapters 10–13. Oxford: Blackwell Scientific.

REFERENCES

Amos RJ, Amess JAL, Hinds CJ & Mollin DL (1982) Incidence and pathogenesis of acute megaloblastic bone-marrow change in patients receiving intensive care. *Lancet* ii: 835–839.

Ashbaugh DG & Petty TL (1973) Positive end-expiratory pressure. Physiology indications and contraindications. *Journal of Thoracic and Cardiovascular Surgery* 65: 165–170.

Aubier M, Murciano D, Legogguic Y et al (1985) Effect of hypophosphataemia on diaphragmatic contractility in patients with acute respiratory failure. *New England Journal of Medicine* 313: 420–424.

Beach T, Millen E & Grenvik A (1973) Hemodynamic response to discontinuance of mechanical ventilation. *Critical Care Medicine* 1: 85–90.

Beyer J, Beckenlechner P & Messmer K (1982) The influence of PEEP ventilation on organ blood flow and peripheral oxygen delivery. *Intensive Care Medicine* **8:** 75–80.

Bjorneboe M, Ibsen B, Astrup P et al (1955) Active ventilation in treatment of respiratory acidosis in chronic diseases of the lungs. *Lancet* **ii:** 901–903.

Boyd AD, Romita MC, Conlan AA, Fink SD & Spencer FC (1979) A clinical evaluation of cricothyroidotomy. *Surgery, Gynecology and Obstetrics* **149:** 365–368.

Brantigan CO and Grow JB (1976) Cricothyroidotomy: elective use in respiratory problems requiring tracheotomy. *Journal of Thoracic and Cardiovascular Surgery* **71:** 72–81.

Browne DRG (1984) Weaning patients from mechanical ventilation. *Intensive Care Medicine* **10:** 55–58.

Cole AGH, Weller SF & Sykes MK (1984) Inverse ratio ventilation compared with PEEP in adult respiratory failure. *Intensive Care Medicine* **10:** 227–232.

Colgan FJ, Nichols FA & DeWeese JA (1974) Positive end expiratory pressure, oxygen transport and the low-output state. *Anesthesia and Analgesia* **53:** 538–543.

Cox D & Niblett DJ (1984) Studies on continuous positive airway pressure breathing systems. *British Journal of Anaesthesia* **56:** 905–910.

Derderian SS, Rajagopal KR & Abbrecht PH et al (1982) High frequency positive pressure jet ventilation in bilateral bronchopleural fistulae. *Critical Care Medicine* **10:** 119–121.

Downs JB & Douglas ME (1981) Intermittent mandatory ventilation: why the controversy? *Critical Care Medicine* **9:** 622–623.

Downs JB, Klein EF Jr, Desautels D, Modell JH & Kirby RR (1973) Intermittent mandatory ventilation: a new approach to weaning patients from mechanical ventilators. *Chest* **64:** 331–335.

Editorial (1981) Artificial ventilation and the heart. *British Medical Journal* **283:** 397–398.

Feeley TW & Hedley-Whyte J (1975) Weaning from controlled ventilation and supplemental oxygen. *New England Journal of Medicine* **292:** 903–906.

Feeley TW, Saumarez R, Klick JM, McNabb TG & Skillman JJ (1975) Positive end-expiratory pressure in weaning patients from controlled ventilation. A prospective randomised trial. *Lancet* **ii:** 725–728.

Gattinoni L, Pesenti A, Rossi GP et al (1980) Treatment of acute respiratory failure with low-frequency positive-pressure ventilation and extracorporeal removal of CO_2. *Lancet* **ii:** 292–294.

Greenbaum DM, Millen JE, Eross B et al (1976) Continuous positive airway pressure without tracheal intubation in spontaneously breathing patients. *Chest* **69:** 615–620.

Grillo HC, Cooper JD, Geffin B & Pontoppidan H (1971) A low-pressure cuff for tracheostomy tubes to minimize tracheal injury. *Journal of Thoracic and Cardiovascular Surgery* **62:** 898–907.

Grindlinger GA, Manny J, Justice R et al (1979) Presence of negative inotropic agents in canine plasma during positive end-expiratory pressure. *Circulation Research* **45:** 460–467.

Hewlett AM, Platt AS & Terry VG (1977) Mandatory minute volume. A new concept in weaning from mechanical ventilation. *Anaesthesia* **32:** 163–169.

Hillman KM & Barber JD (1980) Asynchronous independent lung ventilation (AILV). *Critical Care Medicine* **8:** 390–395.

Jardin F, Farcot J-C, Boisante L et al (1981) Influence of positive end-expiratory pressure on left ventricular performance. *New England Journal of Medicine* **304:** 387–392.

Klain M, Keszler H & Stool S (1983) Transtracheal high frequency jet ventilation prevents aspiration. *Critical Care Medicine* **11:** 170–172.

Klain M, Kalla R, Sladen A & Guntupalli K (1984) High-frequency jet ventilation in weaning the ventilator-dependent patient. *Critical Care Medicine* **12:** 780–781.

Kumar A, Falke KJ, Geffin B et al (1970) Continuous positive-pressure ventilation in acute respiratory failure: effects on hemodynamics and lung function. *New England Journal of Medicine* **283:** 1430–1436.

Kumar A, Pontoppidan H, Baratz RA & Laver MB (1974) Inappropriate response to increased plasma ADH during mechanical ventilation in acute respiratory failure. *Anesthesiology* **40:** 215–221.

Laaksonen VO, Arola MK, Inberg MV et al (1977) Effect of different respirator adjustments on centrol haemodynamics in open-heart surgery patients. *Acta Anaesthesiologica Scandinavica* **21:** 200–210.

Leverment JN, Pearson FG & Rae S (1975) Tracheal size following tracheostomy with cuffed tracheostomy tubes: an experimental study. *Thorax* **30:** 271–277.

Lewis FR, Schlobohm RM & Thomas AN (1978) Prevention of complications from prolonged tracheal intubation. *American Journal of Surgery* **135:** 452–457.

Mathru M, Rao TLK & Venus B (1983) Ventilator-induced barotrauma in controlled mechanical ventilation versus intermittent mandatory ventilation. *Critical Care Medicine* **11:** 359–361.

Michel L, McMichan JC, Marsh HM & Rehder K (1979) Measurement of ventilatory reserve as an indicator for early extubation after cardiac operation. *Journal of Thoracic and Cardiovascular Surgery* **78:** 761–764.

Miller WC, Rice DL, Unger KM & Bradley BL (1981) Effect of PEEP on lung water content in experimental noncardiogenic pulmonary oedema. *Critical Care Medicine* **9:** 7–9.

Moore RA, Allen MC, Wood PJ, Rees LH & Sear JW (1985) Peri-operative endocrine effects of etomidate. *Anaesthesia* **40:** 124–130.

Morgan M & Whitwam JG (1985) Althesin (editorial) *Anaesthesia* **40:** 121–123.

Navaratnarajah M, Nunn JF, Lyons D & Milledge JS (1984) Bronchiolectasis caused by positive end-expiratory pressure. *Critical Care Medicine* **12:** 1036–1038.

Pepe PE, Hudson LD & Carrico CJ (1984) Early application of positive end-expiratory pressure in patients at risk for the adult respiratory distress syndrome. *New England Journal of Medicine* **311:** 281–286.

Petty TL (1981a) Why (not) try PEEP? *Critical Care Medicine* **9:** 67–68.

Petty TL (1981b) Intermittent mandatory ventilation—reconsidered. *Critical Care Medicine* **9:** 620–621.

Price DG (1983) Techniques of tracheostomy for intensive care unit patients. *Anaesthesia* **38:** 902–904.

Qvist J, Pontoppidan H, Wilson RS, Lowenstein E & Laver MB (1975) Hemodynamic responses to mechanical ventilation with PEEP: the effect of hypervolemia. *Anesthesiology* **42:** 45–55.

Rohfling BM, Webb WR & Schlobohm RM (1976) Ventilator-related extra-alveolar air in adults. *Radiology* **121:** 25–31.

Sahn SA & Lakshminarayan S (1973) Bedside criteria for discontinuation of mechanical ventilation. *Chest* **63:** 1002–1005.

Schuster DP, Klain M & Snyder JV (1982) Comparison of high frequency jet ventilation to conventional ventilation during severe acute respiratory failure in humans. *Critical Care Medicine* **10:** 625–630.

Simonneau G, Lemaire F, Harf A, Carlet J & Teisseire B (1982) A comparative study of the cardiorespiratory effects of continuous positive airway pressure breathing and continuous positive pressure ventilation in acute respiratory failure. *Intensive Care Medicine* **8:** 61–67.

Skillman JJ, Malhotra IV, Pallotta JA & Bushnell LS (1971) Determinants of weaning from controlled ventilation. *Surgical Forum* **22:** 198–200.

Sladen A, Guntupalli K & Klain M (1984) High-frequency jet ventilation versus intermittent positive-pressure ventilation. *Critical Care Medicine* **12:** 788–790.

Slavin G, Nunn JF, Crow J & Dore CJ (1982) Bronchiolectasis—a complication of artificial ventilation. *British Medical Journal* **285:** 931–934.

Stauffer JL, Olson DE & Petty TL (1981) Complications and consequences of endotracheal intubation and tracheotomy. *American Journal of Medicine* **70:** 65–76.

Steinhoff HH, Kohlhoff RJ & Falke KJ (1984) Facilitation of renal function by intermittent mandatory ventilation. *Intensive Care Medicine* **10:** 59–65.

Venus B, Jacobs HK & Lim L (1979) Treatment of the adult respiratory distress syndrome with continuous positive airway pressure. *Chest* **76:** 257–261.

Vincken W & Cosio MG (1984) Clinical applications of high-frequency jet ventilation. *Intensive Care Medicine* **10:** 275–280.

Weigelt JA, Mitchell RA & Snyder WH (1979) Early positive end-expiratory pressure in the adult respiratory distress syndrome. *Archives of Surgery* **114:** 497–501.

Weisman LM, Rinaldo JE, Rogers RM & Sanders MH (1983) Intermittent mandatory ventilation. *American Review of Respiratory Disease* **127:** 641–647.

Wilson RS, Sullivan SF, Malm JR & Bowman FO (1973) The oxygen cost of breathing following anesthesia and cardiac surgery. *Anesthesiology* **39:** 387–393.

Zapol WM, Snider MT, Hill JD et al (1979) Extracorporeal membrane oxygenation in severe acute respiratory failure—a randomized prospective study. *Journal of the American Medical Association* **242:** 2193–2196.

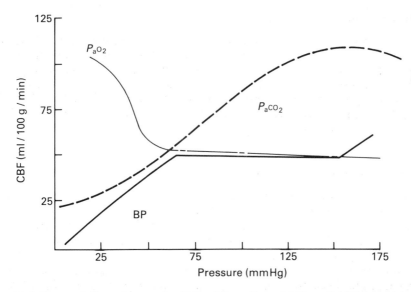

Fig. 14.1 Factors influencing cerebral blood flow. From McDowall (1976), with permission.

Cerebral blood flow is normally closely matched to cerebral oxygen requirements. In comatose head-injured patients, however, wide variations in cerebral blood flow may occur, despite a consistent reduction in the cerebral metabolic rate for oxygen (CMRo$_2$). Thus, in one study 55% of patients exhibited transient cerebral hyperaemia (defined as a normal or increased CBF in the presence of a reduced CMRo$_2$) while in 45% flows were subnormal (Obrist et al, 1984). Moreover, there was little or no evidence of ischaemia in the latter group; rather, they exhibited the normal coupling of CBF and CMRo$_2$. This hyperaemia is probably caused by a loss of vasomotor tone with impaired autoregulation and seems to be at least partly related to the CSF lactacidosis which can occur in head-injured patients.

Hypercarbia increases the concentration of hydrogen ions in the interstitial spaces, causing cerebral vasodilatation and a rise in CBF (Fig. 14.1); severe hypoxaemia (P_ao$_2$ <8 kPa, 60 mmHg) also increases CBF (Fig. 14.1), possibly by a direct effect or via chemoreceptor stimulation and neurogenic influences. Finally, it is important to remember that most inhalational anaesthetic agents cause cerebral vasodilatation.

The phenomena of 'steal' and 'reverse steal', which cause local alterations in the distribution of cerebral blood flow, are also relevant to the management of head-injured patients. Vessels in damaged areas of brain are often relatively unresponsive to the factors which normally influence vascular tone and simply respond passively to alterations in perfusion pressure. In contrast, vessels in intact brain react normally to such stimuli. Thus, hypercarbia will cause dilatation of responsive vessels, diverting blood flow away from areas of cerebral damage and possibly precipitating ischaemia ('steal'). Conversely, hypocarbia will increase flow, and hydrostatic pressure, in damaged vessels and this may potentiate oedema formation ('reverse steal').

Intracranial pressure

The rise in ICP which can occur following severe head injury may be caused by intracranial haemorrhage, an increase in intracranial blood volume, cerebral oedema or a combination of these. In one series, ICP was found to be elevated in 70% of patients who had required craniotomy, but in only 29% of those with diffuse brain injury (Miller et al, 1981). Alterations in intracranial blood volume, associated with the loss of cerebrovascular tone and hyperaemia mentioned previously, are probably largely responsible for intracranial hypertension occurring in the early stages of head injury and for phasic changes in ICP (see below). In one study, there was a highly significant association between hyperaemia and the presence of intracranial hypertension (ICP >20 mmHg, 2.7 kPa) (Obrist et al, 1984). Cerebral oedema develops later and may be caused by vasodilatation, either locally in areas of contusion or globally, associated with a massive increase in capillary hydrostatic pressure and extravasation of fluid into the interstitial spaces. This generates pressure gradients and the oedema then diffuses throughout the brain to produce more generalized swelling.

Not only do haematomas and oedema cause intracranial hypertension which may be associated with serious reductions in cerebral perfusion, but they also produce 'brain shifts'. Thus, unilateral mass lesions above the tentorium cause lateral distortion of the brain with local increases in pressure and impaired perfusion. Initially, the relatively rigid falx cerebri acts as a barrier to mass movements but, eventually, brain may herniate beneath this structure, damaging the corpus callosum. If the supratentorial pressures exceed approximately 40 mmHg (5 kPa), perfusion of the brain stem is jeopardized and compression of the third cranial nerve at the tentorial hiatus will initially produce pupillary constriction, followed by dilatation and absent responses to light.

Intracranial compliance

It is important to appreciate the relationship between the volume of the contents of the skull and the ICP—the 'intracranial compliance curve' (Fig.

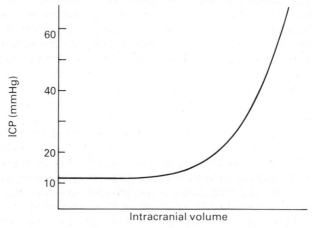

Fig. 14.2 Intracranial compliance curve.

14.2). As intracranial volume increases, there is at first only a gradual rise in ICP because of a compensatory reduction in the volume of blood and CSF within the skull. The CSF is displaced largely into the spinal compartment, where a reduction in the volume of blood within the extradural venous plexuses prevents local increases in pressure. If intracranial volume continues to increase, however, intracranial compliance falls progressively until further compensation is impossible and ICP rises rapidly (Miller et al, 1973). Moreover, when intracranial compliance is reduced, stimuli such as coughing, physiotherapy and endotracheal intubation, which normally cause only small, transient increases in ICP, produce more pronounced and sustained intracranial hypertension.

Immediate care

As discussed earlier, meticulous immediate care of head-injured patients is of vital importance. The airway must be secured and protected, if necessary by endotracheal intubation, and, because patients in traumatic coma are frequently hypoxic (Miller et al, 1981), supplemental oxygen should always be given. In some cases, immediate institution of IPPV will be necessary to control the arterial carbon dioxide tension and reduce acute, severe intracranial hypertension. Restoration of an adequate blood pressure must be achieved as rapidly as possible with intravenous volume replacement and, occasionally, inotropes. At this stage, intravenous mannitol can be administered to control intracranial hypertension. The patient should not be transferred, or undergo investigations, until adequate resuscitation has been completed, and even then should always be accompanied by a suitably qualified doctor.

Investigations

At this stage, skull x-rays should be obtained and may reveal linear or depressed fractures; occasionally, midline shift of a calcified pineal gland is seen on the antero-posterior film. Linear fractures can cause haemorrhage from torn extradural vessels and the presence of a skull fracture is associated with an increased risk of intracranial haematoma (Mendelow et al, 1983), while those with depressed fractures may develop intracranial infection if untreated. Sometimes, there is leakage of CSF through fracture sites and this may be seen as clear fluid trickling from the nose or ear. A positive test for sugar using a Dextrostix will confirm that the fluid is indeed CSF.

Head-injured patients who remain comatose following resuscitation in hospital should be investigated by computed axial tomography (CAT). This can demonstrate cerebral swelling as well as revealing and localizing intracranial haematomas (Fig. 14.3). Compression of the ventricles may also be visible on CAT scan and suggests significantly raised ICP (Fig. 14.4), while midline shift is seen in the presence of significant unilateral mass lesions (Fig. 14.3). However, the absence of an intracranial haematoma on the initial scan does not exclude the possibility that this complication will develop subsequently, particularly if the scan is performed soon after injury. Consequently, frequent neurological assessment, monitoring of ICP and

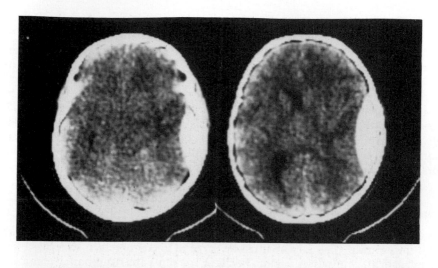

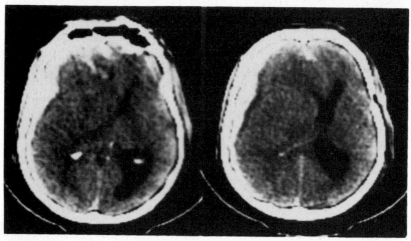

Fig. 14.3 Intracranial haematomata demonstrated by computed axial tomography. Top: Acute extradural haematoma. Biconvex high attenuation collection with associated ipsilateral ventricular compression from oedema. Bottom: Subdural haematoma (acute). High attenuation collection concave outer and convex inner margin. Marked midline shift. (Courtesy of Dr K. Hall.)

repeat scans may all be required to ensure that delayed intracranial haemorrhage is detected.

Because of the dangers of transporting and scanning patients in traumatic coma, it has been suggested that computerized ultrasound is a practical alternative to repeat CAT scans. With this technique, it may be possible to detect midline shift non-invasively at the patient's bedside. Such a finding suggests the presence of a unilateral mass lesion, which can, if time allows, be confirmed by a repeat CAT scan or may, in the presence of significant clinical deterioration, precipitate immediate craniotomy.

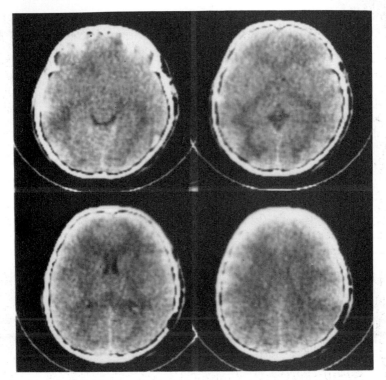

Fig. 14.4 Diffuse cerebral swelling in a patient with severe head injury. Note ventricular compression. (Courtesy of Dr K. Hall.)

Monitoring

Clinical

In the unsedated patient, a clinical assessment of neurological status is possible. The level of consciousness can be graded according to whether the patient is alert and orientated, drowsy but rousable and whether he obeys simple commands or reacts to painful stimuli. A more sophisticated assessment is possible using the Glasgow coma scale. However, this was designed primarily to allow meaningful comparisons between the results obtained in different centres and with alternative treatment regimens; therefore, although this scale is undoubtedly valuable for research, some authorities consider it to be insufficiently sensitive for clinical use. Localizing signs, such as weakness and hypertonicity of the limbs on one side of the body, should also be sought, and the size and reactivity of the pupils assessed. Pupillary signs are late indicators of intracranial compression and the aim should always be to detect deterioration before such changes occur.

Intracranial pressure

Because those head-injured patients admitted to the intensive care unit for controlled ventilation are usually sedated, and often paralysed, the clinical signs of rising ICP and neurological deterioration, except the late pupillary changes, are masked. It is therefore important to measure ICP, both as a guide to therapy aimed at its reduction and control and to detect increasing intracranial compression. If there is a sustained rise in ICP resistant to treatment, a repeat CAT scan may reveal an intracranial haematoma which can then be evacuated. Furthermore, ICP monitoring enables nurses, physiotherapists and medical staff to assess the effects of procedures on intracranial dynamics. As well as the need for IPPV, other suggested indications for ICP monitoring include a Glasgow coma score of <8, the presence of a small haematoma seen on CAT scan, and following decompressive surgery.

ICP may be monitored most sensitively and accurately by introducing a fluid-filled catheter into a lateral ventricle, although this may be difficult in those in whom the ventricles are compressed by cerebral swelling. There is also a risk of introducing infection. An intraventricular catheter does, however, enable the clinician to remove CSF in order to control ICP and to test intracranial compliance (see below). Alternatives include a hollow 'bolt', which can be threaded into the skull to measure extradural or subdural pressure, and catheter tip transducers or fluid-filled catheters inserted subdurally. Regular calibration of these devices is essential to ensure that measurements are accurate and reliable.

Correct interpretation of ICP recordings depends on an appreciation of the intracranial compliance curve (see Fig. 14.2). It is now recognized that even during the initial phase of intracranial volume expansion, compensation is not perfect and ICP in fact rises from a normal value of <10 mmHg (1.3 kPa) to about 25 mmHg (3.3 kPa). Above this level, there is a danger of decompensation, and an ICP of <25 mmHg (3.3 kPa) is therefore often used as a target for treatment aimed at controlling intracranial hypertension (Moss et al, 1983). Nevertheless, the absolute value of the ICP provides only an approximate guide to the degree of cerebral compression. Intracranial compliance can be assessed by injecting a small volume of fluid into the ventricles or can be inferred from the response of the ICP to stimuli such as endotracheal suction (an increase in ICP of >15 mmHg (2 kPa) during the latter manoeuvre indicates that intracranial compliance is markedly reduced). Furthermore, as intracranial compliance falls, there is an increase in the amplitude of the fluctuations in ICP which occur in phase with the pulse and with ventilation. This is a most valuable sign of intracranial compression. Finally, large (60–80 mmHg, 8–10.6 kPa) spontaneous increases in ICP lasting about 20 minutes ('A' waves), as well as rhythmic oscillations at 0.5–2 cycles min^{-1} ('B' waves) and fluctuations related to blood pressure at about 6 min^{-1} ('C' waves), all suggest that intracranial compliance is markedly reduced.

It has been shown that in patients who are unable to obey simple commands, but who do not have an intracranial haematoma, any increase in ICP to above 10 mmHg (1.3 kPa) is associated with a worse outcome whereas, in those with mass lesions, only an ICP above 40 mmHg (5.3 kPa) on admission was associated with a poor outcome (Miller et al, 1977). The presence of A waves is associated with a mortality of about 60% but B and C waves do not imply a worse prognosis (Moss et al, 1983). This relationship between ICP and outcome does not necessarily imply that intracranial hypertension is directly responsible for death, nor that reducing ICP will alter mortality; rather, it is likely that the level of ICP is a reflection of the degree of cerebral damage.

Jugular bulb oxygen content

A thin radiopaque catheter can be inserted percutaneously into the internal jugular vein and passed retrogradely as far as the jugular bulb. Simultaneous sampling of jugular venous and systemic arterial blood allows determination of the cerebral arteriovenous oxygen content difference. Although this provides an assessment of the global balance between cerebral oxygen supply and demand, it will not necessarily detect episodes of regional cerebral ischaemia (Obrist et al, 1984). If cerebral blood flow is also determined (e.g. using the intravenous ^{133}Xe method) $CMRo_2$ can be calculated. At present, these techniques are used mainly for research purposes and their value in the clinical management of head-injured patients has yet to be determined.

Neurophysiological monitoring (Prior, 1985)

A number of neurophysiological techniques can be used to assess the functional state of the nervous system in patients with severe head injury.

Conventional bedside EEGs can be recorded at intervals to obtain diagnostic and prognostic information. They may reveal the presence of seizure activity, can suggest hypoxic/ischaemic damage and will localize any dysfunction as well as indicating its severity and progress. The use of conventional EEGs for continuous monitoring of intensive care patients is, however, both expensive and impractical. Huge amounts of paper tracing are produced, and special skills are required to record and interpret the data. Moreover, neurophysiological monitoring is particularly difficult in the intensive care unit because of interference, for example from electrical equipment, which can give rise to artefact. In order to monitor the EEG for prolonged periods automatically, and to produce information which can be readily interpreted by clinicians after simple instruction, some form of data reduction is required. It is also necessary to reject artefact from the display.

In critically ill patients, the fundamental requirement is to monitor the serial EEG changes which accompany depression and recovery of neuronal function; these are similar whatever their aetiology (drugs, anaesthesia, hypothermia or hypoxia/ischaemia). Depression of neuronal function is accompanied by a reduction in the overall level of cortical electrical activity until electrical silence occurs. The most significant early warning of deterioration is the appearance of 'burst suppression' activity (i.e. the breaking up of previously continuous EEG waves by increasingly long periods of electrical silence). The associated EEG frequency changes are more complex and less consistent, although there is a general tendency for frequencies to decrease.

Both frequency and time domain analyses have been used to extract and display the most clinically relevant features of the EEG. Time domain analyses involve processing the EEG as a continuous signal (e.g. voltage plotted against time), whereas a frequency domain analysis averages the potentials present during a time period ('epoch') and then plots frequency

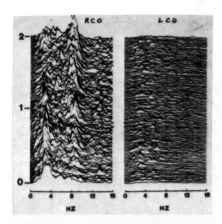

Fig. 14.5 Compressed spectral array recording from right and left centro-occipital regions showing interhemisphere asymmetry. Note the relative lack of activity from the left hemisphere recording compared with the large waves over a relatively wide frequency range on the right. The persistent reduction of left-sided activity in this patient, four days after a head injury, suggests that contusion has led to some permanent left hemisphere damage (unpublished data of A. Bricolo and S. Turazzi, reproduced with permission).

against another variable, such as power. Because the frequency plots provide no time information, serial plots are conventionally displayed sequentially in the 'compressed spectral array' (Fig. 14.5).

Frequency domain analysis. A number of instruments are available which will perform this type of analysis. Although such techniques provide detailed information regarding frequency alterations, the output is relatively complex and difficult to interpret (Fig. 14.5). Moreover, the computing is expensive and it is possible to miss isolated events of short duration, such as a brief seizure discharge or the periods of electrical silence which are characteristic of 'burst suppression'. Frequency-based EEG data are therefore most useful for the detection of subtle changes which may occur, e.g. during sleep or with light levels of anaesthesia.

Time domain analysis. For a more generally applicable monitoring system, a recording of the voltage range and the amount of activity is a better indication of the brain's energy output.

Continuous monitoring of the EEG can be performed, for example, using the cerebral function monitor (CFM). This is a relatively simple, robust and portable apparatus which has been used for almost 20 years. It produces a continuous, filtered and compressed paper trace of cortical electrical activity at $6-30\,cm\,h^{-1}$. This is recorded from two electrodes which are generally positioned over the parietal region on either side, while a third electrode is placed in the midline to help rejection of interference. The recording electrodes are positioned close to the arterial boundary zones, which are particularly vulnerable to reductions in cerebral perfusion, in order to maximize their sensitivity to ischaemic events.

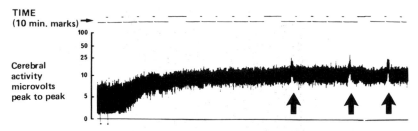

Fig. 14.6 Recording of cortical electrical activity obtained using the cerebral function monitor (CFM). Activity increases as the patient emerges from a period of heavy sedation. Seizure discharges are then seen and are indicated by the arrows.

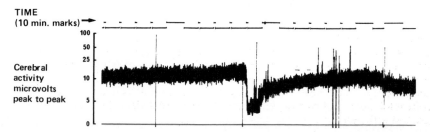

Fig. 14.7 A brief episode of profound cerebral ischaemia occurring in a patient with severe head injury. Rapid institution of measures to improve cerebral oxygenation is associated with partial recovery of cortical electrical activity.

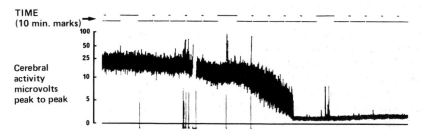

Fig. 14.8 In this cardiac surgery patient postoperative failure of cerebral perfusion culminates in permanent extinction of cortical electrical activity.

The CFM will detect subclinical seizure discharges and status epilepticus (Fig. 14.6) which can then be treated vigorously with anticonvulsants; in a proportion of such cases, a good outcome can then be achieved. Episodes of profound cerebral ischaemia are associated with reductions in CFM voltage (Fig. 14.7) and, if not rapidly corrected, cortical activity is permanently extinguished (Fig. 14.8). The extent of depression of the CFM can be used as a guide to the level of sedation achieved with intravenous anaesthetic agents (Fig. 14.9). Thus, depression of the baseline of the CFM trace to below $5\,\mu$V is generally equivalent to a 'burst suppression' pattern seen on the conventional EEG and indicates that $CMRo_2$ is maximally reduced. Under these circumstances, increasing the level of sedation is unlikely to produce further significant decreases in CBF and ICP (Bingham et al, 1985).

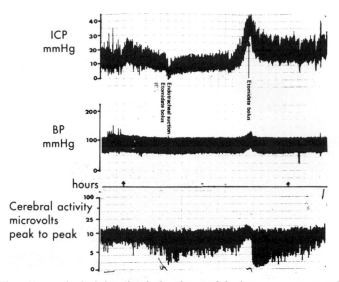

Fig. 14.9 The effects of administering bolus doses of the intravenous anaesthetic agent etomidate (0.2 mg kg^{-1}) on intracranial pressure (ICP) systemic blood pressure (BP) and cortical electrical activity as recorded by the cerebral function monitor (CFM). Etomidate administration reduces ICP on both occasions and this is associated with a fall in the baseline of the CFM trace to below 5 μV. There is also a small reduction in systemic blood pressure. There is no increase in ICP following endotracheal suction subsequent to the first bolus dose of etomidate.

Finally, the CFM recording can provide an indication of prognosis. Thus, if the trace is variable and responsive to noxious stimuli (Fig. 14.10), or sleep-like, a good outcome is likely provided further episodes of cerebral ischaemia and major brain shifts are avoided. If the tracing is monotonous, with the loss of the normal variability and responses to pain, the majority of survivors will be vegetative, while near or total absence of electrical activity (provided this is not due to heavy sedation or hypothermia) is invariably associated with death.

Combined time and frequency domain analysis. An example of this type of analysis is the recently developed cerebral function analysing monitor (CFAM) (Fig. 14.11). This records the amplitude of electrical activity as a mean, together with the 90th and 10th centile values, as well as peaks and troughs which exceed these. In addition, frequency analysis is provided as the percentage of power falling into the traditional frequency bands (beta, alpha, theta and delta). Whether this has any advantage over the CFM in routine clinical practice is at present not clear.

Evoked potentials (Fig. 14.12). Averaged evoked potentials to external sensory stimuli (visual, auditory and somatosensory) also provide useful prognostic information. They are particularly valuable in traumatic coma because the short latency brain stem components of the auditory and somatosensory responses are unaffected by heavy sedation or anaesthesia, even when the EEG has been rendered isoelectric, and they can assess the

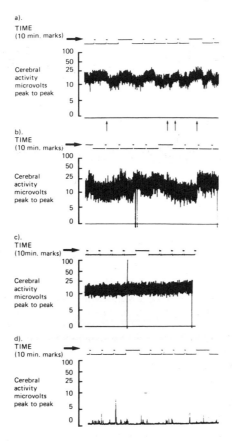

Fig. 14.10 Prognostic information can be derived from the cerebral function monitor (CFM) recording in patients with severe head injury. (a) Variable and responsive trace *or* (b) sleeplike—a good outcome is likely, provided further episodes of cerebral ischaemia and major brain shifts are avoided. (c) Monotonous trace—the majority of survivors will be vegetative. (d) Near or total absence of electrical activity—provided this is not due to heavy sedation or hypothermia, it is invariably associated with death.

functional integrity of lower pathways. They are, however, affected by hypothermia. The most useful are the somatosensory evoked potentials which are obtained by electrical stimulation at a peripheral site, e.g. the median nerve. Auditory brain stem (click) stimuli may also give valuable information. Provided a peripheral response is obtained (this may not be possible, for example, if the eyes or ears have sustained direct traumatic damage), the conduction time through the brain stem to the appropriate cortical site can be measured. Major asymmetries or absence of potentials are associated with serious neurological deficits, vegetative survival or death. Delayed central somatosensory conduction times may indicate a transient functional disturbance due, for example, to white matter oedema.

Electrocardiogram. This may reveal bizarre ST segment, T wave changes such as those shown in Fig. 14.13.

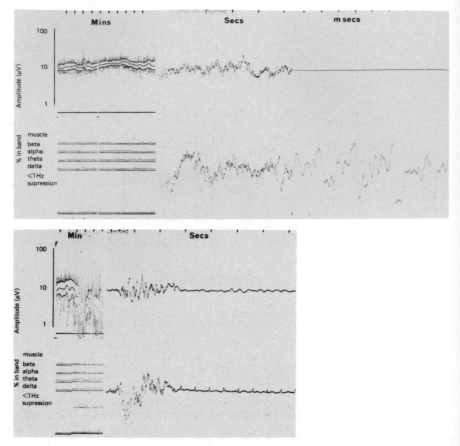

Fig. 14.11 Two samples of monitoring from the CFAM. Upper trace: This was obtained from a lightly anaesthetized normal subject and shows some variability of amplitude (upper part of trace) and a wide range of frequency distributions (lower part of trace). In the middle is a sample of EEG. On the right is a brain stem auditory evoked potential produced by a click stimulus. Lower trace: This was obtained from the same patient when deeply anaesthetized. Note the broad amplitude distribution, including deflections to below 1 μV ('suppressions') alternating with deflections exceeding 10 μV ('bursts'). This 'burst suppression' pattern is well seen in the EEG sample; note ECG picked up from scalp in the lower section. The frequency distribution has shifted and there is a greater percentage of activity in the theta and delta bands with suppression clearly shown.

Management

Intensive care management of severe head injury is aimed at preventing secondary ischaemic cerebral damage and minimizing brain shifts. This is based on maintenance of adequate cerebral perfusion by controlling ICP and optimizing systemic blood pressure. Cerebral metabolic demands should also be minimized and in this respect control of seizure activity is essential. Reduction of raised ICP can be achieved by decreasing intracranial blood volume, reducing cerebral oedema or both.

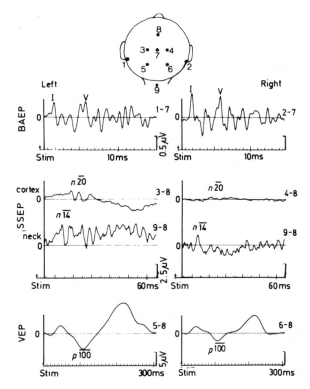

Fig. 14.12 Averaged sensory evoked potentials in traumatic coma. Auditory brain stem potentials (BAEP), somatosensory potentials over second cervical vertebral and contralateral somatosensory cortex following median nerve stimulation at the wrist (SSEP) and visual evoked potentials to binocular flash stimulation (VEP). Note slight delay of BAEP wave I on the right, but otherwise normal BAEP, depressed cortical SSEP and reduced amplitude VEP over the right hemisphere. Six weeks later the patient was conscious and active but with a left hemiparesis. From Prior (1985), with permission.

Reducing intracranial blood volume

This is achieved largely by manipulating cerebral blood flow. Because this produces relatively small alterations in intracranial volume, the change in intracranial pressure is greatest when cerebral compliance is markedly reduced.

Controlled Ventilation. There is no conclusive evidence that IPPV, with or without induced hypocapnia, affects the outcome in those with severe head injury, and in view of the acknowledged difficulties involved in assessing the value of alternative treatments in this situation, the use of controlled ventilation is likely to remain controversial.

Nevertheless, because of the effects of alterations in blood gas tensions on cerebral vascular tone, and because hypoxaemia can precipitate neuronal

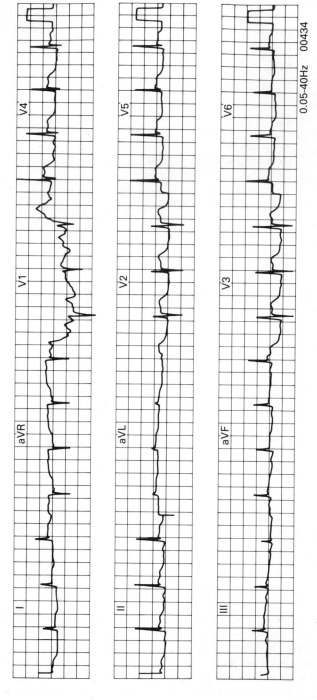

Fig. 14.13 Electrocardiogram recorded from a patient in traumatic coma showing ST segment/T wave abnormalities.

damage in marginally ischaemic areas, it is clearly essential to avoid both hypercarbia and hypoxaemia. It is therefore universally accepted that maintenance of a patent airway with adequate ventilation and oxygenation is vital. This may require endotracheal intubation and, in some cases, controlled ventilation. It is also generally agreed that artificial ventilation should be instituted in head-injured patients who are hypoventilating or have respiratory arrhythmia, and in those with pulmonary dysfunction due, for example, to an associated chest injury, pulmonary oedema (see below), fat embolism or aspiration. Patients who remain hypoxaemic despite administration of supplemental oxygen should also be ventilated, and severely hypoxic patients may benefit from CPPV (see Chapter 13). (The application of PEEP of 5–20 cmH$_2$O (0.5–2 kPa) probably does not affect ICP, provided the patient is in the head-up position and hyperventilated (Frost, 1977).) Some head-injured patients will hyperventilate in response to an increased CSF hydrogen ion concentration caused by cerebral ischaemia and many authorities recommend that IPPV should be instituted in this situation. Other suggested indications for controlled ventilation include spontaneous flexor or extensor posturing, failure to respond to painful stimuli, convulsions and significant intracranial hypertension (e.g. ICP >25 mmHg, 3.3 kPa) (Moss et al, 1983) (Table 14.1).

Table 14.1 Some suggested indications for IPPV in head-injured patients.

Spontaneous extensor posturing
Spontaneous flexor posturing
No response to pain
Repeated convulsions
Spontaneous hyperventilation with $P_a$co$_2$ < 3.5 kPa (25 mmHg)
P_ao$_2$ < 9.0 kPa (70 mmHg) on air *or* P_ao$_2$ < 13 kPa (100 mmHg) on supplemental oxygen
Patients who are underventilating or who show respiratory arrhythmia in the acute phase
Associated pathology, e.g. chest injury, respiratory pathology for which IPPV is indicated
Persistent hyperpyrexia unresponsive to conventional therapy
An intracranial pressure (ICP) of more than 25 mmHg for greater than 25% of a 30-minute period

Potential advantages of controlled ventilation for patients in traumatic coma include avoidance of fluctuations in blood gas tensions, abolition of the work of breathing and greater cardiovascular stability. It also enables the clinician to administer sedative and analgesic drugs (see below) without the risk of precipitating hypercarbia. Elective hyperventilation can be used to induce hypocarbia, thereby achieving a reduction in CBF and ICP. The fall in ICP is, however, often relatively short-lived because interstitial pH, and hence cerebrovascular tone, returns virtually to control levels after four hours (Raichle et al, 1970) and is at its previous value within 12–24 hours. Although it is not certain that these time relations apply in those with head injury, it would seem that hyperventilation is of most benefit as a means of rapidly reducing acutely raised ICP. There are, however, other possible benefits of induced hypocarbia, including the 'inverse steal' phenomenon and correction of cerebral tissue acidosis; the latter may increase neuronal survival and improve autoregulation (Paulson et al, 1972). On the other hand, excessive hypocarbia may produce a massive increase in blood flow through damaged areas of brain and this could enhance oedema formation, precipitate intracerebral haemorrhage and produce local pressure effects. Furthermore, profound vasoconstriction might precipitate cerebral ischaemia.

The aim is therefore to achieve the benefits of moderate hypocarbia without the dangers of extreme cerebral vasoconstriction. An arterial carbon dioxide tension of between 3.5 and 4.5 kPa (25–35 mmHg) is generally considered to be acceptable, although some recommend a lower limit of 4 kPa (30 mmHg). It has been suggested that hyperventilation should be used more selectively in the management of traumatic coma since in those in whom CBF is already reduced, such treatment is more likely to precipitate brain ischaemia. Conversely, patients with hyperaemia, who remain particularly responsive to alterations in carbon dioxide tension, will probably benefit from hyperventilation and are at least risk of developing cerebral ischaemia (Obrist et al, 1984).

Some authorities go so far as to recommend IPPV for all unconscious head injuries. Others consider that in many cases the risks of IPPV and sedation (loss of signs of neurological deterioration, increased risk of pulmonary complications, dangers of tracheostomy and long-term intubation) outweigh the benefits, and it has been suggested that the extensive, unselective, use of controlled ventilation may be associated with a worse outcome (Jennett et al, 1980). Others have suggested, however, that the selective use of controlled ventilation may improve outcome in those with diffuse brain injury (Moss et al, 1983).

Sedation. It is essential that patients with intracranial hypertension do not cough, struggle or resist the ventilator, since this can lead to dangerous rises in ICP. Traditionally, sedation of ventilated patients is achieved using intravenous bolus injections of opiates and benzodiazepines. If necessary, non-depolarizing neuromuscular blocking agents are also administered to assist synchronization with the ventilator (see Chapter 13). However, such treatment has little intrinsic effect on ICP, and bolus-dose administration is associated with fluctuations in the level of sedation.

A number of anaesthetic induction agents can be administered as continuous intravenous infusions to provide a constant, controllable level of sedation. In addition, most have been shown to decrease CBF, probably secondary to a reduction in CMR_{O_2} (Pierce et al, 1962). (An important exception is ketamine, which causes hypertension and a rise in ICP.) It is also possible that the reduction in CMR_{O_2} will protect relatively ischaemic areas of brain from further damage, and seizure activity may be controlled. A disadvantage of all intravenous anaesthetics is that they produce a variable degree of cardiovascular depression and can thereby adversely affect CPP (Prior et al, 1983). Such continuous sedation is normally accompanied by the administration of opiates to provide analgesia. Muscle relaxants can be given to minimize the increases in intrathoracic pressure which may otherwise occur in response to positive pressure ventilation and physiotherapy, as well as to reduce the incidence of coughing and resisting the ventilator. Bolus doses of intravenous anaesthetic agents can also be used to rapidly reduce acutely raised ICP and to prevent surges in ICP in response to noxious stimuli, such as physiotherapy and endotracheal suction (Fig. 14.9) (Prior et al, 1983). This is most effective when combined with muscle relaxation (White et al, 1982). Associated hypotension can on occasions cause worrying reductions in CPP (Prior et al, 1983), although attenuation of the rise in ICP may in itself be beneficial by minimizing intracranial pressure gradients and brain shifts. A beneficial response to the administration of an intravenous anaesthetic agent (a significant reduction in ICP associated with a rise in CPP) is most likely when the baseline voltage of the CFM is greater than 5 µV, the cardiovascular system is stable, the circulating volume is adequate and in the presence of significant intracranial hypertension (ICP >25 mmHg, 3.3 kPa) (Bingham et al, 1985).

Of all the intravenous anaesthetic agents, thiopentone has received most attention, but its use in traumatic coma remains controversial since its effect on functional outcome is unclear (Shapiro, 1985). Although it can undoubtedly control intracranial hypertension and may redistribute blood flow to ischaemic areas, as well as abolishing seizure activity, the reduction in ICP is often transient and its effects on functional neurological outcome are unclear. Furthermore, thiopentone is a particularly potent cardiovascular depressant and continuous infusions of this agent may have to be accompanied by the administration of inotropic agents and monitoring of PCWP in order to maintain haemodynamic stability. A further disadvantage of the barbiturates is that they are redistributed to fat stores and as a consequence their sedative effect may persist for some time (at least 48 hours) after the infusion has been discontinued. Neurological assessment, and in particular examination of brain stem function, must therefore be considerably delayed. Most authorities consider that barbiturates should only be employed when other methods have failed to control severe intracranial hypertension.

Until recently, the short-acting intravenous anaesthetic agents, Althesin and etomidate, were used in a number of centres for sedation and control of ICP in traumatic coma (Moss et al, 1983; Prior et al, 1983). These agents cause less cardiovascular depression than thiopentone and recovery is relatively rapid once the infusion has been discontinued. Unfortunately, neither of these drugs is currently available for prolonged intravenous infusion (see Chapter 13). At present, thiopentone is therefore the only intravenous anaesthetic agent available for use in traumatic coma. Continuous sedation can be provided using intravenous infusions of a benzodiazepine (preferably a short-acting agent such as midazolam) and/or an opiate. Continuous infusions of benzodiazepines, including midazolam, can however be associated with prolonged recovery times.

Cerebral venous drainage. Clearly, intracranial blood volume will rise if cerebral venous drainage is impeded. The importance of adequate muscle relaxation as a means of minimizing venous pressures has already been discussed. In addition, the tapes securing the endotracheal or tracheostomy tube must not constrict the neck veins and the patient's head should be centrally positioned. Traditionally, the head is elevated in order to reduce

ICP, but the response of ICP and intracranial compliance to alterations in head position appear to be variable and it has been recommended that the optimal position should be determined for each patient individually (Ropper et al, 1982).

Control of cerebral oedema

Increases in capillary hydrostatic pressure will exacerbate oedema formation. Control of CBF and systemic blood pressure therefore has the additional theoretical advantage of minimizing cerebral oedema. Most clinicians also restrict intravenous administration of crystalloid solutions, e.g. to $20\,\mathrm{ml\,kg^{-1}}$ $\mathrm{day^{-1}}$ of 5% dextrose.

Diuretics. Traditionally, the fall in ICP which can follow the administration of an osmotic diuretic has been attributed to a reduction in brain water secondary to the creation of an osmotic gradient between the intravascular and interstitial spaces. This effect is transient and its duration depends on the rate at which the gradient is dissipated as osmotically active molecules diffuse into brain tissue; this in turn is influenced by the integrity of the blood–brain barrier. Thus, fluid is removed predominantly from normal areas of brain, thereby accentuating brain shift. Moreover, repeated doses are usually progressively less effective and eventually the increasing concentration of osmotically active molecules in the interstitial space may actually enhance oedema formation—the 'rebound phenomenon'. However, there is no evidence that osmotic agents lower ICP by decreasing brain water content, and it has recently been suggested that the reduction in ICP produced by mannitol is due to cerebral vasoconstriction, possibly as a compensatory response to an increase in CBF produced by the fall in blood viscosity (Muizelaar et al, 1983). The latter mechanism would explain the rapid reduction in ICP which may follow the administration of mannitol.

Although mannitol is the osmotic agent most often used to control intracranial hypertension, urea was popular in the past and some centres favour glycerol. Urea is, however, extremely irritant, can impair coagulation and is associated with particularly severe rebound. Glycerol is probably less effective than mannitol, except in very high doses when it causes haemolysis. With all these agents, there is a danger of precipitating dehydration, electrolyte disturbances and overexpansion of the intravascular compartment. The latter is particularly liable to occur in those with impaired renal function and will be especially dangerous in the presence of heart disease. Hypovolaemia, as well as fluid and electrolyte disturbances, can compromise renal function and may be associated with a metabolic acidosis. Blood pressure and cardiac output must therefore be maintained by infusing colloidal solutions and, if necessary, by administering inotropic agents. Complicated cases may require insertion of a Swan–Ganz catheter.

In order to reduce the risk of rebound and fluid overload, the volume of osmotic agent administered should be carefully controlled. Thus, for example, 20% mannitol $0.3–0.5\,\mathrm{g\,kg^{-1}}$ should be administered not more often than every six hours, and then only if the ICP is unacceptably high. If on any occasion intracranial hypertension fails to respond, or if the plasma osmolality rises to more than $320\,\mathrm{mosmol\,l^{-1}}$, further mannitol should be withheld. If osmotic diuretics and heavy sedation fail to control ICP, it may be worth trying the effect of a 'loop diuretic', such as frusemide or ethacrynic acid.

Steroids. The use of steroids (e.g. dexamethasone 10 mg initially then 4 mg 6-hourly) to control the cerebral oedema associated with severe head injury remains controversial. Although they are thought to reduce the oedema surrounding a space-occupying lesion, such as a cerebral metastasis, recent evidence has shown that they are ineffective in controlling intracranial hypertension, and do not improve outcome, following severe head injury (Cooper et al, 1979; Braakman et al, 1983). Possible complications include salt and water retention, peptic ulceration and reduced resistance to infection. If steroids are used, they should be discontinued gradually in order to avoid a rebound increase in oedema.

In resistant cases, intracranial hypertension may only be controlled by removal of a bone flap or by excising damaged areas of brain. Not only does this allow further expansion of brain substance, but the latter manoeuvre may remove a potential source of oedema fluid.

Finally, if an intraventricular catheter is in situ CSF can be removed intermittently or continuously into a drainage system, although this may not reduce oedema in brain tissue.

In those patients in whom ICP remains low, artificial ventilation can be discontinued after 48–72 hours, provided there are no associated respiratory problems. In more difficult cases, IPPV should be continued until ICP has stabilized at a satisfactory level and respiratory function is adequate.

Neurogenic pulmonary oedema (Editorial, 1985)

In 1918, Moutier published a series of cases of rapidly fatal pulmonary oedema occurring in soldiers who had suffered severe head injury. More recently, pulmonary oedema has been reported in battle casualties in Vietnam who died almost immediately following a major head injury (Simmons et al, 1969). Pulmonary oedema associated with intracranial pathology has also been described in patients with subarachnoid haemorrhage, cerebral emboli, cerebral tumours and cysts, and chronically raised ICP. The differential diagnosis includes cardiac failure, ARDS, overtransfusion and aspiration pneumonitis.

Neurogenic pulmonary oedema develops extremely rapidly, is particularly associated with hypothalamic lesions and does not occur in the presence of cervical cord transection. It is thought to be related to acute hypothalamic dysfunction causing a massive neural discharge. It seems that, initially, this produces marked vasoconstriction and a dramatic rise in pulmonary and systemic arterial pressures, with a fall in cardiac output. As a consequence, there is a shift of circulating volume, pulmonary venous congestion and a rise in left atrial pressure. The transient, but massive, increase in pulmonary capillary pressure disrupts the endothelium, producing a 'permeability' oedema which persists even though intravascular pressures rapidly return to normal.

Management consists of IPPV, with or without PEEP, together with aggressive therapy to reduce ICP. Vasodilatation, for example, using α-blockers or SNP, may be beneficial, although associated hypotension might jeopardize cerebral perfusion. It has been suggested that isoprenaline is the inotrope of choice in these patients because it produces both systemic and pulmonary vasodilatation, as well as increasing cardiac output. Despite these measures, mortality in neurogenic pulmonary oedema remains high.

Prognosis of severe head injury

The Glasgow outcome scale (Jennett and Bond, 1975) can be used to assess recovery from severe head injury in terms of five broad categories (Table 14.2). Although some patients may continue to improve for up to a year or even longer after their injury, the majority reach their ultimate outcome category within three months and 90% fail to improve further beyond six

Table 14.2 Outcome after brain damage (Glasgow outcome scale).

Dead
Persistent vegetative state — Awake but non-sentient
Severe disability — Conscious but dependent
Moderate disability — Independent but disabled
Good recovery — Non-disabling sequelae

months. In a series of 1000 head-injured patients who were in coma for at least six hours, assessment of outcome at six months showed that 49% were dead and 2% were vegetative, 10% were severely disabled, 17% were moderately disabled and 22% made a good recovery (Jennett et al, 1979). Outcome is related to the Glasgow coma score and to the age of the patient (Moss et al, 1983).

BRAIN DEATH AND IRREVERSIBLE CEREBRAL DAMAGE

Brain stem death (Conference of Royal Medical Colleges and Faculties of the United Kingdom, 1976; Jennett, 1982)

If the brain stem is destroyed, consciousness is lost and spontaneous respiration ceases. Independent existence is then impossible and, in the absence of therapeutic intervention, cardiac arrest rapidly supervenes. 'Brain stem death' is therefore now considered to be a definition of death itself. With the advent of artificial ventilation, it became possible temporarily to support such a dead patient, although in all cases cardiovascular failure eventually develops and progresses to cardiac standstill. To continue to artificially support such a patient is therefore futile. Furthermore, it needlessly prolongs the distress to both relatives and staff, is undignified for the patient and is an inefficient and uneconomical use of resources. It is therefore desirable to discontinue artificial ventilation once the diagnosis of brain stem death has been established.

Before considering such a diagnosis it is essential that certain preconditions and exclusions are fulfilled:

Preconditions

1 The patient is in apnoeic coma (i.e. unresponsive and on a ventilator, with no spontaneous respiratory efforts).
2 Irremediable structural brain damage due to a disorder which can cause brain stem death must have been diagnosed with certainty (e.g. head injury, intracranial haemorrhage).

Exclusions

1 The possibility that unresponsive apnoea is the result of poisons, sedative drugs or neuromuscular blocking agents must be excluded. The drug history should be carefully reviewed and adequate time allowed for the persistence of drug effects to be excluded. A nerve stimulator may be used to ensure that the patient is not paralysed. Blood and urine should be tested for the presence of drugs if there is any doubt.
2 Hypothermia must be excluded as a cause of coma. It is recommended that the central body temperature should be more than 35°C.
3 There must be no significant metabolic or endocrine disturbance that could produce or contribute to coma, or cause it to persist. There should be no profound abnormality of the plasma electrolytes, acid–base balance or blood glucose levels.

It is then necessary to establish that all brain stem reflexes are absent. (The tests should not be performed in the presence of seizures or abnormal postures.)
1 The pupils should be fixed and unresponsive to bright light. Both direct and consensual light reflexes should be examined. (Difficulty in interpretation may be experienced when there has been direct trauma to the eye and/or optic nerve, and if topical mydriatics have been used.) Pupil size is irrelevant, although most often they will be dilated.
2 Corneal reflexes should be absent. (Again, there may be difficulty when the eyelids are bruised and oedematous due to trauma.)
3 Oculocephalic reflexes should be absent, i.e. when the head is rotated from side to side, the eyes move with the head and therefore remain stationary relative to the orbit. In a comatose patient whose brain stem is intact, the eyes will rotate relative to the orbit (i.e. doll's eye movements are present).
4 Vestibulo-ocular reflexes should be absent ('caloric testing'). If 20 ml of ice cold water is slowly instilled into the external auditory meatus it will stimulate the tympanic membrane. If the patient's brain stem is intact, reflex eye movements will occur within 20–30 seconds, provided that access to the tympanic membrane is not prevented by, for example, blood or wax in the meatus. This should be checked by direct inspection. It should be remembered that gentamicin can cause end organ poisoning and central pathways may be impaired by drugs. Severe trauma may prevent caloric testing on one side or the other.
5 There should be no motor responses within the cranial nerve territory to painful stimuli applied centrally or peripherally. Spinal reflexes may be present.
6 There must be no gag or cough reflexes in response to pharyngeal, laryngeal or tracheal stimulation.

7 Spontaneous respiration should be absent. This test is crucial to the diagnosis of brain stem death. The patient should be ventilated with 5% CO_2 in 95% oxygen for ten minutes and then disconnected from the ventilator for a further ten minutes. Oxygenation is maintained by insufflation with 100% oxygen at high flows via a catheter placed in the endotracheal tube. The patient is observed for any signs of spontaneous respiratory efforts. A blood gas sample should be obtained during this period to ensure that the P_aCO_2 is sufficiently high to stimulate spontaneous respiration ($>6.7\,kPa$, $50\,mmHg$). It must be remembered that a few patients with severe COAD are dependent on a hypoxic drive to respiration.

The examination should be performed by two doctors a minimum of six hours after the onset of coma, or, if due to cardiac arrest, at least 24 hours after restoration of an adequate circulation. The tests should be performed on two separate occasions, the interval between the two being agreed by all the staff involved. The doctors should be either the consultant in charge of the case and one other (clinically independent of the first and registered for more than five years), or the consultant's deputy, provided he has been registered at least five years and has adequate appropriate experience, and one other. Neither should be a member of the transplant team. A neurologist should be consulted if the underlying diagnosis is in doubt.

In the UK, it is not considered necessary to perform confirmatory tests such as EEG and carotid angiography, since these may be misleading.

Organ donation

In suitable cases, and providing the patient was carrying a donor card and/or the consent of the relatives has been obtained, the organs of those in whom brain stem death has been established may be used for transplantation. In all cases, the coroner's consent must be obtained.

Kidney

The criteria for selecting a suitable kidney donor are shown in Table 14.3. Renal perfusion must be maintained prior to organ donation by appropriate expansion of the circulating volume and, if necessary, a dopamine infusion. Arterial oxygenation, ventilation, body temperature, acid–base status and electrolyte balance must all be maintained. In addition, blood samples should be obtained for screening for hepatitis antigen and HLTV-III, blood group determination and tissue typing. The kidneys must be removed by a surgeon who has examined the donor and is satisfied with the diagnosis of brain stem death. The procedure must be performed under full operating conditions in theatre.

Heart and heart–lung

The criteria for selecting a suitable donor are shown in Table 14.3. Investigations and management are as for kidney donors but, in addition, a chest x-ray and 12-lead ECG should be obtained.

Table 14.3 Selection of suitable donors (details of these criteria may vary slightly in different centres).

Kidney	Brain stem dead 5–70 years old Warm Adequately perfused and hydrated Artificially ventilated
	Free from: hepatitis antigen and HLTV-III malignant disease (except primary brain tumour) septicaemia chronic urinary tract infection (acute urinary tract infection related to catheterization is not a contraindication) renal disease
	The following are not necessarily contraindications: diabetes pneumonia hypertension hypotension
Heart or heart–lung	Brain stem dead Preferably under 40 years old (males) or less than 45 years old (females) Apyrexial Adequately perfused and hydrated Artificially ventilated
	Free from: hepatitis antigen and HLTV-III malignant disease (except primary brain tumour) septicaemia diabetes ischaemic heart disease cardiac murmurs
	In male donors over 35 years old and female donors over 40 years old coronary angiograms may rarely be requested by the transplant team. If there is any doubt about the suitability of a potential donor, it is advisable to contact the transplant team.

Liver

Most suitable kidney donors are also suitable liver donors.

Cornea

All adults are suitable donors provided there is no history of eye disease, intra-ocular surgery, syphilis, hepatitis, or postinfectious polyneuritis. The eyes can be removed up to 12 hours after cardiorespiratory arrest, but preferably within one hour.

Irreversible cerebral damage

Once the diagnosis of brain stem death has been firmly established, there is no ethical dilemma involved in discontinuing artificial ventilation. A much more difficult problem arises when the brain stem remains intact but the cerebral cortex ceases to function, either because of direct ischaemic/hypoxic damage, for example, following cardiac arrest, or because of severe disruption of the white matter, such as may occur following head injury. These patients may breathe adequately unaided and can survive for long periods in a vegetative state. Many would now accept that treatment other than basic medical and nursing care is inappropriate under these circumstances. An even more difficult ethical dilemma is presented by the patient who is severely disabled, but better than vegetative, and there is as yet no consensus on the correct management of such cases (see also Chapter 1).

STATUS EPILEPTICUS

This is a common medical emergency which can be defined as persistent or recurrent motor seizures without intervening periods of consciousness. The interval between fits is usually in the order of 5–15 minutes. The term can also be applied to continuous seizures lasting at least 30 minutes, even when consciousness is not impaired.

Major, or grand-mal, status epilepticus presents with typical tonic and clonic convulsions involving the whole body. Sometimes, however, exhaustion or structural lesions within the central nervous system, partially terminate the convulsions which may then become purely clonic or asymmetrical. In some cases, the location of the seizures varies, while in others the only manifestations are loss of consciousness with spasmodic twitching or flickering of the eyelids. These modified forms of status epilepticus are commonly encountered in critically ill patients.

In partial status epilepticus, there is repetitive focal twitching but this may sometimes become secondarily generalized with loss of consciousness. Some patients suffer a particularly prolonged 'grand mal' seizure in which the protracted clonic and tonic phases can cause extreme hypoventilation and hypoxaemia. In others, there are frequent convulsive episodes but consciousness is regained between seizures. Treatment is nevertheless equally urgent.

Unremitting myoclonic jerks may occur in isolation and are almost exclusively related to degenerative, hypoxic, toxic or metabolic encephalopathies. The twitching may be generalized or localized, rhythmic or disorganized, infrequent or occurring in bursts. They may arise spontaneously or be triggered by external stimuli.

Causes and precipitating factors

Status epilepticus is unusual in patients with chronic epilepsy but may be precipitated by trauma, lack of sleep, fasting, excessive alcohol or intercurrent infection. Failure to take antiepileptic medication, or interference with the absorption or metabolism of these agents (liver failure, renal failure, pregnancy, interaction with other drugs) can also precipitate status.

When patients with no previous history of epilepsy present in status epilepticus, an underlying cause should be suspected. There are many possibilities, including head injury, cerebral tumour (primary or secondary), brain abscess, cerebrovascular accident, meningitis, fat embolism, toxins, withdrawal syndromes, ischaemic cerebral damage, hypoglycaemia, water intoxication and extreme dehydration.

Pathophysiology

Major, prolonged seizures can cause significant brain damage. Not only are the metabolic requirements of discharging neurones increased, but their oxygen supply is often impaired. Hypoxaemia may be caused by airway obstruction, apnoeic episodes or an aspiration pneumonitis, while cerebral blood flow can be decreased by hypotension and cardiac dysrhythmias. Hypercarbia and the accumulation of lactic acid produce an intracerebral acidosis. ICP rises and, in the most severe cases, cerebral oedema may develop as a consequence of impaired autoregulation, venous congestion, neuronal hypoxia and an increase in the permeability of the blood–brain barrier.

Initially, patients in status epilepticus are usually hyperglycaemia but later blood sugar levels may be low. A lactic acidosis develops in severe cases. In some patients, life-threatening autonomic dysfunction supervenes with hyperthermia, excessive sweating, dehydration, hypertension and, later, hypotension. The violent muscular contractions may produce myolysis, myoglobinuria and, in some cases, renal failure.

Management (Delgado-Escueta et al, 1982)

Seizure activity must be controlled immediately and vital functions preserved. Remedial underlying disorders must be identified and treated.

General aspects

The patient must be protected from injury, without using excessive restraint, and should be placed in the lateral position. The airway must be cleared and, if it is available, oxygen should be administered. Endotracheal intubation may be required to secure the airway and protect the lungs from aspiration; in these cases, the nasal route is preferred since this avoids the danger of the patient biting on the tube. An intravenous infusion should be established and at this time blood can be obtained for determination of anticonvulsant levels, blood glucose, urea and electrolytes, and a full blood count. If necessary, the circulating volume is then expanded in order to restore the systemic blood pressure.

Abnormalities of fluid and electrolyte balance, as well as hyperglycaemia, hypoglycaemia, hypocalcaemia and hypomagnesaemia, must be corrected. The acidosis usually resolves spontaneously but may require correction if it persists. It is important to avoid fluid overload in those receiving a continuous infusion of anticonvulsant.

Artificial ventilation is indicated if there is respiratory depression (often induced by large doses of anticonvulsant), refractory hypoxaemia, increasing acidosis, cerebral oedema, hyperpyrexia and if the seizures are not controlled within 50–60 minutes. Muscle relaxation may be required in the latter instance but it is then essential to monitor the EEG (e.g. by using a CFM) in order to detect continued seizure activity.

Hyperpyrexia can exacerbate cerebral damage and should be vigorously treated with fanning, tepid sponging, axillary ice packs and nasogastric or rectal antipyretics. It may be reasonable to administer mannitol to those with prolonged status in whom cerebral oedema is suspected. Attempts to prevent acute renal failure in those with DIC and/or myoglobinuria may involve the administration of mannitol, frusemide and low-dose dopamine (see Chapter 15).

Further investigations may include a CAT scan to identify intracranial space occupying lesions, and a lumbar puncture when meningoencephalitis, subarachnoid haemorrhage or an intracranial abscess is suspected. An EEG can identify and localize seizure activity and may assist in the diagnosis of the underlying disorder.

Anticonvulsants

Convulsive status should not be allowed to continue; if it persists for more than 60 minutes, severe permanent brain damage may occur. Specific treatment is therefore urgent and should be instituted as soon as the airway has been secured and intravenous access has been established.

Benzodiazepines. Intravenous diazepam is rapidly effective in most forms of status and is the first-line treatment. Repeated boluses, or an infusion, are required to maintain the effect, and, in protracted status, the efficacy of these agents may decline progressively. In adults, 10–20 mg of diazepam can be given intravenously over a few minutes, followed by a continuous infusion (50 mg in 500 ml 5% dextrose initially at $40\,\mathrm{ml\,h^{-1}}$).

Phenytoin (diphenylhydantoin). This agent is additive with diazepam. A single loading dose to a total of $18\,\mathrm{mg\,kg^{-1}}$ can be given slowly intravenously ($50\,\mathrm{mg\,min^{-1}}$). Although the onset of effect may be delayed for 20–30 minutes, serum levels are maintained in the therapeutic range for 24 hours. Some authorities recommend that phenytoin should be given simultaneously with the first dose of diazepam. The main danger is myocardial toxicity.

Barbiturates. Thiopentone is an effective anticonvulsant at doses lower than those normally required to induce anaesthesia. Nevertheless, there is a risk of cardiovascular and respiratory depression, and endotracheal intubation is usually necessary. Many patients will require IPPV. Thiopentone is indicated when the patient fails to respond to diazepam and phenytoin and should be given as an initial bolus of 1–$3\,\mathrm{mg\,kg^{-1}}$ intravenously. This should be followed by a continuous infusion titrated to control seizure activity; this may require more than 3 mg min^{-1} in some cases. Blood thiopentone levels should be monitored.

Chlormethiazole. This is an effective anticonvulsant and is occasionally used for the treatment of refractory status epilepticus. It must be given as a continuous infusion, usually in a mean hourly dose of 0.5–0.7 g.

Prognosis

Currently, mortality rates should not exceed 10–12%.

TETANUS (Kerr, 1979)

The advent of effective prophylactic immunization has virtually eliminated tetanus in the developed world. In these countries, this condition now occurs mainly in those who have failed to maintain an adequate level of immunity; in England and Wales, for example, only 17 cases were reported in 1977. On the other hand, tetanus is common in most Third World countries, where several hundred thousand die of this disease every year, many of the victims being neonates and young children. In Europe, the disease is particularly common in France and Portugal where it occurs most frequently in women and in the elderly. Often, the site of entry is a trivial wound and in some cases may even be invisible. In others, the organism gains access via varicose ulcers, areas of ischaemic gangrene (particularly in diabetics) or following intra-abdominal, pelvic or obstetric surgery. In the Third World, uterine and neonatal tetanus are relatively frequent, as is tetanus associated with injuries to the feet.

Aetiology

Tetanus is caused by *Clostridium tetani*, an anaerobic, gram-positive, spore-bearing bacillus found mainly in cultivated soil and as an inhabitant of the lower gastrointestinal tract. This organism produces a potent exotoxin (tetanospasmin) which is responsible for the clinical manifestations of the disease. Exotoxin travels from the site of infection to the spinal cord, mainly via the perineurium of motor nerves, but also sometimes within autonomic and sensory nerve fibres, at a rate of approximately 75 mm day^{-1}. It then accumulates preferentially in the ipsilateral ventral root of the spinal cord where it passes into the presynaptic terminals of the inhibitory spinal interneurones and blocks release of the transmitter substance. Gamma motor neurones, interneurones and gamma segments of the medulla are therefore disinhibited and discharge spontaneously. Simultaneous contraction of both agonist and antagonist muscle groups produces the characteristic spasms.

Clinical features

The incubation period for tetanus varies between 4 and 15 days and tends to be shorter in the more severe cases. Nevertheless, severe attacks can also occur following a long incubation period.

Investigations are generally unhelpful in identifying cases of tetanus and the diagnosis is made clinically. The majority of patients present with classical trismus ('lockjaw'). Initially, there is only some slight difficulty in opening the mouth, but this may progress until the patient is unable to eat and develops a characteristic 'risus sardonicus'. Dysphagia may also be present at this stage. More unusual presentations include cephalic tetanus, in which a wound in the head and neck region is associated with local cranial nerve involvement, or local tetanus, where spasms are confined to the injured area. The differential diagnosis includes local causes of trismus (e.g. an abscess), hysteria and dystonic reactions to phenothiazines.

All these forms of tetanus may then progress, at a variable rate, through the various grades of severity. Usually, the paroxysms gradually become more generalized to involve the muscles of the neck, the trunk and, to a lesser extent, the limbs. During contractions, the neck may become rigid and hyperextended, while spasm of the paravertebral muscles can produce a marked lumbar lordosis (opisthotonus). Ventilation may be seriously impaired and respiratory arrest can occur, either due to involvement of the thoracic and abdominal musculature or because of glottic spasm. Moreover, swallowing becomes impossible and this contributes to the risk of asphyxia. Limb involvement usually consists of tonic spasms occurring particularly on the same side as the offending wound.

In severe cases, there may be continuous, but fluctuating, overactivity of the sympathetic nervous system (Kerr et al, 1968). This is associated with profuse sweating, salivation, paroxysmal hypertension, tachycardia, dysrhythmias, vasoconstriction, pyrexia and gastrointestinal stasis. Occasionally, dangerous episodes of bradycardia and hypotension occur, either spontaneously or in response to stimuli such as endotracheal suction, and these may culminate in cardiac arrest. The signs of autonomic dysfunction usually develop 2–4 days after the patient first requires muscle relaxants and resolve within 7–10 days. It has been suggested that the appearance of an unexplained tachycardia may be a useful early indication of autonomic involvement (Benedict and Kerr, 1977).

Treatment

Eradication of infection

The source of infection is identified in only about two-thirds of tetanus cases and many appear very trivial (e.g. an ingrowing toenail). Nevertheless, potentially infected wounds must be incised, cleaned, laid open and all the dead tissue excised. Frequently, even apparently minor puncture sites are explored, and a deep-seated necrotic area will be found, often surrounding a foreign body. When tetanus develops following an abortion, dilatation and curettage or a hysterectomy should be performed while in cases associated with limb ischaemia, amputation may be required. Benzylpenicillin (penicillin G) should be administered in a dose of 3–6 mega units day^{-1}, or more, for at least one week. Erythromycin can be used as an alternative in those allergic to penicillin. Hyperbaric oxygen is probably of little value.

Neutralization of toxin

Patients at risk of developing tetanus who have previously been immunized should receive a booster dose of tetanus toxoid. Such active immunization must be combined with thorough wound debridement and antibiotic prophylaxis, as outlined above. The rare at-risk patient who has never been vaccinated will require passive immunization with homologous, or heterologous antitoxin, as well as receiving the first dose of tetanus toxoid.

Most authorities recommend that patients with established tetanus should be passively immunized with either heterologous (equine) or homologous (human anti-tetanus immunoglobulin) antitoxin administered intravenously or intramuscularly. This may reduce the mortality, possibly by neutralizing circulating toxin, thereby preventing relapse or further deterioration. Others consider that systemic passive immunization is unhelpful in the established case, since toxin is already fixed within the spinal cord; for this reason, intrathecal administration has been recommended as being more efficacious. Unfortunately, those preparations currently available commercially are stabilized using phenol byproducts and are not suitable for subarachnoid injection. There is a relatively high incidence of adverse reactions to equine serum and, although more expensive, human anti-tetanus immunoglobulin is now generally preferred. There appears to be no advantage in using high doses of antitoxin. A reasonable approach is to give 30 iu per kg of 'Humotet' anti-tetanus serum intramuscularly, as well as a dose of tetanus toxoid. A slow intravenous infusion is probably safe, but experience with this route of administration is limited.

Intensive care

All patients with tetanus should be admitted to an intensive care unit for observation, assessment and treatment. The priorities are to control the spasms and prevent aspiration and/or asphyxia by endotracheal intubation or tracheostomy.

Those with isolated trismus should be disturbed as little as possible to avoid precipitating a paroxysm. In particular, oral fluids should not be permitted, nor should a nasogastric tube be passed since both can precipitate laryngeal spasm. Sedatives, preferably diazepam, should be given to control muscle spasms and the patient should be closely observed. Facilities for emergency intubation must be immediately available at the bedside.

Patients with generalized tetanus will require endotracheal intubation or tracheostomy combined with sedation to control spasms. Diazepam has excellent muscle relaxant properties, with minimal cardiovascular effects, and is the sedative of choice in this situation. It can be administered as a continuous intravenous infusion, although it is important to remember that active metabolites of diazepam are cumulative. If this fails, intravenous opiates should be added to the regimen. Barbiturates, e.g. an intravenous dose of thiopentone followed by regular phenobarbitone, may also be effective. All these agents can cause respiratory depression; therefore, controlled ventilation is often required. Chlorpromazine, which produces some α-adrenergic blockade, may also prove valuable.

If this regimen is unsuccessful (spasms lasting more than 15–20 seconds persist), the patient should be paralysed, preferably using a continuous infusion of a non-depolarizing muscle relaxant. Pancuronium has been used most frequently, but atracurium or vecuronium may prove to be suitable alternatives. Because neuromuscular blockade and IPPV may have to be maintained for 15–20 days, this is a potentially hazardous technique and should only be used in those unresponsive to alternative measures.

Autonomic disturbances are minimized by heavy sedation, and the use of adrenergic blocking agents has been shown to be, a satisfactory means of controlling the cardiovascular disturbance (Prys-Roberts et al, 1969). β-Blockers (usually propranolol) can be used to control tachycardias and dysrhythmias but α-blockers are now rarely used because of the risk of severe hypotension. Labetalol has been used successfully in this situation (Dundee and Morrow, 1979). Episodes of hypotension may resolve if the patient is stimulated, e.g. by endotracheal suction, vigorous passive limb movements or allowing the arterial carbon dioxide tension to rise.

The general principles of managing the immobile, ventilated intensive care patient are outlined in Chapter 13. Patients with tetanus lose relatively large quantities of salt and water as a result of excessive sweating and salivation. These losses are difficult to quantify and careful daily assessment of fluid and electrolyte balance is particularly important. Tetanus victims are often hypovolaemic when first seen and this may be unmasked by sedation and/or IPPV; rapid volume expansion is then required. Nutritional support can usually be provided via the enteral route, but constipation can be a problem and paralytic ileus may occur in those receiving muscle relaxants. Occasionally, therefore, parenteral feeding is necessary. Prophylactic subcutaneous heparin should be given to all patients.

Prognosis

The acute phase of tetanus persists for 3–4 weeks, and complete recovery may take up to a further four weeks. The disease is most severe during the first week, plateaus during the second and wanes in the third. Provided patients receive extensive rehabilitation, a full recovery without neurological sequelae can be anticipated. However, some patients will have sustained crush fractures of one or more vertebral bodies as a result of their spasms.

In one series of adult patients with tetanus, the mortality rate was 11% and the majority of deaths (38.4%) were related to unexpected cardiac arrest (Trujillo et al, 1980). Other causes of death include secondary infection, particularly pneumonia, pulmonary embolism and complications of tracheostomy. Occasionally, severe generalized tetanus develops extremely rapidly with continuous spasms, high fever, hypertension and tachycardia. In such cases, death usually follows within 24–48 hours, due to major circulatory disturbances.

MYASTHENIA GRAVIS (Scadding and Havard, 1981)

Myasthenia gravis is relatively rare, with an incidence of approximately 1 in 30 000. It is commonest in young females, two-thirds of all cases being women, with a peak onset in the twenties. Men tend to develop the disease later in life, and most of those who present when more than 50 years old are males.

Pathogenesis

This is an autoimmune disorder in which there is a reduction in the effective number of acetylcholine receptors at skeletal muscle motor end plates. In many patients (between 87 and 93% of cases) antibodies to these receptors can be detected and, although there is a poor correlation between absolute antibody levels and the severity of the disease, they are almost certainly important in the pathogenesis of myasthenia gravis. Antibodies to striated muscle are detected in approximately one-third of patients with myasthenia, usually in those with a thymic tumour, but are also found in association with thymic tumours in the absence of muscle weakness. It is therefore unlikely that their presence is of pathogenic significance.

Clinical features

The muscle weakness in myasthenia gravis is typically exacerbated by exertion and improved by rest. It has a characteristic distribution affecting, in descending order of frequency, the extra-ocular, bulbar, neck, limb girdle, distal limb and trunk muscles. In those patients with thymitis, there appears to be an association between myasthenia and certain specific HLA subgroups while in those with thymoma, there is no clear HLA association. Patients with thymitis who are less than 40 years old tend to have other associated autoimmune diseases and respond well to thymectomy. In some cases, weakness is confined to the extra-ocular muscles and these patients do not benefit from thymectomy, although they may respond to steroids.

A number of myasthenic syndromes have been described and may be encountered on the intensive care unit when such a patient fails to breathe following an anaesthetic during which muscle relaxants were used. For example, the Eaton–Lambert syndrome (Lambert et al, 1956) occurs in association with small cell bronchial carcinoma and is characterized by muscle weakness with aching and stiffness which, in contrast to true myasthenia, improves on exertion and spares the ocular and bulbar muscles. Nevertheless, these patients are also exquisitely sensitive to non-depolarizing muscle relaxants, and anticholinesterases have little beneficial effect. Oral guanidine and steroids may improve muscle strength, and plasma exchange may be effective.

Tensilon test

The diagnosis of myasthenia gravis can be established, and the adequacy of treatment assessed, using an intravenous test-dose of the short-acting anticholinesterase, edrophonium. To perform this 'Tensilon test' an intravenous cannula should be inserted, the ECG should be continuously monitored and atropine should be available to counteract bradycardia. An indicator of muscle function, appropriate for the particular patient, should be chosen for assessment before and after edrophonium. Usually, the most severely affected muscle group is selected. Thus, if extra-ocular muscle weakness is most prominent, eye movement and/or diplopia can be evaluated, while straight arm raising time can be used for those with predominantly limb involvement. Many of the patients admitted to the intensive care unit will have respiratory muscle weakness and in these cases, forced vital capacity provides an excellent objective indicator of the response to an anticholinesterase. Edrophonium should be administered slowly intravenously, initially in a dose of 2 mg, followed one minute later by a further 3 mg, provided no adverse effects are seen. Muscle function should be assessed one and ten minutes later.

Treatment

Anticholinesterases

Oral pyridostigmine bromide (60 mg tablets) is the treatment of choice; initially, 60 mg four times daily and then gradually increased to achieve the optimal response. If required, pyridostigmine can be taken during the night, but the maximum dose is 20 tablets a day. In difficult cases, pyridostigmine can be combined with neostigmine (15 mg tablets), which has a more rapid onset of action and can therefore be particularly useful first thing in the morning. It may not be possible to abolish muscle weakness completely, and if the dose of anticholinesterase is progressively increased in an attempt to achieve complete relief of symptoms a 'cholinergic crisis' may be precipitated.

Anticholinergics

These may be required to control side effects such as salivation, lachrymation, colic and diarrhoea. In general, however, these drugs are best avoided in the routine management of myasthenia since they may mask the onset of a cholinergic crisis.

Immunosuppressives

Steroids may be useful in those who fail to improve following thymectomy, or preoperatively in the most seriously ill patients. They are also valuable in ocular myasthenia and in those who are unsuitable for surgery. The administration of steroids may be associated with initial, sometimes severe, deterioration and any improvement may not be apparent for several weeks. Steroids can precipitate hypokalaemia by increasing urinary potassium excretion, and this can exacerbate the muscle weakness. Plasma potassium levels should be maintained in the upper normal range. Azathioprine can be used in those with severe myasthenia unresponsive to other measures, but can also produce an initial deterioration. Improvement may be delayed for up to 6–12 weeks, and is maximal at 6–15 months. Azathioprine can cause bone marrow depression and liver dysfunction.

Plasma exchange

In some patients, plasma exchange produces a dramatic, but temporary, improvement associated with a fall in antibody levels. Exchange is usually performed on five successive days, the maximal response is normally seen at 7–10 days and improvement persists for about one month. Plasma exchange can be a useful technique for managing acute problems, e.g. during the perioperative period, or to allow weaning from ventilatory support. Azathioprine can be used to prevent a rebound increase in antibody levels.

Thymectomy

This is being performed increasingly frequently, most often for young adults with severe disease of short duration and in older patients refractory to medical treatment. Remission or improvement occurs in approximately 80% of those without a thymic tumour, although the response may be delayed, sometimes for several years. The explanation for this improvement is unclear. Thymectomy or radiotherapy can also be used to treat thymoma, but the prognosis is worse in these cases and radiotherapy may be associated with a deterioration in the myasthenia.

Intensive care

As a result of improvements in the medical management of myasthenia, respiratory support is required less frequently, although an increasing number of patients are admitted for postoperative care following thymectomy.

As mentioned previously, deterioration may occur following administration of steroids, azathioprine or radiotherapy. Furthermore, hormonal changes, such as occur during menstruation or pregnancy and in thyrotoxicosis, as well as intercurrent infection and surgery, can exacerbate muscle weakness. A number of drugs can precipitate deterioration, including respiratory depressants, diuretics (probably as a result of hypokalaemia) and the aminoglycosides (which can inhibit acetylcholine release). Laxatives can decrease the absorption of anticholinesterases, while antiarrhythmics such as procainamide, lignocaine, propranolol, quinidine (and quinine, present in tonic water) reduce the excitability of muscle membrane and probably also inhibit neuromuscular transmission.

It may be difficult to distinguish between an exacerbation of myasthenia and a cholinergic crisis; both can result in respiratory failure, bulbar palsy and virtually complete paralysis. Respiratory difficulty may be exacerbated by excessive secretions in a cholinergic crisis. In severe cases, immediate endotracheal intubation and controlled ventilation will be required, while in others a Tensilon test can be performed to establish the aetiology of the crisis.

The indications for artificial ventilation and weaning in myasthenia and other neuromuscular causes of ventilatory failure are discussed in Chapters 12 and 13. When IPPV is initiated, anticholinesterases should be withdrawn and reintroduced 24–48 hours later, if necessary guided by the response to edrophonium. Some believe that a period without anticholinesterase therapy allows the motor end plate to regain its sensitivity, but the evidence for this is scanty. If the response to anticholinesterases is unsatisfactory, the use of plasma exchange, with or without azathioprine, or steroids should be considered. Secretions must be controlled with frequent physiotherapy and, if necessary, anticholinergics; some patients will require tracheostomy, particularly if bulbar muscles are involved. Plasma potassium and magnesium levels should be maintained in the high normal range and adverse drug effects (see above) must be avoided in those requiring prolonged IPPV. Subcutaneous heparin should be administered as prophylaxis against thromboembolic complications. Ventilatory function, as assessed by the forced vital capacity (FVC), is the best guide to the ability to wean from controlled ventilation, while the adequacy of bulbar muscle function largely determines the timing of extubation and the need for a tracheostomy.

The appropriate management for patients admitted to intensive care following thymectomy depends on the severity, and distribution, of their preoperative muscle weakness. Thus, mild myasthenics, without respiratory or bulbar muscle involvement, may be extubated immediately. Those with more severe disease will require elective postoperative ventilation until respiratory function is adequate (vital capacity more than $10–15\,\mathrm{ml\,kg^{-1}}$). The endotracheal tube should remain in place until both respiratory and bulbar muscle function are considered to be satisfactory and the risk of unexpected deterioration is minimal (i.e. approximately 48 hours postoperatively). Nasal endotracheal tubes are generally preferred in these cases because they are more easily tolerated by the alert patient. Some centres have rigid protocols for postoperative care following thymectomy; others adjust their treatment regimen to suit the individual patient.

ACUTE INFLAMMATORY POLYNEUROPATHY (Hughes, 1978)

In 1916, Guillain, Barré and Strohl described two cases of paralysis with muscle tenderness and areflexia, associated with a high protein content, but normal white cell count, in the CSF. Both patients eventually recovered. Landry had previously described a similar case in 1859, although he had not obtained CSF, and the condition should therefore properly be called the Landry–Guillain–Barrée–Strohl syndrome. However, common practice is to omit the names of both Landry and Strohl from this eponym. The term acute inflammatory polyneuropathy (AIP) encompasses this well-known syndrome as well as other causes of acute polyneuritis not associated with an identifiable preceding infection or CSF changes. Acute neuropathies due to toxic, metabolic or nutritional causes, as well as those associated with collagen diseases and vasculitis, are excluded from this definition.

The frequency of AIP is approximately 1.6 per 100 000 of the population per annum. The sex incidence is equal, with a slight preponderance of cases between the ages of 16 and 25 years. A precipitating event can be identified in approximately two-thirds of cases, often a minor viral upper respiratory tract infection. AIP is particularly associated with cytomegalovirus infections but may also follow mycoplasma, or even bacterial, infections as well as immunization and surgery.

Pathology

Cellular infiltrates, consisting predominantly of lymphocytes, are found throughout the peripheral nervous system. These are associated with segmental demyelination and marked slowing of conduction times. Only Schwann-cell-derived myelin is attacked, while that originating from oligodendrocytes within the CNS is spared. Although motor involvement is clinically most conspicuous, AIP affects the dorsal roots and dorsal root ganglia as well as the ventral roots. It is possible that neuronal damage is caused by humoral factors, as well as being cell-mediated, since raised antibody titres against myelin have been identified in patients with AIP. The pathogenesis of this disease may therefore be either cross-antigenicity between the infecting organism and the myelin sheath or the organism itself may be incorporated into, and persist within, the myelin sheath. An alternative explanation is that the precipitating infection inhibits the suppressor cells which normally prevent the development of autoimmune phenomena. The relative frequency of preceding mycoplasma infection, which is known to cause other autoimmune phenomena, suggests that cross-antigenicity is the most likely mechanism. Raised antibody titres against other organisms, in particular a variety of viruses, may also be demonstrated but their relationship to the onset of AIP is unclear.

An elevated CSF total protein concentration ($>0.4\,\mathrm{g\,l^{-1}}$), with a normal white cell content ($<10\,\mathrm{ml^{-1}}$), is characteristic of the Guillain–Barré syndrome, but is not invariable in AIP. Sometimes, the protein content rises later in the course of the illness, but in some cases the concentration remains normal throughout.

Clinical features

Weakness is normally distal initially, and may be asymmetrical, but ascending paralysis often progresses rapidly to involve proximal muscle groups, including the respiratory and bulbar muscles. Although motor involvement predominates, sensory symptoms such as paraesthesiae and numbness are common and marked sensory loss is occasionally seen. In some cases, muscle pain and tenderness is severe, while sphincter function is usually preserved.

Sometimes, a patient will present with cranial nerve involvement; for example, the combination of ophthalmoplegia, ataxia and areflexia is a well-recognized variant of AIP. The presence of muscle fibrillation indicates complete denervation and suggests that recovery will be delayed or incomplete.

The autonomic nervous system may also be involved in AIP (Lichtenfeld, 1971), most commonly in those with extensive disease or cranial nerve involvement. The manifestations of the autonomic neuropathy are complex and can be lethal. Sinus tachycardia is a common feature and may be punctuated by periods of profound bradycardia or even asystole occurring either spontaneously or in response to stimulating procedures such as endotracheal suction. These episodes are often accompanied by sweating and flushing. Blood pressure is unstable and prolonged periods of hypertension may occur. These are associated with vasoconstriction and may be interspersed with episodes of hypotension, with or without tachycardia. Associated ECG abnormalities include flattening of T waves, ST segment depression, an increased QRS voltage, left axis deviation and prolongation of the Q–T interval. Gastrointestinal disturbances may also occur, as may profuse sweating and salivation. Hallucinations are sometimes associated with these autonomic disturbances.

Management

The administration of steroids to patients with AIP appears to delay recovery and may increase the incidence of residual disability and relapse (Hughes et al, 1978). Steroids and other immunosuppressant agents, e.g. azathioprine and cyclophosphamide, are therefore no longer recommended in AIP.

Current evidence does, however, support the use of plasma exchange in patients with severe Guillain–Barré syndrome who require artificial ventilation. In experienced units, this seems to be a safe procedure which can accelerate recovery and thereby shorten the period on IPPV, as well as the time spent in hospital, sufficiently to justify the costs. Approximately one-third of patients fail to respond to plasma exchange and the technique is most likely to be successful when performed early in the course of the disease (within two weeks of its onset). The mechanism for the beneficial effect of plasma exchange in Guillain-Barré syndrome remains uncertain (Hughes, 1985).

Respiratory and bulbar muscle function must be closely monitored so that controlled ventilation can be instituted before lung function deteriorates or respiratory arrest supervenes. The FVC should be measured at least twice a day in all cases, and more frequently in those who develop respiratory muscle weakness. As well as the absolute value of FVC, the speed with which ventilatory impairment progresses influences the decision to intervene. If lung function is also impaired, for example, due to recurrent aspiration or secondary pneumonia, the patient may require artificial ventilation before the FVC has fallen below the conventional $10-15\,\mathrm{ml\,kg^{-1}}$ (see also Chapter 13). Artificial ventilation should also be considered if the patient complains of breathlessness and must be instituted immediately if the arterial carbon dioxide tension is elevated. The presence of abdominal paradox (indrawing of the abdominal wall during inspiration) and respiratory difficulty when supine are indicative of significant diaphragm weakness.

Autonomic disturbances can be minimized by achieving and maintaining an adequate circulating volume, by ensuring satisfactory oxygenation, especially during endotracheal suction, and by adequate sedation. β-Blockade can be used to control episodes of hypertension and tachycardia, although high doses may be required. Chlorpromazine and phentolamine have also been used as antihypertensives. Insertion of a pacemaker should be considered in those with significant bradycardia and is essential if the patient suffers an episode of asystole. Atropine may alleviate the situation until the pacemaker is in place. Because severe autonomic disturbances can occur suddenly and unexpectedly, some centres routinely administer regular atropine and a β-blocking agent to all patients with AIP who require intensive care. Others simply treat the haemodynamic abnormalities appropriately as they arise.

Potentially lethal complications of AIP include thromboembolism and pulmonary infection, as well as autonomic dysfunction. These complications are theoretically preventable. Prophylactic subcutaneous heparin, and frequent passive limb movements, minimize the risk of deep vein thrombosis and pulmonary embolism. Antacid prophylaxis (see Chapter 8) and measures to reduce the risk of aspiration, atelectasis and pulmonary infection (see Chapters 6 and 13) are also important aspects of the care of patients with severe AIP.

Prognosis

Evolution of the disease is usually complete within three weeks, but the speed of recovery is variable. Some improvement is generally seen within a few days of the period of maximum disability, but sometimes several weeks elapse before recovery begins. About half the survivors will have improved substantially within three to six months, and 60% will have completely recovered within one year. Approximately 10% will have a significant, permanent residual handicap, while about 5% relapse. It is possible to achieve an overall mortality rate of around 5% or less.

RABIES

This is an acute viral encephalitis transmitted to man by animal bites, usually from vampire bats, dogs or foxes. Traditionally, rabies is considered to be invariably fatal, but it is possible that some patients may survive if they can be successfully supported during the acute phase of the illness.

Rabies is relatively common in Third World countries, but a few cases also occur in the USA. In Europe, animal rabies is spreading westwards through northern Europe and Germany into eastern France.

Following inoculation, the incubation period of rabies varies between 20 days or less and more than 90 days. The clinical manifestations consist of painful muscle contractions and spasms, particularly affecting the larynx, oropharynx and respiratory muscles. Hydrophobia is common and even the sight of water may provoke intense spasm of oropharyngeal and laryngeal muscles. Respiratory function is frequently impaired due to the effects of aspiration, muscle spasms and abnormal patterns of ventilation caused by lesions in the brain stem. It is possible that viral pneumonia also contributes to the impairment of lung function. Other neurological features include convulsions, upper motor neurone syndromes, monoplegia, paraplegia and an acute ascending motor neuropathy. An acute myocarditis may explain the cardiac dysrhythmias and ECG abnormalities.

Prophylaxis

The wound should be thoroughly cleaned, debrided and laid open. Anti-rabies serum can be introduced into the wound and infiltrated into the surrounding area. Immunization requires the administration of 7–21 daily injections of vaccine and can be combined with human anti-rabies γ-globulin. Although serotherapy can impede the development of an immune response, this can be avoided by administering booster doses 10, 20 and 90 days after the vaccination programme is completed. If rabies is established, serum should be given, but vaccination is of no value.

Intensive care

This follows the same principles as outlined above for the treatment of tetanus and involves the administration of sedatives, muscle relaxants and anticonvulsants. Tracheostomy and IPPV may also be required. Personnel in

contact with the patient must be vaccinated and should wear protective
gowns, gloves and masks.

FURTHER READING

Brain Failure and Resuscitation (1981) *Clinics in Critical Care Medicine 2*. New York:
  Churchill Livingstone.
Jennett B & Teasdale G (1977) Prognosis of neurosurgical patients requiring intensive
  care. In Ledingham IMcA (ed.) *Recent Advances in Intensive Therapy*, pp 33–45.
  Edinburgh: Churchill Livingstone.
McDowall DG (1983) Management of severe head injury. In Ledingham IMcA &
  Hanning CD (eds) *Recent Advances in Critical Care Medicine*, pp 129–142.
  Edinburgh: Churchill Livingstone.

REFERENCES

Adams JH, Graham DI, Scott G, Parker LS & Doyle D (1980) Brain damage in fatal
  non-missile head injury. *Journal of Clinical Pathology* **33**: 1132–1145.
Benedict CR & Kerr JH (1977) Assessment of sympathetic overactivity in tetanus.
  British Medical Journal **ii**: 806.
Bingham RM, Procaccio F, Prior PF & Hinds CJ (1985) Cerebral electrical activity
  influences the effects of etomidate on cerebral perfusion pressure in traumatic
  coma. *British Journal of Anaesthesia* **57**: 843–848.
Braakman R, Schouten HJA, Blaauw-van Dishoeck M & Minderhoud JM (1983)
  Megadose steroids in severe head injury. Results of a prospective double-blind
  clinical trial. *Journal of Neurosurgery* **58**: 326–330.
Brierley JB, Brown AW, Excell BJ & Meldrum BS (1969) Brain damage in the rhesus
  monkey resulting from profound arterial hypotension. I. Its nature, distribution
  and general physiological correlates. *Brain Research* **13**: 68–100.
Conference of Medical Royal Colleges and their Faculties in the United Kingdom
  (1976) Diagnosis of brain death. *British Medical Journal* **ii**: 1187–1188.
Cooper PR, Moody S, Kemp Clark W et al (1979) Dexamethasone and severe head
  injury. A prospective double-blind study. *Journal of Neurosurgery* **51**: 307–316.
Delgado–Escueta AV, Wasterlain C, Treiman DM & Porter RJ (1982) Management
  of status epilepticus. *New England Journal of Medicine* **306**: 1337–1340.
Dundee JW & Morrow WF (1979) Labetalol in severe tetanus. *British Medical Journal*
  i: 1121–1122.
Editorial (1985) Neurogenic pulmonary oedema. *Lancet* **i**: 1430–1431.
Frost EAM (1977) Effects of positive end-expiratory pressure on intracranial pressure
  and compliance in brain-injured patients. *Journal of Neurosurgery* **47**: 195–200.
Guillain G, Barré JA & Strohl A (1916) Sur un syndrome de radiculo-névrite avec
  hyperalbuminose du liquide encéphalo-rachidien sans réaction cellulaire. *Bulletins
  et mémoires de la Société Medicale des Hôpiteaux de Paris* **40**: 1462–1470
  (translated *Archives of Neurology* (1968) **18**: 450–452)
Hughes RAC (1978) Acute inflammatory polyneuropathy. *British Journal of Hospital
  Medicine* **20**: 688–693.
Hughes RAC (1985) Plasma exchange for Guillain–Barré syndrome. *British Medical
  Journal* **291**: 615–616.
Hughes RAC, Newsom-Davis JM, Perkin GD & Pierce M (1978) Controlled trial of
  prednisolone in acute polyneuropathy. *Lancet* **ii**: 750–753.
Jennett B (1982) Brain death. *Intensive Care Medicine* **8**: 1–3.

Jennett B & Bond M (1975) Assessment of outcome after severe brain damage. A practical scale. *Lancet* **i:** 480–484.

Jennett B & MacMillan R (1981) Epidemiology of head injury. *British Medical Journal* **282:** 101–104.

Jennett B, Teasdale G, Braakman R et al (1979) Prognosis of patients with severe head injury. *Neurosurgery* **4:** 283–289.

Jennett B, Teasdale G, Fry J et al (1980) Treatment for severe head injury. *Journal of Neurology, Neurosurgery and Psychiatry* **43:** 289–295.

Kerr J (1979) Current topics in tetanus. *Intensive Care Medicine* **5:** 105–110.

Kerr JH, Corbett JL, Prys-Roberts C, Crampton Smith A & Spalding JMK (1968) Involvement of the sympathetic nervous system in tetanus. *Lancet* **ii:** 236–241.

Lambert EH, Eaton LM & Rooke ED (1956) Defect of neuromuscular conduction associated with malignant neoplasm. *American Journal of Physiology* **187:** 612–613.

Lichtenfeld P (1971) Autonomic dysfunction in the Guillain–Barré syndrome. *American Journal of Medicine* **50:** 772–780.

McDowall DG (1976) Neurosurgical anaesthesia and intensive care. In Hewer CL & Atkinson RS (eds) *Recent Advances in Anaesthesia and Analgesia 12*. Edinburgh: Churchill Livingstone.

Mendelow AD, Teasdale G, Jennett B et al (1983) Risks of intracranial haematoma in head injured adults. *British Medical Journal* **287:** 1173–1176.

Miller JD, Garibi J & Pickard JD (1973) Induced changes of cerebrospinal fluid volume. Effects during continuous monitoring of ventricular fluid pressure. *Archives of Neurology* **28:** 265–269.

Miller JD, Becker DP, Ward JD et al (1977) Significance of intracranial hypertension in severe head injury. *Journal of Neurosurgery* **47:** 503–516.

Miller JD, Butterworth JF, Gudeman SK et al (1981) Further experience in the management of severe head injury. *Journal of Neurosurgery* **54:** 289–299.

Moss E, Gibson JS, McDowall DG & Gibson RM (1983) Intensive management of severe head injuries. *Anaesthesia* **38:** 214–225.

Moutier F (1918) Hypertension et mort par oedème pulmonaire aigu, chez les blessés cranio-encéphaliques. *Presse Medical* **26:** 108–109.

Muizelaar JP, Wei EP, Kontos HA & Becker DP (1983) Mannitol causes compensatory cerebral vasoconstriction and vasodilation to blood viscosity changes. *Journal of Neurosurgery* **59:** 822–828.

Obrist WD, Langfitt TW, Jaggi JL, Cruz J & Gennarelli TA (1984) Cerebral blood flow and metabolism in comatose patients with acute head injury. Relationship to intracranial hypertension. *Journal of Neurosurgery* **61:** 241–253.

Old GE & Jensen FT (1978) Cerebral autoregulation in unconscious patients with brain injury. *Acta Anaesthesiologica Scandinavica* **22:** 270–280.

Paulson OB, Olesen J & Christensen MS (1972) Restoration of autoregulation of cerebral blood flow by hypocapnia. *Neurology* **22:** 286–293.

Pierce EC, Lambertsen CJ, Deutsch S et al (1962) Cerebral circulation and metabolism during thiopental anesthesia and hyperventilation in man. *Journal of Clinical Investigation* **41:** 1664–1671.

Prior PF (1985) EEG monitoring and evoked potentials in brain ischaemia. *British Journal of Anaesthesia* **57:** 63–81.

Prior JGL, Hinds CJ, Williams J & Prior PF (1983) The use of etomidate in the management of severe head injury. *Intensive Care Medicine* **9:** 313–320.

Prys-Roberts C, Corbett JL, Kerr JH, Crampton Smith A & Spalding JMK (1969) Treatment of sympathetic overactivity in tetanus. *Lancet* **i:** 542–546.

Raichle ME, Posner JB & Plum F (1970) Cerebral blood flow during and after hyperventilation. *Archives of Neurology* **23:** 394–403.

Ropper AH, O'Rourke D & Kennedy SK (1982) Head position, intracranial pressure and compliance. *Neurology* **32:** 1288–1291.

Rose J, Valtonen S & Jennett B (1977) Avoidable factors contributing to death after head injury. *British Medical Journal* **ii:** 615–618.

Scadding GK & Havard CWH (1981) Pathogenesis and treatment of myasthenia gravis. *British Medical Journal* **283:** 1008–1012.

Shapiro HM (1985) Barbiturates in brain ischaemia. *British Journal of Anaesthesia* **57:** 82–95.

Simmons RL, Martin AM, Heisterkamp CA & Ducker TB (1969) Respiratory insufficiency in combat casualties. II. Pulmonary edema following head injury. *Annals of Surgery* **170:** 39–44.

Trujillo MJ, Castillo A, Espana JV, Guevara P & Eganez H (1980) Tetanus in the adult: intensive care and management experience with 233 cases. *Critical Care Medicine* **8:** 419–423.

White PF, Schlobohm RM, Pitts LH & Landauer JM (1982) A randomized study of drugs for preventing increases in intracranial pressure during endotracheal suction. *Anesthesiology* **57:** 242–244.

15
Acute Renal Failure

Because of its enormous vascular supply and metabolic activity, the kidney is particularly susceptible to the effects of underperfusion and hypoxaemia. Although acute renal failure (ARF) may occasionally result from a single identifiable event, such as hypotension or drug toxicity, it occurs most frequently in patients with multiple organ failure and overwhelming sepsis. The outcome in this latter category of patient is poor, particularly in those with respiratory failure.

The prevention of ARF is therefore a fundamental aspect of intensive care practice. This entails meticulous cardiovascular support, including rapid expansion of the circulating volume and the judicious use of inotropes when indicated, as well as careful maintenance of crystalloid balance, aggressive treatment of sepsis and the avoidance of nephrotoxic drugs. Constant vigilance for the early signs of impaired renal function, followed by immediate corrective measures when required, is also essential. In some circumstances, the use of specific preventive therapy is warranted (see below).

DEFINITION AND CAUSES (Table 15.1)

ARF can be defined as a sudden (and usually reversible) failure of the kidneys to excrete the waste products of metabolism, and may be broadly categorized as prerenal, renal or postrenal.

Prerenal failure, in which there is no intrinsic renal damage, is due to impaired renal perfusion, usually related to an episode of shock or hypovolaemia. Prerenal uraemia can also result from excessive production of waste products which may then accumulate in those with pre-existing mild renal impairment. Postrenal failure is caused by urinary tract obstruction.

Table 15.1 Causes of acute renal failure.

Acute tubular necrosis (ATN)

Glomerular disease
   crescentic nephritis
   systemic lupus erythematosus (SLE)
   polyarteritis nodosa (PAN)
   Goodpasture's syndrome

Acute interstitial nephritis

Vascular lesions

The terms 'acute renal failure' and 'acute tubular necrosis' (ATN) have become virtually synonymous. The latter strictly refers to necrosis of kidney tubules but is now used to describe the clinical syndrome of reversible acute renal failure which can follow an episode of shock (vasomotor nephropathy) or exposure to a nephrotoxin. It accounts for the majority of cases of ARF encountered in intensive care units. Nephrotoxins which can precipitate ATN include a variety of drugs (e.g. aminoglycosides) and myoglobin released from damaged muscle in patients with severe crush injuries or non-traumatic rhabdomyolysis (e.g. alcohol withdrawal, barbiturate poisoning or uncontrolled seizure activity).

ARF may also, but less commonly, be due to a variety of glomerular lesions, e.g. a rapidly progressive crescentic nephritis or a glomerulonephritis related to a systemic illness such as systemic lupus erythematosus (SLE), polyarteritis nodosa (PAN) or Goodpasture's syndrome. Acute interstitial nephritis is now recognized as an unusual but important cause of ARF and is usually a result of an acute or subacute 'allergic' reaction to drugs. While classically described in association with methicillin, or other penicillins, numerically the non-steroidal anti-inflammatory drugs are now becoming an increasingly important cause of this condition.

Hyperuricaemia is another relatively uncommon cause of ARF, the basis of which is uric acid deposition in the distal tubules and collecting ducts. Hyperuricaemic ARF is now seen most frequently as a complication of chemotherapy for lymphomas or leukaemias.

Renal failure due to vascular lesions may be embolic (e.g. from a mural thrombus) or thrombotic (e.g. following trauma or vascular surgery) or in association with atheroma or polyarteritis nodosa.

Finally, ARF is a common complication of liver disease, including fulminant hepatic failure (FHF), decompensated cirrhosis and obstructive jaundice, but the term 'hepatorenal syndrome' is non-specific and should probably be avoided.

Pathogenesis of acute intrinsic renal failure (Table 15.2)

Except for those cases caused by nephrotoxins, the onset of ATN is almost always related to an episode of reduced renal blood flow and is precipitated by the vasomotor response to hypotension and hypovolaemia. The reduction in renal blood flow is associated with marked selective cortical ischaemia, probably related to preglomerular vasoconstriction (Hollenberg et al 1973; Reubi et al, 1973). Although it has been suggested that systemic activation of the renin–angiotensin system is an important mediator of these alterations in renal blood flow, it seems more likely that intrarenal renin release, with local angiotensin-induced afferent arteriolar constriction, is responsible (Myers and Moran, 1986).

Table 15.2 Pathogenesis of acute renal failure.

Renal ischaemia
Decreased glomerular ultrafiltration coefficient
Tubular backleak of filtrate
Tubular obstruction

Renal blood flow usually remains low throughout the oliguric phase, even when volume deficits have been replaced and blood pressure restored, but then returns to normal during recovery of renal function. Some therefore attribute the continued reduction in glomerular filtration rate (GFR) to persistent afferent arteriolar constriction or to occlusion of small blood vessels by ischaemic cell swelling (Flores et al, 1972). Renal cortical ischaemia does not always persist, however, and, using an ischaemic model of ARF, it has been shown that the tubules remained collapsed despite restoration of renal blood flow to supranormal values, suggesting a defect in glomerular filtration (Cox et al, 1974). This may be explained in part by a loss of the normal ultrafiltration capacity of the glomerulus, although tubular injury, involving predominantly the proximal tubules, may be of central importance in the development of oliguria (Myers and Moran, 1986). Tubular obstruction by endothelial cell swelling and/or casts as well as leakage of tubular fluid across necrotic epithelium into the interstitium may also contribute to oliguria.

In critically ill patients, ARF commonly occurs in association with major sepsis and septicaemia, and this may be in part related to the direct or indirect effects of endotoxin. This is known to impair renal blood flow in experimental animals, even in the absence of hypotension (Hinshaw et al, 1959), and can initiate intravascular coagulation, as well as triggering a number of other potentially damaging events (see Chapter 10).

Obstructive jaundice may be incriminated in the development of ARF when there is no other obvious cause, but the precise mechanism is unclear. Although the toxic effects of circulating endotoxin or bile have been held responsible for the renal haemodynamic disturbances observed in these patients, others have suggested that jaundice renders the kidneys more sensitive to ischaemia (Dawson, 1964).

ARF is also common in FHF; in one study, approximately 80% of those in grade III or IV coma had some impairment of renal function (Wilkinson et al, 1974). Although most cases are due to identifiable prerenal factors, or to vasomotor nephropathy associated with hypotension, gastrointestinal haemorrhage, or septicaemia, in a few the mechanism is unclear. In decompensated cirrhosis, ARF is probably caused by a redistribution of renal blood flow, with a reduction in total flow and GFR occurring only as late events. This redistribution of flow may largely account for the intense sodium retention which occurs in cirrhosis, with hyperaldosteronism playing a less important role. The ability to handle a water load, concentrate urine and excrete hydrogen ions is also impaired in cirrhotics. ARF may then be precipitated by an episode of gastrointestinal bleeding, a sudden increase in ascites or overvigorous diuretic administration.

In summary, therefore, although it has been suggested that renal cortical ischaemia is the main pathogenic event in ARF, it seems likely that in most cases more than one mechanism is involved, and that the factors which initiate the damage are not necessarily the same as those which perpetuate renal dysfunction.

DIAGNOSIS AND INVESTIGATIONS

In intensive care patients, oliguria (urine output $< 0.5\,ml\,kg^{-1}h^{-1}$) is usually the first indication that renal function is impaired; the diagnosis is then confirmed by a progressive rise in blood urea and creatinine levels, associated with a metabolic acidosis and hyperkalaemia, as well as salt and water retension. Occasionally, an unexpected increase in plasma potassium concentration is the earliest sign of impaired renal function, particularly in the presence of tissue injury. Oliguria is not, however, an essential prerequisite for the diagnosis of ARF, since when renal concentrating ability is reduced even the production of 2–3 litres of urine a day may not reflect a sufficiently high GFR to excrete the nitrogenous metabolic waste products, particularly if the patient is hypercatabolic.

In all cases, and particularly if the patient is anuric or has intermittent complete anuria, bladder outflow obstruction must be excluded as a cause of ARF. This possibility should be suspected in patients with previous symptoms of prostatic enlargement and in those who have suffered recent trauma or surgery to the pelvic area. Examination may reveal an enlarged bladder. If there is any doubt, aseptic bladder catheterization should be performed or, if a urinary catheter is already in place, it should be examined for obstruction. If bladder outflow obstruction is excluded, the urethral catheter should be removed after instilling 50 ml noxythiolin to minimize the risk of urinary tract infection. Rectal and vaginal examinations should be performed and the external genitalia must be inspected.

Anuria is an ominous sign in patients who have recently undergone surgery to the aorta in close proximity to the renal arteries. If loss of vascular supply to the kidneys is a serious possibility, then the implications for management are profound. Early renography, followed by direct renal arteriography if no perfusion is shown, is indicated.

Once bladder outflow obstruction has been excluded, it is important to define whether the patient has prerenal, renal or postrenal failure.

The history can provide a clue to the aetiology and may establish whether there was any pre-existing renal impairment. Many critically ill patients will be unable to communicate, but relatives or close friends can be interviewed and documented case histories will often be available from the admitting team or referring hospital. It is important to establish whether there is any evidence of previous renal disorders (childhood nephrotic syndrome, haematuria, nocturia, renal colic, hypertension, failed medical examinations for insurance purposes or for entry into the armed forces) as well as to ask about recognized aetiological factors, such as analgesic abuse (particularly in patients with arthritis or migraine), 'mainlining' of drugs, ingestion of non-steroidal anti-inflammatory drugs (NSAIDs), diabetes and recent infections, surgery or trauma. The family history may suggest the possibility of polycystic disease. Finally, it is important to enquire about any recent exposure to unusual chemicals or solvents at work or in the home.

Old case-notes should be scrutinized for the results of previous urine testing (proteinuria, haematuria), urea and creatinine determinations and blood pressure recordings. Plain abdominal films, intravenous urograms or ultrasound examinations may also be available and can give an indication of kidney size and the presence of stones. Recent notes may reveal an episode of hypotension (e.g. on the anaesthetic chart) or sepsis, as well as providing a record of drugs administered (look particularly for gentamicin, NSAIDs and contrast media).

In prerenal failure, the excretory function of the kidneys is impaired by shock, hypovolaemia or crystalloid depletion; this causes oliguria and a reduction in GFR, with maximal tubular reabsorption of salt and water. Proteinuria is usually absent. In general, blood urea rises more than creatinine and the urine is concentrated (osmolality > 500 mmol l^{-1}) with a low sodium content (< 20 mmol l^{-1}). In some cases, however, there may be a renal 'leak' of sodium in which case urinary sodium content may be > 30 mmol l^{-1} and oliguria is less marked or absent. Classically, the urine/plasma ratios of osmolality, urea and creatinine are greater than 2, 30 and 15 respectively. Unfortunately, in many intensive care patients, values for the urine/plasma ratios of osmolality, urea and creatinine are borderline or misleading, especially in non-oliguric renal failure, when diuretics have been administered, and in those with pre-existing renal or hepatic disease, cardiac failure or electrolyte disturbances (particularly hypokalaemia). Consequently, they are rarely of value and the distinction can only be made on the basis of a clinical assessment of the state of hydration (oedema, neck veins, blood pressure, postural hypotension) and the response to a volume challenge, guided as necessary by measurements of CVP and/or PCWP.

The diagnosis of intrinsic ARF is suggested by demonstrating that urine and plasma are iso-osmolar, that the urinary sodium concentration is high (> 30–50 mmol l^{-1}) and that the urinary potassium concentration is low (< 10 mmol l^{-1}). Proteinuria is present. The differential diagnosis then includes ATN, glomerular lesions (acute glomerulonephritis, vasculitis), acute interstitial nephritis, renal vascular lesions, and an acute exacerbation of chronic renal disease.

Once prerenal failure has been excluded, the most immediate problem is the exclusion or identification of urinary tract obstruction. Renal size must also be determined since small kidneys are indicative of underlying chronic renal disease. In most patients, ultrasound scanning can reliably identify obstruction, as well as providing a reasonable estimate of kidney size. If ultrasound is inconclusive, high-dose intravenous urography provides the same information and very occasionally may define the site of the obstruction. Usually, however, when obstruction is detected, antegrade or retrograde ureterography is necessary to define the site. Obstruction requires skilled urological assessment with a view to urgently establishing free drainage of urine.

The possibility that ARF is due to glomerular disease should be considered, particularly when there are extrarenal signs such as skin lesions (especially purpura), arthritis, neurological manifestations (e.g. mononeuritis) or pulmonary involvement. Hypertension is usual in these cases. Serum complement levels may be reduced and, in some, circulating immune complexes are identified. Examination of the urine may reveal red cell casts and proteinuria, whereas in vasomotor nephropathy the urinary sediment will contain only tubular cells with a few granular casts. If the presentation suggests the possibility of a treatable lesion, renal biopsy may be indicated. There is, however, a significant risk of complications with this procedure, particularly haemorrhage, and these should be weighed against the likely benefits.

When glomerular disease presents as ARF, it is usually due to an acute process, such as a rapidly progressive crescentic nephritis, or a systemic disease such as PAN, SLE or Goodpasture's syndrome. The latter should be suspected when there is pulmonary involvement with haemorrhage and the diagnosis can be confirmed by demonstrating linear deposits of IgG along the glomerular basement membrane and by identifying circulating anti-glomerular basement membrane antibody.

Renal cortical necrosis usually presents as ARF and cannot normally be distinguished from vasomotor nephropathy in the acute stage. The aetiological factors are often the same and include severe shock, major surgery, transfusion reactions, infections and burns. However, cortical necrosis occurs particularly in association with obstetric disasters, especially later in pregnancy (Kleinknecht et al, 1973). It has been suggested, therefore, that cortical necrosis occurs especially in those with a hypercoagulable state in whom development of DIC may cause particularly severe renal ischaemia. Cortical necrosis may simply be a more severe form of ATN, with less chance of recovery, and should be suspected if oliguria is prolonged. The diagnosis is likely if the kidney size is found to be decreasing and cortical calcification, which appears in approximately half the patients after about six weeks, is virtually diagnostic. In such cases, a renal biopsy may be performed in order to confirm the diagnosis.

Acute interstitial nephritis may be associated with a rash, fever and joint involvement with marked eosinophilia and raised serum IgE levels. Large numbers of eosinophils may be identified in the urine. Renal biopsy confirms the diagnosis.

Renal vascular lesions present as sudden oliguria, or often complete anuria, accompanied by hypertension and loin pain. Vascular obstruction may be due to embolism, e.g. from a mural thrombus, or thrombosis, e.g. following trauma, due to vascular surgery, or related to PAN or atheroma. The diagnosis can be confirmed by radio-isotope scan or direct renal arteriography. The latter will be required to define the site of the lesion.

MANAGEMENT AND CLINICAL COURSE

Prerenal failure

This should be treated by optimizing the circulating volume, replacing fluid and electrolyte deficits and restoring the blood pressure. If cardiac output and blood pressure remain low despite volume expansion, an inotrope may be required, in which case dopamine is the agent of choice (see Chapter 10). Hypoxaemia, hypercarbia and, in some cases, metabolic acidosis, should also be corrected (see Chapter 4). Diuretics should not be given to patients with prerenal oliguria and in this respect it is important to appreciate that there may be a delay of several hours between completion of these measures and restoration of the urine output.

Incipient renal failure

Although the treatment of acute renal failure is largely supportive, a number of active measures are usually employed based on the premise that there may be an incipient phase of ATN which can be reversed by prompt intervention. While this is a popular concept, the evidence that such a phase exists is largely anecdotal and the efficacy of measures designed to abort or limit the severity of subsequent established ARF is still debated. Nevertheless, in most units one or more of the following measures are usually employed:

Mannitol. It has been suggested that this osmotic diuretic may have a protective effect when used prophylactically in those with obstructive jaundice (Dawson, 1964), and during surgery on the abdominal aorta (Barry et al, 1961), but it is unclear whether this agent can influence the course of ARF when given after the initiating event. There is some experimental evidence that mannitol can produce potentially beneficial effects in ARF, including prevention of cellular swelling (Flores et al, 1972), improved renal haemodynamics (Johnston et al, 1979) and attenuation or prevention of tubular obstruction by increasing proximal intratubular pressures and urine flow rates (Cronin et al, 1978). However, although there is some uncontrolled clinical evidence that early administration of mannitol can abort or at least limit the severity of ARF (Luke et al, 1965), this has yet to be substantiated. Furthermore, its use may be complicated by circulatory overload and pulmonary oedema, particularly if a diuresis does not follow its administration, as well as cellular dehydration. Nevertheless, some authorities recommend administering intravenous mannitol (e.g. 20g of a 20% solution) within up to 48 hours after the renal insult.

Frusemide. This loop diuretic can increase renal cortical blood flow (Birtch et al, 1967) and may specifically improve the glomerular filtration rate, possibly partly by a tubular effect (De Torrente et al, 1978). Nevertheless, the clinical value of frusemide in ARF remains uncertain. Minuth and his colleagues (1976) performed a retrospective, non-randomized study and claimed that a response to frusemide decreased the need for dialysis, although it did not appear to affect mortality. Some authorities therefore feel that frusemide may be valuable because it converts oliguric renal failure to non-oliguric renal failure, thereby minimizing the risks of hyperkalaemia and fluid overload, facilitating nutritional support and decreasing dialysis requirements. Others believe that frusemide only produces a diuresis in those in whom ARF would in any case have been rapidly reversible. Indeed, a number of controlled studies have shown frusemide to be ineffective (Kleinknecht et al, 1976), while Lucas and his colleagues (1977) showed that administration of frusemide produced a marked diuresis but did not improve renal blood flow or the glomerular filtration rate, nor did it prevent the subsequent development of established ARF. Moreover, there are theoretical objections to the use of this agent since it may increase the nephrotoxicity of some antibiotics and could actually precipitate ARF when used in the presence of hypovolaemia. Nevertheless, it is still recommended by many clinicians, usually in high doses (e.g. 250–500mg in 100ml 5% dextrose infused over 20 minutes) or as an infusion (e.g. $0.02–0.06 \, \text{mg} \, \text{kg}^{-1} \, \text{min}^{-1}$ to a maximum of $4 \, \text{mg} \, \text{kg}^{-1}$ in adults over 3–6 hours). Some suggest that plasma levels should be measured in order to reduce the risk of ototoxicity, especially if the patient is also receiving aminoglycosides, but this is usually not possible. If there is no response within 4–8 hours, frusemide should be discontinued.

Dopamine (see also Chapter 10). Dopamine has been shown to increase renal plasma flow, glomerular filtration rate and sodium excretion (McDonald et al, 1964) and might therefore be useful in the management of the early phase of ARF.

In an uncontrolled study, Henderson et al (1980) administered low-dose dopamine ($1\,\mu g$ kg^{-1} min^{-1}) to patients in early oliguric ARF, with urine:plasma osmolality ratios of <1.1 : 1.0, who had failed to respond to a large dose of frusemide. They demonstrated a significant increase in urine output, which was subsequently maintained in 7 of the 11 patients after the dopamine was discontinued. Their impression was that by producing a diuresis, dopamine decreased dialysis requirements, simplified management and may have improved the outcome. In another study (Parker et al, 1981), dopamine 1.5–2.5 μg kg^{-1} min^{-1} increased urine output, creatinine clearance, osmolar clearance and the excreted fraction of filtered sodium, without affecting haemodynamics or free water clearance. Again, dialysis requirements were reduced. Moreover, there is some experimental evidence that the combination of frusemide and dopamine may act synergistically in this situation (Lindner, 1983), possibly because the vascular effects of dopamine facilitate penetration of frusemide to its site of action in the macula densa. Since such low doses of dopamine are free of side effects (Henderson et al, 1980) its use would seem to be justified at present in oliguric patients when prerenal causes have been excluded. If a diuresis ensues, low-dose dopamine should be continued in order to maintain the urine output and simplify subsequent management. However, it has yet to be established whether this regimen can abort incipient ARF.

Early oliguric phase

In this phase, most patients are fluid overloaded due to delayed recognition of the onset of ARF, often exacerbated by 'volume challenges' administered in an attempt to restore urine output. Although the plasma sodium concentration may be low, total body sodium is usually normal or increased. In extreme cases, the combination of salt and water overload can produce peripheral and pulmonary oedema, sometimes with hypertension, and these constitute an indication for early dialysis. It is therefore important to fluid restrict patients as soon as the diagnosis of intrinsic ARF is certain. Intravenous fluids should be limited to that required to replace insensible losses. In general, administration of sodium and potassium should be avoided, except in order to exactly replace specific, identified losses. Drug doses must be modified appropriately at this time.

Although the rising blood urea and creatinine levels seldom create a problem at this stage, dangerous hyperkalaemia can occur early, particularly if intravenous potassium continues to be administered after the onset of renal impairment. A combination of factors contribute to hyperkalaemia, including reduced renal excretion and increased cellular release of potassium. The latter may be attributable to direct tissue trauma, haemolysis, protein catabolism, infection, steroids and the effects of acidosis. The rate of increase in plasma potassium, as well as the rise in urea and creatinine levels, therefore depends largely on the degree of catabolism and the extent of any tissue damage; it is therefore particularly rapid in those with severe trauma or sepsis. Hyperkalaemia produces characteristic ECG abnormalities (elevated and pointed T wave, flattened or absent P wave followed by widened QRS complex) and if unchecked can culminate in cardiac arrest in diastole. Although the rise in potassium levels may be attenuated by the use of calcium exchange resins (30–60g 6-hourly orally or rectally), dangerous hyperkalaemia should be treated with dextrose and insulin (e.g. 50ml 50% dextrose with 10 units soluble insulin) and/or correction of the acidosis with 8.4% sodium bicarbonate (in order to encourage cellular uptake of potassium). In more urgent cases, 10–20ml 10% calcium chloride can be used to counteract the effects of hyperkalaemia on the myocardium. These measures will only alleviate the situation temporarily and preparations for dialysis should be instituted immediately. In extreme cases with marked bradycardia or asystole, isoprenaline or cardiac massage may sustain the patient until hyperkalaemia can be corrected by dialysis.

Because metabolic acidosis develops relatively slowly, and is compensated by hypocarbia, it is not usually a problem at this stage unless it was a significant component of the precipitating illness (e.g. septicaemia, low cardiac output or diabetic ketoacidosis). Administration of bicarbonate (which will exacerbate salt and water overload, may precipitate hypocalcaemia and causes a left shift of the oxyhaemoglobin dissociation curve) is therefore rarely indicated, except to counteract hyperkalaemia and when acidosis is extreme.

Occasionally, severe malignant hypertension complicates the early oliguric phase of ARF and this should be controlled using, for example, hydralazine or an infusion of sodium nitroprusside.

Established acute renal failure

In this phase, the measures outlined above must be combined with the removal of uraemic toxins and with nutritional support.

Derangement of other functions of the kidney, such as erythropoietin production, the formation of 1,25-dihydroxycholecalciferol and the catabolism of parathyroid hormone, are of limited clinical relevance in established ARF. It is not necessary to administer allopurinol since the risks of uric acid induced interstitial nephritis are negligible. Similarly, the administration of Aludrox in order to reduce serum phosphate levels is unnecessary because metastatic calcification is extremely unlikely.

Complications of established ARF and uraemia (Kleinknecht et al, 1972)

Many of the systemic manifestations of uraemia may be due to 'middle molecules'; blood urea and creatinine levels are only an approximate guide to blood levels of these 'middle molecules' and other toxic substances.

Gastrointestinal disturbances are prominant and include stomatitis, anorexia, nausea, vomiting, hiccups and diarrhoea or constipation. The introduction of routine antacid prophylaxis, better nutrition and more aggressive dialysis may all have contributed to the virtual disappearance of gastrointestinal haemorrhage as an immediate cause of death (Cameron, 1986).

Central nervous system effects may progress from mild confusion, with decreased responsiveness, to agitation, disorientation, hyperreflexia, twitching, irritability and, occasionally, frank convulsions. The EEG changes usually indicate a non-specific metabolic disturbance. These central nervous system manifestations tend to occur only in severe uraemia and may resolve slowly, even when uraemia has been controlled with dialysis.

Acute uraemic fibrinous pericarditis, which can cause cardiac tamponade, is now rarely encountered because of the availability of dialysis techniques.

Haemopoietic disturbances are common. Erythropoiesis is depressed, presumably by uraemic toxins and this, sometimes exacerbated by haemolysis and blood loss, is responsible for the inevitable normocytic, normochromic anaemia in which the haemoglobin concentration falls inexorably to around 7g per 100ml. This anaemia is not, in itself, an indication for blood transfusion. Coagulopathies, manifested as a purpuric rash or frank haemorrhage, are also common and are usually caused by a defect in platelet function, although they may occasionally be related to DIC (see Chapter 10). The platelet defect is probably due to retained toxins since the abnormality can be corrected by dialysis (Lindsay et al, 1975). These haematological abnormalities resolve during the diuretic phase, when the patient may require supplements of iron, folic acid or, rarely, vitamin B_{12}.

Finally, uraemic patients are very susceptible to infection; in one study, 74% of cases of acute tubular necrosis developed an infection and this caused 54% of the deaths (McMurray et al, 1978). The infection may have been present initially (e.g. related to trauma or surgery) or may arise during the period of ARF (e.g. peritonitis). Pulmonary infections are also common, particularly in those requiring mechanical ventilation.

A number of events may precipitate respiratory failure in those with ARF, including pulmonary oedema, pulmonary infection, a variety of cerebral disorders such as hypertensive encephalopathy and cerebral oedema, the effects of marked uraemia or the accumulation of sedative drugs. The combination of acute respiratory failure and acute renal failure is extremely difficult to manage and is associated with a poor prognosis.

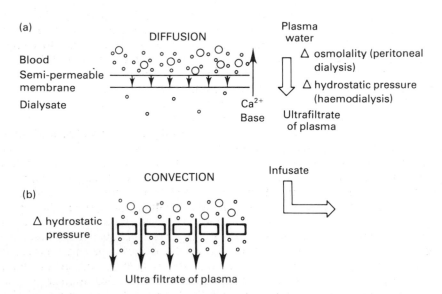

Fig. 15.1 Principles of blood purification. (a) Diffusion—solutes are removed by diffusion across a semi-permeable membrane (synthetic in haemodialysis, peritoneum in peritoneal dialysis) according to their concentration gradient. Fluid is removed by hydrostatic pressure (haemodialysis) or osmosis (peritoneal dialysis). (b) Convection—the ultrafiltrate is replaced by a sterile electrolyte solution which has a similar composition to the dialysate used in haemodialysis.

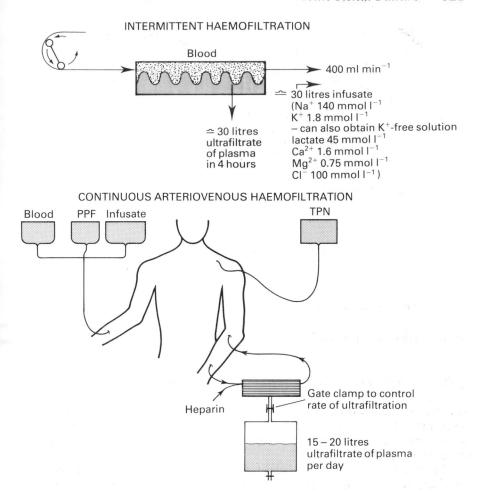

Fig. 15.3 Principles of intermittent haemofiltration and continuous arteriovenous haemofiltration.

Haemofiltration (Fig. 15.3). This technique relies on massive convection of plasma water across a porous membrane and its replacement with electrolyte solution. Solutes are removed only in proportion to their concentration in plasma and large volumes of ultrafiltrate must therefore be produced in order to control uraemia and hyperkalaemia. The pores in the membrane only allow the passage of molecules with molecular weights of up to 30 000; therefore, albumin and other proteins are not lost from the circulation.

When performed intermittently (Fig. 15.3a) a flow rate of 400 ml min^{-1} can produce approximately 30 litres of ultrafiltrate in about four hours. The length of each session is determined by the volume of ultrafiltrate required to control uraemia, while the volume of infusate used to replace the fluid loss is adjusted to achieve the appropriate fluid balance. This technique is relatively expensive and usually requires the creation of an arteriovenous shunt to provide the high blood flow.

Continuous arteriovenous haemofiltration (CAVH) is becoming an increasingly popular technique for use in critically ill patients (Fig. 15.3b). This entails creation of an arteriovenous shunt (or percutaneous cannulation of the femoral artery and vein) via which the haemofilter is connected to the patient's circulation. The flow of blood through the haemofilter, and the transmembrane pressure gradient, is determined by the patient's systemic arterial pressure. Provided this is adequate, flow rates through the filter are sufficient to produce 15–20 litres of ultrafiltrate per day. These volume losses are then replaced as required with crystalloid, blood, plasma and nutrients. CAVH has been shown to be a safe and effective method of fluid removal in critically ill septic patients with ARF, although additional intermittent haemodialysis may be required to control uraemia (Ossenkoppele et al, 1985). If required, the volume of ultrafiltrate produced can be controlled by using a gate clamp and may be reduced to only a few litres a day. This 'continuous ultrafiltration' is a useful means of creating 'space' for parenteral nutrition between dialysis sessions.

The relative ease with which CAVH can be instituted belies the fact that this is a potentially dangerous technique which requires considerable expertise and is labour intensive unless augmented by electromechanical weighing devices or a computer to assist in monitoring fluid balance. Furthermore, filtration is dependent on the patient's arterial pressure, which may be insufficient in those unstable patients who are most at risk of severe hypotension in response to haemodialysis.

Nutritional support (see also Chapter 5)

The provision of adequate nutritional support is essential for the successful management of ARF. Hyperalimentation may reduce mortality rates, particularly in high-risk patients with infectious or haemorrhagic complications, and may even shorten the period of impaired renal function (Abel et al, 1973). In general, patients should receive sufficient nourishment, either enterally or parenterally, to maintain a positive nitrogen balance, regardless of the volume of fluid administered in order to achieve this. Dialysis or haemofiltration should then be employed to prevent fluid overload.

General management considerations

Meticulous mouth care is required to prevent oral candidiasis; the urethral catheter should be removed in order to minimize the risk of urinary tract infection and all patients should receive antacid prophylaxis. Careful adjustment of drug doses, in particular H_2-receptor antagonists and antibiotics, has already been mentioned. If possible, the patient should be weighed daily in order to assess fluid balance although, in practice, this can be difficult in intensive care patients. Finally, it is clearly essential to treat the underlying condition, e.g. by performing a laparotomy in those with intra-abdominal sepsis.

Diuretic phase

In those with acute tubular necrosis, kidney function will normally recover spontaneously. This is heralded by the onset of a diuresis, usually 5–20 days after the initial insult, although in some cases this may occur within 48 hours or be delayed for many weeks.

Initially, the glomerular filtration rate remains relatively low and consequently blood urea and creatinine levels may continue to rise for a few days after the onset of a diuresis. Because tubular function is still impaired, the patient may lose large quantities of sodium, potassium and water, as well as phosphate and magnesium, although in some cases the diuresis may simply represent mobilization of accumulated solutes and water. Urinary losses must therefore be closely monitored; as an approximate guide, half the total fluid and electrolytes excreted should be replaced. However, frequent, careful assessment of each individual is essential in order to avoid water and electrolyte (particularly potassium) depletion on the one hand, or persistent polyuria due to excessive fluid administration on the other.

Non-oliguric ARF (Anderson et al, 1977)

This probably represents a less severe form of vasomotor nephropathy in which the glomerular filtration rate is maintained at approximately 2–5 ml min^{-1}, urine continues to be produced and the urinary sodium concentration is approximately 50 mmol l^{-1}. This non-oliguric form of ARF is becoming more common, possibly due to the use of dopamine and diuretics, as well as the increasing number of cases of tubular necrosis induced by toxic drugs. Dialysis is required less frequently, or not at all, complications (gastrointestinal bleeding, sepsis, acidosis, and neurological disturbances) are reduced, recovery is more rapid and the mortality is lower.

Management of some specific types of ARF

Acute interstitial nephritis

When nephritis is due to an acute hypersensitivity reaction to a drug, removal of the offending agent may prevent further deterioration in renal function. Recovery may, however, be slow and incomplete although the administration of steroids may be of some benefit.

Hyperuricaemic ARF

Treatment consists of rehydration and haemodialysis, followed by alkalinization and the administration of allopurinol.

ARF due to glomerular disease

Most cases of acute crescentic glomerulonephritis progress rapidly and inexorably to end-stage renal failure. This is also generally the case in Goodpasture's syndrome, although high-dose steroids, immunosuppressants and plasma exchange may be beneficial. Although the combination of these measures can usually rapidly control pulmonary haemorrhage, the outcome of the renal lesion is clearly related to the severity of renal impairment at presentation. In over half of the patients, glomerular basement membrane antibody had disappeared from the circulation at two months, and this appears to be permanent (Lockwood et al, 1981).

Vascular ARF

Acute renal artery occlusion requires immediate surgery or fibrinolytic therapy, followed by heparinization. In acute renal vein thrombosis, the patient should be heparinized and/or receive streptokinase.

ARF due to obstruction

It is imperative to relieve the obstruction as quickly as possible, particularly in the presence of infection which might otherwise spread retrogradely and cause renal destruction or septicaemia. Surgery can be preceded by dialysis. Following relief of the obstruction, there may be a massive diuresis, due to the accumulation of urea and other osmotically active molecules, as well as a defect in tubular function.

PROGNOSIS OF ARF (Kleinknecht et al, 1972; McMurray et al, 1978; Cameron, 1986)

The final outcome of ARF depends on the aetiology; mortality rates range from approximately 35–60% in medical, surgical or trauma patients, 0–30% in those cases related to obstetric disasters and 75% or more in burns victims. When renal failure is the only problem, mortality rates may be as low as 8%, but in the remainder (i.e. those patients likely to require intensive care), the average mortality is >60%. The presence of sepsis, particularly intra-abdominal, also adversely affects the prognosis, although age does not. Another factor affecting outcome is the site of surgery, mortality rates being particularly high following gastrointestinal surgery, especially when the bowel rather than the stomach is involved (Cameron, 1986).

   Although the overall mortality has remained unchanged over the last 20 years or so, this may be partly explained by changes in the type of patients being treated. Improvements in resuscitation, evacuation of casualties and surgical techniques have resulted in the survival of more seriously ill patients, while there has been a reduction in the number of obstetric cases with ARF (who have the best prognosis) and an increase in those associated with generalized sepsis, liver failure and cardiac arrest. It is worth noting that most patients now die as a result of the precipitating cause, rather than as a direct result of the renal failure.

   In those who do recover, there is usually no obvious residual renal impairment and kidney function has normally recovered to about 80% of normal after one year. This justifies an aggressive approach to the management of ARF unless associated conditions render the outlook hopeless.

FURTHER READING

Chapman A (ed.) (1980) Acute Renal Failure. *Clinics in Critical Care Medicine.* Edinburgh: Churchill Livingstone.

Kanfer A, Kourilsky O, Sraer, JD & Richet G (1983) Acute renal failure. In Tinker J & Rapin M (eds) *Care of the Critically Ill Patient*, pp 433–455. Berlin: Springer-Verlag.

Robson JS (1977) Pathogenesis of acute renal failure. In Ledingham I McA (ed.) *Recent Advances in Intensive Therapy*, pp 203–215. Edinburgh: Churchill Livingstone.

REFERENCES

Abel RM, Beck CH, Abbott WM et al (1973) Improved survival from acute renal failure after treatment with intravenous essential L-amino acids and glucose. *New England Journal of Medicine* **288:** 695–699.

Anderson RJ, Linas SL, Berns AS et al (1977) Non-oliguric acute renal failure. *New England Journal of Medicine* **296:** 1134–1138.

Barry KG, Cohen A, Knochel JP et al (1961) Mannitol infusion II: the prevention of acute functional renal failure during resection of an aneurysm of the abdominal aorta. *New England Journal of Medicine* **264:** 967–971.

Birtch AG, Zakheim RM, Jones LG & Barger AC (1967) Redistribution of renal blood flow produced by furosemide and ethacrynic acid. *Circulation Research* **21:** 869–878.

Cameron JS (1986) Acute renal failure in the intensive care unit today. *Intensive Care Medicine* **12:** 64–70.

Cox JW, Bechler RW, Sharma H et al (1974) Studies on the mechanism of oliguria in a model of unilateral acute renal failure. *Journal of Clinical Investigation* **53:** 1546–1558.

Cronin RE, DeTorrente A, Miller PD et al (1978) Pathogenic mechanisms in early norephinephrine-induced acute renal failure: functional and histological correlates of protection. *Kidney International* **14:** 115–125.

Dawson JL (1964) Jaundice and anoxic renal damage: protective effect of mannitol. *British Medical Journal* **i:** 810–811.

De Torrente A, Miller PD, Cronin RE et al (1978) Effects of furosemide and acetylcholine in norephinephrine-induced acute renal failure. *American Journal of Physiology* **235:** F131–F136.

Flores J, Di Bona DR, Beck CH & Leaf A (1972) The role of cell swelling in ischemic renal damage and the protective effect of hypertonic solute. *Journal of Clinical Investigation* **51:** 118–126.

Henderson IS, Beattie TJ & Kennedy AC (1980) Dopamine hydrochloride in oliguric states. *Lancet* **ii:** 827–828.

Hinshaw LB, Bradley GM & Carlson CH (1959) Effect of endotoxin on renal function in the dog. *American Journal of Physiology* **196:** 1127–1139.

Hollenberg NK, Sandor T, Conroy M et al (1973) Xenon transit through the oliguric human kidney: analysis by maximum likelihood. *Kidney International* **3:** 177–185.

Johnston PA, Bernard DB, Donohoe JF, Perrin NS & Levinsky NG (1979) Effect of volume expansion on haemodynamics of the hypoperfused rat kidney. *Journal of Clinical Investigation* **64:** 550–558.

Kleinknecht D, Jungers P, Chanard J, Barbanel C & Ganeval D (1972) Uremic and non-uremic complications in acute renal failure: evaluation of early and frequent dialysis on prognosis. *Kidney International* **1:** 190–196.

Kleinknecht D, Grunfeld JP, Gomez PC, Morea JF & Gardia-Torres R (1973) Diagnostic procedures and long-term prognosis in bilateral renal cortical necrosis. *Kidney International* **4:** 390–400.

Kleinknecht D, Ganeval D, Gonzales-Duque LA & Fermanian J (1976) Furosemide in acute oliguric renal failure. A controlled trial. *Nephron* **17:** 51–58.

Lindner A (1983) Synergism of dopamine and furosemide in diuretic-resistant, oliguric acute renal failure. *Nephron* **33:** 121–126.

Lindsay RM, Moorthy AV, Koens F & Linton AL (1975) Platelet function in dialyzed and non-dialyzed patients with chronic renal failure. *Clinical Nephrology* **4:** 52–57.

Lockwood CM, Pusey CD, Rees AJ & Peters DK (1981) Plasma exchange in the treatment of immune complex disease. *Clinics in Immunology and Allergy* **1:** 433–455.

Lucas CE, Zito JG, Carter KM, Cortez A & Stebner FC (1977) Questionable value of furosemide in preventing renal failure. *Surgery* **82:** 314–320.

Luke RG, Linton AL, Briggs JD & Kennedy AC (1965) Mannitol therapy in acute renal failure. *Lancet* **i:** 980–982.

McDonald RH, Goldberg LI, McNay JL & Tuttle EP (1964) Effects of dopamine in man: augmentation of sodium excretion, glomerular filtration rate and renal plasma flow. *Journal of Clinical Investigation* **43:** 1116–1124.

McMurray SD, Luft FC, Maxwell DR et al (1978) Prevailing patterns and predictor variables in patients with acute tubular necrosis. *Archives of Internal Medicine* **138:** 950–955.

Minuth AN, Terrell JB & Suki WN (1976) Acute renal failure: a study of the course and prognosis of 104 patients and of the role of furosemide. *American Journal of Medical Science* **271:** 317–324.

Myers BD, Moran SM (1986) Hemodynamically mediated acute renal failure. *New England Journal of Medicine* **314:** 97–105.

Ossenkoppele GJ, van der Meulen J, Bronsveld W & Thijs LG (1985) Continuous arteriovenous hemofiltration as an adjunctive therapy for septic shock. *Critical Care Medicine* **13:** 102–104.

Parker S, Carlon GC, Isaacs M, Howland WS & Kahn RC (1981) Dopamine administration in oliguria and oliguric renal failure. *Critical Care Medicine* **9:** 630–632.

Reubi FC, Vorburger C & Tuckman J (1973) Renal distribution volumes of indocyanine green, [^{51}Cr]EDTA, and ^{24}Na in man during acute renal failure after shock. Implications for the pathogenesis of anuria. *Journal of Clinical Investigation* **52:** 223–235.

Shaldon S, Baldamus CA, Koch KM & Lysaght MJ (1983) Of sodium, symptomatology and syllogism. *Blood Purification* **1:** 16–24.

Wilkinson SP, Blendis LM & Williams R (1974) Frequency and type of renal and electrolyte disorders in fulminant hepatic failure. *British Medical Journal* **i:** 186–189.

16
Acute Liver Failure

CAUSES

Fulminant hepatic failure (FHF)

This can be defined as a clinical syndrome developing as a result of massive necrosis of liver cells, or any other sudden and severe impairment of hepatic function (Trey and Davidson, 1970). There should be no history or evidence of pre-existing liver disease and the signs of encephalopathy must appear within eight weeks of the onset of illness. The mortality of FHF remains very high; this condition therefore represents an important challenge because, although rare, it is a disease which affects young people and from which those who survive will make a complete recovery.

Subacute hepatic necrosis

This diagnosis is made when the onset of encephalopathy is delayed beyond eight weeks from the onset of illness. It may represent part of the spectrum of acute non-A, non-B viral hepatitis occurring in an older age group (Gimson and Williams, 1983). It is associated with a very poor prognosis (<10% survival) and, at present, artificial liver support does not seem to be either effective or appropriate for this group of patients. In general, bilirubin levels are less elevated and the prothrombin time less prolonged than in FHF, while the liver is small and ascites may be present.

Acute-on-chronic liver failure

This occurs when an acute illness causes decompensation of pre-existing chronic liver disease (usually hepatic cirrhosis, but occasionally alcoholic or chronic active hepatitis). Recognized precipitating factors include shock, surgery, anaesthesia, infection, metabolic disturbances and drugs (e.g. excessive diuretic administration). In patients with hepatic cirrhosis, gastrointestinal haemorrhage is a common cause of sudden deterioration. When such patients develop the syndrome of FHF, the prognosis is extremely poor, partly because there is little potential for hepatic regeneration.

Ischaemic/hypoxic hepatocellular damage

This can occur in acute or chronic cardiac failure, as well as following an episode of severe shock and, now very rarely, as a complication of cardiac surgery. In these cases there may be hepatomegaly and a marked rise in transaminases (>1000 iu l^{-1}) with a prolonged prothrombin time, but bilirubin levels are usually only moderately elevated (< 500 mmol l^{-1}). FHF is, however, rare following ischaemic liver damage and, when it does occur, the prognosis is poor.

FULMINANT HEPATIC FAILURE (FHF)

Causes

The most common cause of FHF in the UK is paracetamol hepatotoxicity, which, in one series, accounted for 48% of cases. Viral hepatitis was responsible for 37%, with hepatitis A being diagnosed in 32% and hepatitis B in 24% of these cases (Gimson and Williams, 1983). Epstein–Barr virus, cytomegalovirus, and herpes simplex virus cause liver failure only rarely, but may contribute to the death of immunocompromised patients. Outside the UK, viral hepatitis is the most frequent cause of FHF, while drug-induced liver failure is slightly less common. As well as paracetamol hepatotoxicity, idiosyncratic reactions to antituberculosis drugs (especially isoniazid), monoamino oxidase inhibitors and methyldopa can cause FHF.

Severe hepatic necrosis may also occasionally follow halothane anaesthesia (Walton et al, 1976); the incidence is higher in females, the elderly and the obese and is increased by multiple exposure. Moreover, approximately 20% of patients undergoing repeated halothane anaesthesia have been found to have less severe forms of liver injury (Wright et al, 1975). The diagnosis of halothane-associated hepatitis should be suspected when the signs of severe hepatocellular necrosis, often accompanied by fever and chills, develop within two weeks of exposure.

FHF occurring during pregnancy (Williams and Ede, 1981) may be related to viral hepatitis or acute fatty liver. Acute fatty liver usually presents as nausea, repeated vomiting and abdominal pain developing between the 30th and 38th week of pregnancy. Severe hepatic dysfunction may also occasionally be related to toxaemia of pregnancy and be caused by localized or systemic DIC.

Poisoning with carbon tetrachloride, yellow phosphorus, mushrooms (*Amanita phalloides*) and alcohol can also be complicated by the development of FHF, while in children and young adults it is worth remembering that Wilson's disease can present acutely, although usually there is evidence of underlying chronic liver disease (chronic active hepatitis, cirrhosis).

Mechanisms of FHF

It is unclear why only some of those with viral hepatitis develop FHF while in others the infection pursues a more benign course. Hepatitis B virus has no direct cytopathic effect and the onset of massive hepatocellular necrosis does not appear to be related either to the strain of virus or the size of the inoculum. There is, however, some evidence to suggest that those who develop liver failure produce an enhanced immune response to all three antigenic determinants of the virus and that the excess antibody leads to the formation of immune complexes. The latter may then obstruct hepatic sinusoids and cause ischaemic necrosis of liver cells. In contrast, cellular damage following hepatitis A or non-A, non-B infection is probably due to a direct cytopathic effect of the virus and in these cases it is likely that an impaired immune response contributes to the fulminant course.

The exact mechanism of halothane-induced FHF remains unclear (Editorial, 1986). Nevertheless, it is known that in the presence of local hypoxia, halothane is metabolized in the liver by the reductive pathway to produce unstable radicals which can damage liver cells. This hepatotoxicity may be enhanced when the hepatic microsomal enzyme cytochrome P450 has been induced by prior exposure to drugs such as phenobarbitone, or halothane itself. A number of features of halothane-associated FHF suggest that a hypersensitivity reaction is involved. For example, the syndrome is rare, it occurs after more than one exposure, and in many patients there is a history of a previous adverse reaction to halothane anaesthesia. It has been suggested, therefore, that FHF due to exposure to halothane is precipitated by a hypersensitivity reaction to liver cell components rendered antigenic by interaction with halothane or one of its metabolites. However, although a specific halothane-related antibody can be detected in a proportion of patients, this is not always the case and it seems that some cases of 'halothane-associated hepatitis' are related to a viral infection (Neuberger et al, 1983), possibly exacerbated by the immunosuppression which can follow surgery and anaesthesia. Furthermore, the antibody to 'halothane-altered hepatocytes' may simply arise as a secondary response to hepatocellular damage, rather than being the cause of cellular destruction.

It is now known that hepatocellular damage following paracetamol overdose is related to the production of a toxic metabolite which accumulates when hepatic glutathione has been overwhelmed (Black, 1980), but individuals vary considerably in their susceptibility to liver damage induced by this agent. A number of specific antidotes are available and management of paracetamol overdose is discussed further in Chapter 17. In other drug- or toxin-related causes of FHF, there is direct interference with cellular metabolism.

Clinical presentation and diagnosis

The syndrome of FHF is characterized by an encephalopathy which presents as an acute mental disturbance, usually progressing rapidly to stupor or coma, in the absence of signs of chronic liver disease. Often, the initial changes are subtle, e.g. a change in personality, lack of attention to personal detail, perhaps with euphoria or depression and some slowing of mentation. Later, the patient may become confused and begin to behave inappropriately. Drowsiness is a prominant feature and some patients will sleep continually, although at this stage they can be roused. Difficulty with writing and an inability accurately to reproduce shapes (e.g. a star) are characteristic (constructional apraxia) and these skills can be tested repeatedly in order to follow the patient's progress. A 'flapping' tremor (asterixis) can often be demonstrated at this stage and is associated with a rigid facies, muscle stiffness and dysarthria. Many patients will then lose consciousness and progress to deep coma with hypertonia, decerebrate/decorticate posturing and disturbances of vital reflexes. Traditionally, hepatic encephalopathy is classified clinically into four grades as shown in Table 16.1. In practice,

Table 16.1 Hepatic encephalopathy.

Grade I	Fluctuant mild confusion, euphoria, slowed mentation, disordered sleep rhythm
Grade II	Increasing drowsiness and inappropriate behaviour
Grade III	Severe confusion, semi-stuporose but rousable and responsive to simple commands
Grade IV	Comatose but may respond to painful stimuli

however, this is complicated by spontaneous fluctuations in coma grade and the necessity to administer sedatives to patients who are aggressive or to enable invasive procedures to be performed. The EEG changes (Fig. 16.1) correlate with the degree of cerebral dysfunction and, although not necessary to establish the diagnosis, serial EEGs can be performed, together with regular clinical assessment of the grade of encephalopathy, in order to follow the patient's progress.

These signs of encephalopathy are usually accompanied by rapidly increasing jaundice and a characteristic 'hepatic fetor' (an unpleasant, sweetish smell due to exhalation of mercaptans). The rise in serum bilirubin concentration is associated with the appearance of bilirubin and its breakdown products in the urine. However, the diagnosis may be difficult if the mental disturbance precedes the development of clinical jaundice. This occurs particularly in children with FHF and in adults who have taken a paracetamol overdose. In some cases, the patient may present with abdominal pain suggestive of an 'acute abdomen'.

Serum aminotransferase levels are initially nearly always markedly elevated, often to more than 2000 iu l^{-1}, but the alkaline phosphatase level is

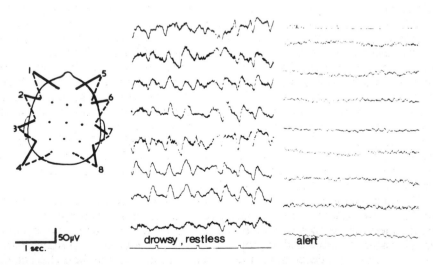

Fig. 16.1 Electroencephalographic changes in hepatic coma. High voltage slow waves with some triphasic components best seen at the front of the head.

usually only moderately raised. Serum albumin, because of its long half-life, generally remains normal until later in the illness. A fall in aminotransferase levels, despite increasing hyperbilirubinaemia, indicates total destruction of liver cells and is associated with a very poor prognosis. The prothrombin time is always markedly prolonged, reflecting reduced hepatic synthesis of clotting factors, and thrombocytopenia is common. Blood ammonia levels are usually increased. Other components of the clinical syndrome may include hypoglycaemia, renal and respiratory failure, electrolyte and acid–base disturbances, and sepsis.

In the early stages, the liver may be palpable, although later in the illness it becomes small, and when FHF follows the more protracted course typical of non-A, non-B hepatitis, both spider naevi and ascites may occur.

Pathogenesis of encephalopathy (Crossley et al, 1983; Editorial, 1984)

Reductions in cerebral energy production, abnormal neurotransmitter function, direct effects on neuronal membranes or, most likely, a combination of these factors, are thought to be responsible for the disturbance of neurotransmission which precipitates hepatic encephalopathy. These abnormalities are in turn largely related to the accumulation of toxic substances normally metabolized by the liver. Although there are many similarities between the clinical and biochemical features of encephalopathy in FHF and chronic liver impairment, there are also a number of respects in which they differ; in particular, cerebral oedema is a common and important complication of FHF but is extremely rare in chronic liver disease. In both cases, the disturbance of cerebral function is often exacerbated by hypoglycaemia, alterations in acid–base homeostasis, fluid and electrolyte abnormalities, hypoxia and increased sensitivity to sedatives.

Examples of recognized toxins which accumulate in liver failure include ammonia, fatty acids, mercaptans (derived from methionine), phenols and various aromatic aminoacids. Although bile acids are also retained, it seems unlikely that these play a major role in the production of encephalopathy.

Blood levels of ammonia and short-chain fatty acids are elevated in hepatic failure and both can produce coma, although there is a poor correlation between the blood ammonia concentration and the degree of coma. Moreover, the clinical picture of ammonia intoxication differs from that of hepatic encephalopathy. The mercaptans are well-recognized cerebral toxins and can induce reversible coma (Zieve et al, 1974), and it has been proposed that they may exert a synergistic effect with both ammonia and free fatty acids (Zieve et al, 1974). One suggested mechanism of action for these toxins, and phenols, is inhibition of Na^+, K^+ ATPase on the neuronal membrane. This could impair membrane repolarization, and might also disrupt the integrity of the blood–brain barrier.

The serum aminoacid profile is abnormal in both chronic liver impairment and FHF. In patients with chronic liver disease and superimposed acute insults, there is an increase in blood levels of the aromatic amino acids phenylalanine, tyrosine and tryptophan, as well as methionine, glutamate and aspartate and a reduction in the concentrations of the branched-chain aminoacids valine, leucine and isoleucine (Rosen et al, 1977). This abnormality is probably the result of increased catabolism, as well as impaired liver function. Circulating levels of aromatic amino acids are also markedly increased in FHF, but in this situation the concentration of branched-chain amino acids is normal (Rosen et al, 1977). It is thought that this altered amino acid profile is caused by massive hepatocellular necrosis with release of amino acids into the circulation and that catabolism plays a less important role. The high circulating levels of aromatic amino acids, combined with their enhanced uptake by active carrier systems and disruption of the blood–brain barrier, lead to increased intracerebral concentrations of phenylalanine, tyrosine and tryptophan. The excess tyrosine is converted to octopamine, while phenylalanine is metabolized first to phenylethylamine and then phenylethanolamine. These substances are thought to act as weak (or 'false') neurotransmitters, displacing some of the normal transmitter compounds such as dopamine and noradrenaline. Furthermore, tryptophan is converted into the inhibitory neurotransmitter serotonin and the intracerebral formation of normal excitatory transmitters may be reduced by competition for enzyme systems. Finally, ammonia stimulates brain glutamine synthesis, which results in a rapid exchange of brain glutamine for neutral plasma amino acids; this provides a possible link between the neurotoxicity of ammonia and the false neurotransmitter hypothesis (James et al, 1979).

There is, however, some evidence against the false transmitter theory, and a number of other mechanisms have been postulated. For example, in experimental FHF blood levels of γ-aminobutyric acid (GABA) are markedly increased, probably because of reduced hepatic metabolism of the GABA normally synthesized by gut bacteria. Moreover, the number of postsynaptic binding sites for GABA in the brain is increased (Schafer and Jones, 1982). Since the blood–brain barrier is disrupted in FHF, the concentration of GABA within the brain will rise, thereby contributing to neural inhibition. The increase in GABA binding sites may also partly explain the enhanced sensitivity of these patients to sedatives.

It has also been suggested that middle molecular weight substances may contribute to the development of encephalopathy (Bloch et al, 1978). These have been identified in the serum of patients with FHF, as well as chronic encephalopathy and can inhibit leukocyte sodium transport (Sewell et al, 1982). There is evidence that this occurs within the brain where it could interfere with neurotransmission and might contribute to the formation of cerebral oedema by increasing intracellular sodium content (Seda et al, 1984). This hypothesis is supported by the finding that haemodialysis with a polyacrylonitrile membrane (which is permeable to larger solutes than the standard cuprophane membrane) can improve encephalopathy in FHF.

Management

General aspects

In the great majority of those who survive an episode of FHF, liver architecture returns essentially to normal and the development of cirrhosis is very unusual (Karvountzis et al, 1974). Aggressive management of FHF is therefore based on the premise that if the patient is supported through the acute illness, regeneration of the liver will be associated with complete recovery. Currently, there is some support for the hypothesis that a number of hepatocytes survive the initial insult but are functionally impaired by persisting ischaemia/hypoxia, perhaps related in part to vascular obstruction. Reversal of haemodynamic and respiratory abnormalities is therefore a fundamental aspect of supportive care for the patient with FHF. It is likely, however, that, at least in some cases, hepatic necrosis will be so extensive that liver regeneration is not possible.

Patients with FHF should be admitted to an intensive care unit as soon as their conscious level deteriorates and should then, if possible, be transferred to a specialist centre once they have been resuscitated and stabilized. Successful management then depends largely on the quality of supportive care, combined with an awareness of the potential complications, so that they can be either prevented, or recognized early and treated appropriately.

Cross infection

Measures to prevent cross infection and minimize the dangers to staff should be instituted in all cases of viral hepatitis, or when the aetiology of liver failure is uncertain. Particular care is required when handling blood, urine or faeces and it is most important to avoid contamination of conjunctivae, cuts or abrasions, as well as self-inoculation. Saliva and tears are also potentially infective. Staff should wear an impermeable apron and gloves when performing medical or nursing procedures, and protective goggles may be used when the risk of conjunctival inoculation is considered to be high. Excreta should be disposed of immediately. Hypochlorite is the disinfectant of choice and a hypochlorite detergent (1000 parts per million) should be used for cleaning.

Hypoglycaemia

This is common and may be due to raised plasma insulin levels combined with a failure of hepatic gluconeogenesis. Hypoglycaemia can be avoided by giving a continuous intravenous infusion of 10 or 20% dextrose, supplemented as necessary by bolus doses of 50 ml 50% dextrose, to maintain the blood sugar level above 4 mmol l^{-1}. There is also, however, a danger of precipitating hyperglycaemia because of impaired glucose uptake by the liver.

Bleeding

Patients with FHF inevitably develop a coagulopathy. Prolongation of the prothrombin time is related to impaired hepatic synthesis of clotting factors (II, V, VII, IX and X) which, if the illness is prolonged, may later be compounded by a fall in fibrinogen levels. Thrombocytopenia is common and may be due to hypersplenism, bone marrow depression or DIC, although the latter is not usually clinically significant and the use of heparin is not recommended. Functional platelet abnormalities have also been described in association with morphological changes.

Correction of the clotting factor deficiency with infusions of fresh frozen plasma (FFP) does not appear to influence the overall mortality and may precipitate sodium overload or, possibly, DIC. Platelet transfusions are rarely indicated but vitamin K, 10mg, should be administered daily, although the latter generally has little demonstrable effect.

Upper gastrointestinal haemorrhage is a potentially lethal complication of FHF and may be related to an oesophagitis, gastric erosions or duodenal ulceration. It has been shown that this complication can be virtually eliminated if gastric pH is maintained above 5 by the administration of an H_2-receptor antagonist (MacDougall et al, 1977) (see also Chapter 4).

Electrolyte disturbances

In the absence of renal failure there is a marked tendency to hypokalaemia; this necessitates the infusion of large quantities of potassium chloride. Hyponatraemia is also common, especially later in the course of FHF and is due to redistribution of sodium into the cells combined with increased renal retention of water. Hypernatraemia, on the other hand, is unusual but can be precipitated by the sodium load in transfusions of FFP or plasma protein fraction and is sometimes exacerbated by dehydration due to hyperglycaemia or diuretic administration. Hypocalcaemia may occur. A fall in serum organic phosphate levels may lead to a reduction in red cell 2, 3-DPG concentration and a decrease in oxygen availability (see Chapter 4).

Hypotension, unrelated to any obvious cause, is common and is associated with vasodilation rather than primary cardiac failure (Trewby and Williams, 1977). Even when blood pressure is normal, severe tissue hypoxia may be present, as evidenced by a metabolic acidosis and raised blood lactate levels. Furthermore, there is an inverse correlation between the mixed venous lactate concentration and both the systemic vascular resistance and the oxygen extraction ratio, suggesting that the fall in peripheral resistance reflects a diversion of blood flow away from respiring tissues (Bihari et al, 1985).

Because of a generalized increase in capillary permeability, hypovolaemia is common in patients with FHF and is often combined with relative hypovolaemia due to the vasodilatation just described. Adequate expansion of the circulating volume is therefore essential, guided by the CVP, the urine output and, in some cases, the PCWP. If this fails to restore the blood pressure, one should not hesitate to use an inotrope since, in the presence of raised ICP, hypotension can precipitate cerebral ischaemia. Dopamine is the agent of choice, although high doses may be necessary in order to produce some vasoconstriction. Occasionally, adrenaline or noradrenaline is required.

Dysrhythmias are also common and may be related to hypoxia, acid–base disturbances or electrolyte abnormalities. In one series, ectopic beats occurred in 20% and heart block or bradycardia in 18%. ST segment and T wave abnormalities were seen in one-third of cases (Weston et al, 1976). At post mortem, macroscopic changes included petechial haemorrages, pericardial effusions and fatty ventricular muscle.

Respiratory dysfunction

A respiratory alkalosis due to hyperventilation is common in the early stages of FHF (Record et al, 1975) and may be a result of stimulation of the respiratory centre by toxins or an intracellular acidosis. Later, hypoxic depression of the respiratory centre may supervene and sudden, unexpected respiratory arrest may occur, in some cases related to severe intracranial hypertension.

Many patients with FHF will be hypoxaemic and this may be due to infection, intrapulmonary shunts or pulmonary oedema. The commonest abnormality is non-cardiogenic pulmonary oedema (ARDS, see Chapter 13) which occurred in 37 of a series of 100 patients with FHF reported by Trewby and his colleagues (1978). These authors were unable to demonstrate any correlation between the onset of ARDS and the presence of endotoxaemia, hypoalbuminaemia or renal failure. It has been suggested that precapillary arteriolar dilatation disrupts pulmonary capillaries by exposing them to an increased hydrostatic pressure. Alternatively, the development of ARDS may simply be a manifestation of the generalized increase in capillary permeability.

Control of the airway and protection of the lungs from aspiration of blood or stomach contents is essential, and these patients should be intubated early—certainly as soon as the airway protective reflexes are depressed. Hypoxaemia and hypercarbia should be avoided by early artificial ventilation, although it is important to remember that the institution of IPPV may be associated with a marked reduction in hepatic perfusion if cardiac output is allowed to fall. In those with refractory hypoxaemia, PEEP may be required and the underlying pulmonary abnormality should be treated as outlined in Chapters 12 and 13.

Renal disorders

Renal impairment is common in patients with FHF (Wilkinson et al, 1975) (see Chapter 15). Even though the development of renal failure is not necessarily related to the severity of liver impairment (e.g. ATN may occur without encephalopathy), its onset is associated with an extremely high mortality. Haemodialysis should be instituted early. Most authorities consider that associated hypotensive episodes are rarely sufficiently severe to preclude the use of this technique, although a few recommend peritoneal dialysis. Continuous haemofiltration may prove to be a valuable technique in some cases.

Impaired host defences

A number of abnormalities have been identified which contribute to the increased susceptibility of patients with FHF to infection. These include a deficiency of complement factors involved in both the classical and alternative pathways (Wyke et al, 1980), a reduced chemoattractant activity of patient's sera for normal polymorphonuclear leukocytes (Wyke et al, 1982a) and a reduction in plasma fibronectin levels (Gonzalez-Calvin et al, 1982). Consequently, bacteraemia is relatively common and is most often due to gram-positive organisms (mainly streptococci and *Staphylococcus aureus*), whereas *E. coli* is the commonest type of gram-negative organism isolated (Wyke et al, 1982b). Because bacteraemia usually occurs within 48 hours of the onset of grade IV coma, and may be associated with a deterioration in liver function, broad-spectrum antibiotic prophylaxis is now recommended when patients develop grade III coma. Benzylpenicillin should be combined with tobramycin or a third-generation cephalosporin.

Cerebral oedema

This has been demonstrated in post mortem studies of patients dying with FHF (Silk et al, 1977) and may be due to intermediate molecular weight substances altering the permeability of the blood–brain barrier or to intracellular accumulation of sodium and water related to inhibition of Na^+, K^+ APTase (Seda et al, 1984).

Although monitoring ICP can assist in the early detection and rational treatment of intracranial hypertension, some authorities feel that the complications, in particular bleeding and deterioration during transfer to and from the operating theatre, may outweigh the benefits. The administration of steroids is of no value in controlling the cerebral oedema associated with FHF, but mannitol is extremely effective in reducing ICP and may improve survival in those with intracranial hypertension (Canalese et al, 1982). In those with renal failure, continuous arteriovenous haemofiltration may create 'space' for the administration of mannitol. In the absence of ICP monitoring, intracranial hypertension should be suspected, and treated, if the pupils become unequal or cease to react to light and in the presence of decorticate/decerebrate posturing, hyperventilation, profuse sweating or opisthotonus. Other measures to control intracranial hypertension can be instituted as outlined in Chapter 14. ICP monitoring is essential in those who require mechanical ventilation with muscle paralysis.

Encephalopathy

Identifiable precipitating factors, such as fluid and electrolyte disturbances, hypoxaemia and hypercarbia must be corrected. Sedatives may also precipitate or exacerbate coma, as well as hypotension, and should in general be avoided. If sedation is essential, small doses of a benzodiazepine are recommended. Alternatives include promethazine, chlormethiazole or phenobarbitone. Convulsions are relatively common and should be treated with diazepam; under these circumstances, it is usually necessary to paralyse and ventilate the patient.

Although it is traditional to institute measures designed to minimize the nitrogenous load absorbed from the bowel, this practice is based on the observable improvement which is produced in chronic hepatic encephalopathy and there are no controlled data to suggest that such treatment is beneficial in FHF. Nevertheless, it is conventional to withdraw protein from the diet and, if blood is suspected in the gastrointestinal tract, the bowel is emptied with an enema (e.g. 80 ml magnesium sulphate in 50% solution w/v). Lactulose is also given in a starting dose of 60 ml, followed by 30 ml 8-hourly or more frequently, in order to produce two soft bowel motions a day. It is not necessary to produce diarrhoea. Lactulose is a non-absorbable synthetic disaccharide which is not metabolized in the small bowel. It is hydrolysed in the colon to lactic and acetic acid, thereby causing a fermentative diarrhoea, and may act by trapping ammonia in the bowel by virtue of the fall in pH of the colonic contents. A second-generation disaccharide (lactitol) is available in more convenient powder form and is more palatable than lactulose, while being equally effective in chronic stable encephalopathy. Oral neomycin 1 g 6-hourly can be used to sterilize the bowel but because significant amounts of this drug are absorbed, there is a risk of ototoxicity in those with renal impairment and some centres have now discontinued its routine prescription.

It was at one time suggested that manipulation of the abnormal plasma amino acid profile might be beneficial in hepatic encephalopathy. This was achieved by intravenous infusion of branched-chain amino acids, but although early trials indicated some benefit, subsequent controlled studies have failed to demonstrate any clinical improvement.

Temporary liver support

This is based on the principle that removal of the toxins which accumulate in FHF may prevent the development of cerebral oedema and provide a more favourable environment for hepatic regeneration (Zieve et al, 1985).

Initially, techniques were employed which were designed to replace some of the synthetic functions of the liver, as well as removing the accumulated toxins. These included exchange transfusions or plasmapheresis, cross-circulation with healthy volunteers or patients in irreversible coma, and extracorporeal perfusion of isolated animal (or human) livers. Cross-circulation with healthy humans is, of course, only applicable to those with FHF of non-infectious origin and even then exposes the volunteer to some risk; its use has been abandoned. Although these techniques can produce temporary improvements in the patient's conscious level, there is no evidence that they influence long-term survival and, because they are generally expensive, technically demanding and difficult to perform on a daily basis, their use has been superseded by artificial methods of liver support.

Artificial liver support

Because these techniques remove not only toxins, important substances normally produced by the liver, e.g. clotting factors, may have to be replaced by appropriate intravenous infusions.

Charcoal haemoperfusion. In the past there was considerable enthusiasm for the use of charcoal haemoperfusion. Activated charcoal adsorbs a wide range of water-soluble substances, including those of middle molecular weight. Initial attempts to use this technique were hampered by severe thrombocytopenia, charcoal embolization and hypotension. By covering the charcoal with an acrylic hydrogel, platelet damage and charcoal embolization were initially largely prevented, without reducing its adsorptive capacity, although later these complications recurred. Subsequently, the use of prostacyclin as an anticoagulant, combined with heparin, resolved these problems and in one series remarkable results were obtained by instituting charcoal haemoperfusion early (i.e. in grade III encephalopathy) (Gimson et al, 1982). More recent evidence from a large study, however, suggests that charcoal haemoperfusion does not significantly influence overall survival (J.G. O'Grady and R. Williams, personal communication).

Haemodialysis. Haemodialysis with a polyacrylonitrile membrane allows a more rapid transfer of middle molecular weight substances than is possible with a standard cuprophane membrane, as well as removing compounds of higher molecular weight. Although initially improved survival rates were reported (Silk et al, 1977), this technique is no longer used.

At present, therefore, the use of artificial liver support cannot be recommended except, possibly, as part of a research programme within specialist units.

Prognosis

The mortality of FHF is closely related to the depth and duration of coma, but decorticate/decerebrate states are potentially reversible and recovery is possible even when the EEG is isoelectric. Nevertheless, the mortality of those who progress to grade III encephalopathy is between 70 and 80% (Editorial, 1984), whereas approximately two-thirds of those who only progress to grade II survive. Over the last 10–15 years, there has been some reduction in mortality rates, almost certainly largely related to improvements in the standards of general intensive care (e.g. control of cerebral oedema, dialysis, artificial ventilation) rather than specific interventions. Not surprisingly, the prognosis is better when coma has an identifiable precipitating cause, such as the administration of sedatives. Younger patients have a better chance of recovery (Gazzard et al, 1975), while halothane-associated FHF has a particularly bad prognosis in all age groups. In patients with viral hepatitis, the prognosis is influenced by the infecting agent, since those with hepatitis A have a lower incidence of cerebral oedema and improved survival (43%) compared with both hepatitis B and presumed non-A, non-B hepatitis (17% and 8% survival) (Gimson and Williams, 1983). Clearly, the development of serious complications, such as respiratory failure, renal failure or haemorrhage, will adversely affect the outcome.

Standard liver function tests are of no value in assessing the prognosis, although the prothrombin time at presentation and the direction and rapidity of its change provide a reasonable clinical guide to the likely outcome.

Causes of death

In one series of 132 consecutive patients in grade IV encephalopathy, autopsy was performed in 96 of the 105 who died. In only 25 of these was death considered to be solely attributable to massive hepatic necrosis. In 36% of cases, cerebral oedema was considered to be the main contributory factor, while in 28 patients death was due to major gastrointestinal haemorrhage and in 12 patients sepsis was a contributory factor. Most importantly, in ten of these patients liver function appeared to be improving at the time of death, suggesting that if these major complications could be prevented, or successfully treated, a number of patients might have survived (Gazzard et al, 1975).

ACUTE DECOMPENSATION OF CHRONIC LIVER DISEASE

Most often, acute decompensation of chronic cirrhosis requiring admission to the intensive care unit is the result of gastrointestinal haemorrhage, although other precipitating factors include infection (particularly with *E. coli* and spontaneous bacterial peritonitis) and the excessive use of diuretics.

Management

Measures to reduce the absorption of nitrogenous compounds from the bowel should be instituted and combined with general supportive care as outlined above for FHF. Infection must be identified and treated appropriately.

The source of gastrointestinal haemorrhage must be positively identified by fibre-optic endoscopy since bleeding may originate not only from oesophageal varices but also from gastroduodenal ulceration and acute gastric or oesophageal mucosal erosions. In some cases, conservative management with replacement of the circulating volume, and administration of FFP or platelets where indicated, may be all that is required. However, bleeding may be recurrent and torrential. If it persists and is arising from peptic ulceration, emergency surgery may be indicated in those in mild coma who are otherwise fit. Management of those with mucosal erosions is more difficult. Although perfusion of the coeliac axis with vasopressin is occasionally successful, the incidence of complications is high and some prefer to administer an H_2-receptor antagonist.

When the bleeding originates from varices, most authorities would initially attempt to control the haemorrhage by sclerotherapy. If this fails, a Sengstaken tube can be inserted. Initially, only the gastric balloon should be inflated and 1 kg of traction applied. If the patient continues to bleed, the oesophageal balloon should be inflated to a pressure of 40 mmHg measured with a Tycos gauge. There are a number of hazards associated with the use of these devices, including avascular necrosis of the oesophagus if the balloons remain inflated for more than 24–48 hours, laryngeal obstruction if the tube is dislodged and aspiration of saliva. The oesophageal balloon is deflated for five minutes each hour, the pharynx is kept dry by continuous low pressure suction on the pharyngeal lumen and the stomach is aspirated regularly. An alternative means of controlling haemorrhage is to administer vasopressin (20 units diluted in 100 ml 5% dextrose) intravenously over 20 minutes. A maximum of three doses can be given in one hour; if defecation does not occur, the dose is probably inadequate.

Once haemorrhage has been controlled, subsequent management of oesophageal varices usually involves sclerotherapy (e.g. using injections of ethanolamine via a gastroscope). Direct ligation, transection and resuturing of the lower oesophagus, and decompression of the portal system are rarely required, except in those with gastric varices which are difficult to control with sclerotherapy.

Control of ascites can be attempted using diuretics (e.g. frusemide 40 mg combined with amiloride 10 mg daily), although there is a danger of sodium depletion with excessive diuretic administration and, traditionally, rapid mobilization of ascitic fluid is avoided. Nevertheless, when severe ascites is causing respiratory embarrassment, paracentesis of up to 3–5 litres a day can be performed and appears to be safe. It can be accompanied by intravenous administration of albumin solutions. The sodium intake should be restricted to less than 50 mmol day^{-1}, or even 20 mmol day^{-1} in massive ascites. Ultrafiltration or insertion of a Levine shunt may be of value in resistant cases.

Finally, some cases may be suitable for liver transplantation.

FURTHER READING

Murray WR & MacSween RNM (1983) Hepatobiliary disturbances. In Ledingham IMcA & Hanning CD (eds) *Recent Advances in Critical Care Medicine 2*, pp 143–159. Edinburgh: Churchill Livingstone.

Murray-Lyon IM & Trewby PN (1977) Hepatic failure. In Ledingham IMcA (ed.) *Recent Advances in Intensive Therapy 1*, pp 125–144. Edinburgh: Churchill Livingstone.

Trewby PN & Williams R (1978) The management of hepatic failure. In Hanson GC & Wright PL (eds) *Medical Management of the Critically Ill*, pp 99–115. London: Academic Press.

REFERENCES

Bihari D, Gimson AES, Lindridge J & Williams R (1985) Lactic acidosis in fulminant hepatic failure. Some aspects of pathogenesis and prognosis. *Journal of Hepatology* **1**: 405–416.

Black M (1980) Acetaminophen hepatotoxicity. *Gastroenterology* **78**: 382–392.

Bloch P, Delorme, ML, Rapin JR et al (1978) Reversible modifications of brain neurotransmitters of the brain in experimental acute hepatic coma. *Surgery, Gynecology and Obstetrics* **146**: 551–558.

Canalese J, Gimson AES, Davis C et al (1982) Controlled trial of dexamethasone and mannitol for the cerebral oedema of fulminant hepatic failure. *Gut* **23**: 625–629.

Crossley IR, Wardle EN & Williams R (1983) Biochemical mechanisms of hepatic encephalopathy (editorial). *Clinical Science* **64**: 247–252.

Editorial (1984) Hepatic encephalopathy today. *Lancet* **i**: 489–491.

Editorial (1986) Halothane associated liver damage. *Lancet* **i**: 1251–1252.

Gazzard BG, Portmann B, Murray-Lyon IM & Williams R (1975) Causes of death in fulminant hepatic failure and relationship to quantitative histological assessment of parenchymal damage. *Quarterly Journal of Medicine* **44**: 615–626.

Gimson AES & Williams R (1983) Acute hepatic failure: aetiological factors, pathogenic mechanisms and treatment. In Thomas H & MacSween R (eds) *Recent Advances in Hepatology*, Vol. 1, pp 57–69. Edinburgh: Churchill Livingstone.

Gimson AES, Braude S, Mellon J, Canalese J & Williams R (1982) Earlier charcoal haemoperfusion in fulminant hepatic failure. *Lancet* **ii**: 681–683.

Gonzalez-Calvin J, Scully MF, Sanger Y et al (1982) Fibronectin in fulminant hepatic failure. *British Medical Journal* **285**: 1231–1232.

James JH, Ziparo V, Jeppsson B & Fischer JE (1979) Hyperammonaemia, plasma amino acid imbalance and blood–brain amino acid transport: a unified theory of portal systemic encephalopathy. *Lancet* **ii**: 772–775.

Karvountzis GG, Redeker AG & Peters RL (1974) Long-term follow-up studies of patients surviving fulminant viral hepatitis. *Gastroenterology* **67**: 870–877.

MacDougal BRD, Bailey RJ & Williams R (1977) H$_2$ receptor antagonists and antacids in the prevention of acute gastrointestinal haemorrhage in fulminant hepatic failure. *Lancet* **i**: 616–619.

Neuberger J, Gimson AES, Davis M & Williams R (1983) Specific serological markers in the diagnosis of fulminant hepatic failure associated with halothane anaesthesia. *British Journal of Anaesthesia* **55:** 15–19.

Record CO, Iles RA, Cohen RD & Williams R (1975) Acid–base and metabolic disturbances in fulminant hepatic failure. *Gut* **16:** 144–149.

Rosen HM, Yoshimura M, Hodgman JM & Fisher JE (1977) Plasma amino acid patterns in hepatic encephalopathy of differing etiology. *Gastroenterology* **72:** 483–487.

Schafer DF & Jones EA (1982) Hepatic encephalopathy and the γ-aminobutyric acid neurotransmitter system. *Lancet* **i:** 18–20.

Seda HWM, Hughes RD, Gove CD & Williams R (1984) Inhibition of rat brain Na/K ATPase activity by serum from patients with fulminant hepatic failure. *Hepatology* **4:** 74–79.

Sewell RB, Hughes RD, Poston L & Williams R (1982) Effects of serum from patients with fulminant hepatic failure on leucocyte sodium transport. *Clinical Science* **63:** 237–242.

Silk DBA, Hanid, MA, Trewby PN et al (1977) Treatment of fulminant hepatic failure by polyacrylonitrile membrane haemodialysis. *Lancet* **ii:** 1–3.

Trewby PN & Williams R (1977) Pathophysiology of hypotension in patients with fulminant hepatic failure. *Gut* **18:** 1021–1026.

Trewby PN, Warren R, Contini S et al (1978) The incidence and pathophysiology of pulmonary edema in fulminant hepatic failure. *Gastroenterology* **74:** 859–865.

Trey C & Davidson CS (1970) The management of fulminant hepatic failure. In Popper H & Schaffner F (eds) *Progress in Liver Disease*, Vol. 3, pp 282–298. New York: Grune and Stratton.

Walton B, Simpson BR, Strunin L et al (1976) Unexplained hepatitis following halothane. *British Medical Journal* **i:** 1171–1176.

Weston MJ, Talbot IC, Howorth PJN et al (1976) Frequency of arrhythmias and other cardiac abnormalities in fulminant hepatic failure. *British Heart Journal* **38:** 1179–1188.

Wilkinson SP, Portmann B, Hurst D & Williams R (1975) Pathogenesis of renal failure in cirrhosis and fulminant hepatic failure. *Postgraduate Medical Journal* **51:** 503–505.

Williams R & Ede RJ (1981) Hepatitis in pregnancy. *British Medical Journal* **283:** 1074–1075.

Wright R, Eade OE, Chisholm M et al (1975) Controlled prospective study of the effect on liver function of multiple exposures to halothane. *Lancet* **i:** 817–820.

Wyke RJ, Rajkovic IA, Eddleston ALWF & Williams R (1980) Defective opsonisation and complement deficiency in serum from patients with fulminant hepatic failure. *Gut* **21:** 643–649.

Wyke RJ, Yousif-Kadaru AGM, Rajkovic IA, Eddleston ALWF & Williams R (1982a) Serum stimulatory activity and polymorphonuclear leucocyte movement in patients with fulminant hepatic failure. *Clinical and Experimental Immunology* **50:** 442–449.

Wyke RJ, Canalese JC, Gimson AES & Williams R (1982b) Bacteraemia in patients with fulminant hepatic failure. *Liver* **2:** 45–52.

Zieve L, Doizaki WM & Zieve FJ (1974) Synergism between mercaptans and ammonia or fatty acids in the production of coma: a possible role for mercaptans in the pathogenesis of hepatic coma. *Journal of Laboratory and Clinical Medicine* **83:** 16–28.

Zieve L, Shekleton M, Lyftogt C & Draves K (1985) Ammonia, octanoate and a mercaptan depress regeneration of normal rat liver after partial hepatectomy. *Hepatology* **5:** 28–31.

17
Acute Poisoning

More than 100 000 people are admitted to hospital each year in the UK suffering from the effects of acute poisoning and this now accounts for over 10% of all medical admissions. Although only approximately 15% of poisoning victims require intensive observation and supportive care (with or without active treatment), management of such patients may account for up to one-third of admissions to a multidisciplinary intensive care unit.

The vast majority of adult cases of acute poisoning are self-administered, although most of these are manipulative or represent 'a cry for help' rather than a genuine attempt at suicide. Thus, the mean age of patients admitted to hospital with an overdose is approximately 25 years, with a female to male ratio of 1.5:1, whereas the mean age of successful suicides is about 50 years. Other cases of acute poisoning may be accidental (especially in 1–5-year-olds, in which case medicinal, domestic or cosmetic agents are ingested, or related to industrial mishaps), experimental (usually in young adults), part of the syndrome of child abuse or homicidal.

Because the hospital mortality of acute poisoning is less than 1%, active measures to hasten the elimination of the poison (which are associated with a significant morbidity and, in some cases, mortality) can only be recommended in a few exceptional instances; indeed, the 'Scandinavian method' of elective supportive care was originally introduced because of the dangers associated with the use of analeptics in patients in barbiturate coma.

Above all else, therefore, the management of acute poisoning involves the application of the principles of supportive care detailed elsewhere in this book, including maintenance and protection of the airway, respiratory support, expansion of the circulating volume and, occasionally, the judicious use of inotropic agents. Moreover, fluid and electrolyte balance must be maintained, adequate nutritional support should be provided and hypothermia treated or prevented. Skilled nursing care is of paramount importance.

DIAGNOSIS

The quantity and nature of the substances taken must be determined, and in this respect it is important to appreciate that in many instances a mixture of drugs will have been ingested, often including alcohol and a benzodiazepine.

In most cases, a history can be obtained from the patient, although this is frequently misleading and about half will exaggerate or, less often, minimize the severity of poisoning (Wright, 1980). Sometimes patients refuse to divulge any information, while others are incoherent or unconscious. In all cases, therefore, the history should be corroborated by interviewing witnesses, such as relatives, friends and ambulancemen, as well as by contacting the general practitioner when appropriate. Bottles, pills or other substances found on or about the patient may provide important clues as to the nature of the poisoning, although these can also be misleading (e.g. drugs may have been stored in incorrectly labelled bottles). Tablets can often be identified using the *Chemist and Druggist Directory* and in some cases it may be appropriate to send a sample of the substance ingested to the laboratory for analysis. When possible, samples of gastric aspirate, blood and urine should be obtained for laboratory identification of the poisons involved. Assistance is always available from the local poisons information service.

Other important aspects of the initial enquiry include a history of previous psychiatric disorders and self-poisoning episodes, as well as evidence of complicating illnesses, such as liver or renal disease, which might impair the patient's ability to handle poisons. A detailed physical examination should be performed and when indicated body temperature should be recorded with a low reading rectal thermometer. An assessment of the patient's conscious level is particularly important; this should be repeated at regular intervals in order to follow progress and, in some cases, indicate the need for active intervention. A simple clinical grading of conscious levels suitable for use in cases of acute poisoning is shown in Table 17.1.

Table 17.1 Clinical grading of conscious level in acute poisoning.

Grade 0	Fully conscious
Grade I	Drowsy but responsive to verbal commands
Grade II	Unconscious but responding to painful stimuli
Grade III	Unconscious but responding only to maximal painful stimulus
Grade IV	Unconscious, not responding to pain

Baseline determinations of haemoglobin concentration, blood sugar, urea and electrolyte levels should be performed in all cases. Blood gas analysis is also routine and may reveal hypercarbia due to respiratory depression or hypoxaemia related to pulmonary pathology such as infection, atelectasis, aspiration or oedema. A chest x-ray should also be obtained.

MAINTENANCE OF VITAL FUNCTIONS

A number of patients will require immediate endotracheal intubation to secure and protect their airway, while artificial ventilation should be instituted in those with respiratory failure. Blood pressure can usually be restored by expanding the circulating volume, although inotropic support will occasionally be necessary. Convulsions may be related to poisoning with convulsant drugs or cerebral hypoxia and should initially be treated with intravenous diazepam (see Chapter 14, pp. 292–295).

Very few specific antidotes are available and some of these may themselves have toxic effects; consequently, they are rarely indicated. Analeptics must never be used.

PREVENTION OF FURTHER ABSORPTION OF POISON

Gastric aspiration and lavage

When performed in seriously poisoned patients, gastric aspiration and lavage is associated with a considerable risk of complications, such as pulmonary aspiration, seizures, dysrhythmias and perforation of the stomach. It should therefore only be undertaken by experienced personnel, with the facilities available to treat any complications, and then only if potentially dangerous amounts of a toxic substance have been ingested within six hours of admission. This time limit can be extended up to 12 hours in cases of poisoning with agents which delay gastric emptying, such as salicylates and tricyclic antidepressants.

Gastric aspiration and lavage is effective for the majority of solid poisons, but it is debatable whether it should be performed when corrosive substances have been taken. Aspiration of kerosene, or its derivatives, can produce a particularly destructive form of lipoid pneumonia and the technique should be avoided in such cases.

Procedure

Gastric aspiration and lavage should only be performed if the patient has an adequate cough reflex or has an endotracheal tube in place with the cuff inflated. The use of an intravenous anaesthetic agent and muscle relaxation to allow endotracheal intubation of a semi-comatose patient is only justified when gastric lavage is clearly indicated; in the majority of cases, it is not. The patient should be positioned head down, lying on the left side. Facilities for pharyngeal suction must be immediately available. Foreign matter should be removed from the mouth and pharynx before introducing a wide-bore tube into the mouth which the patient is then persuaded to swallow (a large tube is less likely to enter the trachea and allows aspiration of particulate matter). The stomach contents are then aspirated and retained for analysis, following which lavage is performed with 250 ml warmed tap water. This procedure is repeated until the aspirate is clear of debris. Some authorities suggest that activated charcoal should be introduced in order to adsorb any residual poison in the stomach or upper intestine, but there is no evidence that this practice is beneficial. On the other hand, gastric instillation of Fuller's earth in paraquat poisoning and of desferrioxamine in iron poisoning are generally accepted measures (see below). Subsequently, the wide-bore tube is replaced by a Ryle's tube which is aspirated hourly.

In children, induction of vomiting with ipecacuanha is occasionally of value but this practice is contraindicated in poisoning with corrosives, petroleum products or antiemetics. Ipecacuanha paediatric emetic draught BP is administered in a dose of 10 ml in those 6–18 months old and 15 ml in those between 18 months and 5 years old, followed by 200 ml water. This dose can be repeated once only if vomiting does not occur after 20–25 minutes. Apomorphine should be avoided since it may induce protracted vomiting.

When the skin or eyes have been contaminated (often the result of an industrial accident) copious irrigation should be performed.

ACCELERATED ELIMINATION OF POISON

Active measures to increase the elimination of a poison are only indicated if the patient is seriously ill and deteriorating, if significant amounts of the poison can be removed and if this is likely to produce worthwhile improvement.

Forced diuresis

This is based on the principle that an increase in urine volume will reduce the concentration difference between renal tubular and interstitial fluid, thereby minimizing reabsorption of the poison or its active metabolite(s). The technique is therefore only applicable to cases of poisoning in which either the drug itself or its active metabolites are excreted in the urine in significant amounts. Urinary excretion can be further enhanced by altering the pH of the urine in order to increase the degree of ionization of the substance and reduce its lipid solubility. Thus, in the case of weak acids (e.g. salicylates) the urine should be rendered alkaline, while for weak bases an acidic urine is required. Forced acid diuresis is very rarely indicated but may be considered in severe chlorpromazine poisoning. Suitable regimens are shown in Table 17.2.

Table 17.2 Forced diuresis regimens.

Alkaline diuresis

500 ml sodium bicarbonate 1.26% or 1.4%
1 litre 5% dextrose
500 ml normal saline + potassium chloride 20 mmol

This regimen should be administered for three successive hours.

(Some authorities recommend that this regimen should be repeated until the patient regains consciousness or, in salicylate overdose, the blood level is reduced to less than $60 \, mg \, 100 \, ml^{-1}$.)

Acid diuresis

500 ml 5% dextrose + 1.5 g ammonium chloride
500 ml 5% dextrose
500 ml normal saline

This regimen should be administered at a rate of $1 \, l \, h^{-1}$ and repeated four times over a four-hour period.

Forced diuresis is associated with a considerable risk of fluid overload and pulmonary oedema, especially in the elderly and those with renal impairment or heart disease. Electrolyte disturbances may also occur. It is therefore essential to ensure that a diuresis ensues and to monitor plasma and urinary electrolytes, as well as urine pH. The technique is probably best avoided in those at risk of fluid overload, but if it is considered essential, the volumes infused should be reduced appropriately. The use of mannitol is particularly liable to produce electrolyte disturbances, while acetazolamide can precipitate a metabolic acidosis and frusemide may compete for tubular secretion of salicylic acid. These diuretics should therefore be avoided, although frusemide may be required to treat pulmonary oedema.

Haemodialysis, peritoneal dialysis and haemoperfusion

The value of these procedures is dubious. Theoretically, haemoperfusion will remove large amounts of both short- and long-acting barbiturates, but will not significantly influence the elimination of tricyclic antidepressants since, although adsorbed on to charcoal, they are distributed throughout the body water and in fat stores. Similarly, haemoperfusion will remove only small quantities of dangerous cytoplasmic poisons such as paraquat or paracetamol. On the other hand, haemoperfusion might be of value in patients poisoned with sedative drugs such as barbiturates or meprobamate who are in grade IV coma and deteriorating. The technique is, however, relatively complex and associated with a significant risk of complications (see Chapter 16). Moreover, the mortality of poisoning with these agents is virtually nil with aggressive supportive care.

Peritoneal or haemodialysis may be considered in those with renal failure or refractory acid–base disturbances. It is occasionally indicated when a patient is deteriorating despite adequate supportive care as a result of poisoning with a dialysable substance.

Exchange transfusion

This technique may very occasionally be useful in life-threatening poisoning due to toxins with a high plasma distribution (e.g. phosphorus and methanol).

MANAGEMENT OF SPECIFIC POISONS

Barbiturates

There has been a considerable reduction in the availability of these drugs, which should now only be prescribed as anticonvulsants. Although this has resulted in a marked decrease in the incidence of barbiturate overdose, this remains a relatively common cause of death from poisoning in the UK.

Barbiturate overdose produces generalized depression of the central nervous system. The conscious level is reduced and this may progress to deep coma with flaccidity and hyporeflexia. The corneal reflex is often absent. The pupillary response to light is sluggish or absent and conjugate eye movement is lost. Unequal pupils suggest hypoxic cerebral damage and this possibility is supported by the presence of other focal neurological signs, which may sometimes be accompanied by seizures.

Profound cardiovascular depression may occur and is caused by a reduction in central vasomotor activity, a decrease in arteriolar tone and myocardial depression. Cardiac output and blood pressure are low, while central venous pressure may be high (in those with myocardial failure) or low (in the presence of relative hypovolaemia). A metabolic acidosis may occur.

Respiratory depression causes hypoventilation with hypercarbia and hypoxaemia. The latter may be exacerbated by an increased capillary permeability leading to the development of ARDS (see Chapter 12) and/or ventilation/perfusion mismatch (Sutherland et al, 1977).

The reduction in muscle tone, combined with cardiovascular depression, causes vascular stasis and tissue hypoxia. Ischaemic muscle damage may be associated with increased circulating levels of creatine kinase, a raised erythrocyte sedimentation rate and a rise in body temperature. The latter is often delayed for up to 72 hours after the overdose. In the long term, this syndrome may be followed by muscle calcification. Local hypoxia may also be responsible for the development of skin blisters, which are seen in approximately 5% of patients with barbiturate poisoning. Although these blisters often develop over pressure areas, they are not necessarily related to trauma and may occasionally occur following even a relatively trivial overdose.

Gastrointestinal motility is often depressed. It is thought that the fluctuations in conscious level which sometimes occur in barbiturate poisoning are due to the intermittent recovery of intestinal function leading to further absorption of the drug.

Hypothermia is a common complication of barbiturate overdose and is a result of impaired hypothalamic function, the reduction in muscle tone and vascular dilatation.

The vast majority of those who reach hospital alive will survive with aggressive supportive care, provided they have not suffered irreversible cerebral damage. Central venous pressure monitoring, and in some cases insertion of a Swan–Ganz catheter, is required in all seriously poisoned patients in order to guide intravenous volume replacement. Hypothermia must be prevented or treated (see Chapter 11).

Because prolonged coma may be complicated by pneumonia, some authorities recommend charcoal or resin haemoperfusion in those who are deeply unconscious, and failing to improve, following a massive overdose of a long-acting barbiturate. However, this technique is most effective for medium- and short-acting agents and its value in the management of poisoning is disputed (Lorch and Garella, 1979). The possible benefits of a reduction in the duration of coma must be offset against the complications of the technique and it should be remembered that many patients will have taken a variety of poisonous substances.

Tricyclic antidepressants

These drugs are extensively prescribed for an 'at risk' population of depressed patients. Furthermore, improvement in mood is often delayed for up to two weeks after the start of treatment. Consequently, acute poisoning with tricyclics is common and the incidence is increasing.

The features of tricyclic overdose are due to a mixture of central excitation and depression, combined with anticholinergic effects. Although the conscious level may be decreased, coma is rare. Both pyramidal and extrapyramidal disturbances may occur and convulsions are common. Some patients hallucinate, and rapid, distorted speech is characteristic. Respiration is frequently depressed. Anticholinergic effects are manifested as widely dilated pupils, dry mouth, absent sweating, urine retention and paralytic ileus. The combination of central depression and an inability to sweat impairs temperature regulation and may lead to hyperthermia. Examination may reveal hyperreflexia and extensor plantar responses. The diagnosis can be confirmed by detecting the drug in the urine.

The cardiovascular effects of tricyclic antidepressants are complex. Sinus tachycardia is common and both hyper- and hypotension may occur. Electrocardiographic changes include a dose-related prolongation of the Q–T interval, widening of the QRS complex, AV block, bundle-branch block, and intraventricular conduction disturbances. A few patients develop dangerous ventricular dysrhythmias and in one case death occurred five days after the overdose (Masters, 1967). On the other hand, a review of 72 consecutive cases of tricyclic overdose suggested that late unexpected complications are very rare and a two-day period of intensive observation is probably sufficient (Stern et al, 1985).

Because stomach emptying may be delayed following an overdose of tricyclics, gastric aspiration and lavage may be worth while up to 12 hours after ingestion. Active measures to hasten elimination of tricyclics are, however, ineffective because these drugs are highly lipid-soluble, strongly protein-bound and only small amounts are excreted in the urine.

Management is therefore supportive. The ECG should be monitored continuously for 48–72 hours following a serious overdose. If ventricular dysrhythmias do occur, they may be resistant to conventional treatment, although some claim that they have experienced no difficulty in defibrillating such patients and that the subsequent infusion of lignocaine successfully prevents recurrence. A prophylactic intravenous infusion of lignocaine is also recommended for those with ventricular ectopics. Phenytoin may be useful since it can control both the ventricular dysrhythmias and any accompanying convulsions. Although it would seem logical to administer an anticholinesterase such as physostigmine, this is unwise in the acute phase since such treatment may precipitate seizures, bradycardia and cardiac failure. Similarly, administration of a β-blocker may cause extreme bradycardia and even asystole.

A few patients may be hypotensive in the absence of dysrhythmias, but expansion of the circulating volume will usually restore the blood pressure. Inotropes should be avoided because of the danger of precipitating dysrhythmias.

Extrapyramidal symptoms can be controlled with benztropine 1–2 mg i.m. or i.v., while the agitation and convulsions which may occur during the recovery phase are best treated with intravenous diazepam.

Paracetamol

The incidence of poisoning with paracetamol has gradually increased over the last 20 years and this is now one of the commonest causes of FHF (see Chapter 16).

Patients who have taken a paracetamol overdose normally remain fully conscious. Clinical features may include pallor, perspiration, epigastric pain, nausea and vomiting. Occasionally, a massive paracetamol overdose may directly damage the myocardium and cause peripheral vasodilatation with shock. Metabolic acidosis may be severe. Erythema, urticaria and mucosal lesions are quite common and, if skin lesions are extensive, hyperthermia may develop. Hyperglycaemia may occur a few days after ingestion. Acute haemolytic anaemia may develop and produce acute renal failure.

These symptoms are not, however, a reliable indication of the severity of poisoning and there is a wide individual variability in tolerance to paracetamol, as well as susceptibility to hepatotoxicity.

In general, serious toxicity can be anticipated if an adult has taken more than 20 500 mg tablets, and if more than 15 g have been ingested (i.e. 30 × 500 mg tablets) an antidote should be given immediately. Plasma levels should always be determined in order to assess the severity of poisoning and, when related to the time since ingestion, they correlate closely with the subsequent risk of liver damage. Thus, in the absence of treatment, a level of more than $250 \mu g \, ml^{-1}$ at four hours, or more than $100 \mu g \, ml^{-1}$ at 12 hours, is usually hepatotoxic (Prescott et al, 1976) (Fig. 17.1), while a level less than $100 \mu g \, ml^{-1}$ at four hours excludes the risk of liver damage.

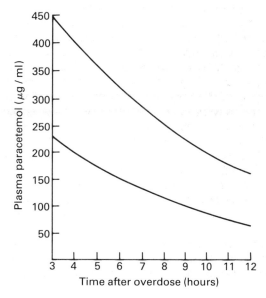

Fig. 17.1 Plasma paracetamol concentrations related to time since ingestion. From Prescott et al (1976), with permission.

Paracetamol hepatotoxicity is due to a toxic metabolite (formed via an oxidative pathway dependent on cytochrome P450) which is normally scavenged by intracellular glutathione. Following an overdose, this mechanism may be overwhelmed and the highly reactive metabolite combines with sulphydryl groups of liver cell proteins, producing a centrilobular necrosis. Preventive treatment is based on the principle that by providing an alternative supply of sulphydryl groups, unstable precursors can be displaced from either glutathione or liver cell protein. A variety of agents have been recommended, including cysteamine, methionine and N-acetylcysteine. Cysteamine (2 g i.v. over 10 min, followed by 3 further 400 mg doses) is effective if given within 12 hours of ingestion but can cause cutaneous vasodilatation, nausea, vomiting and drowsiness which may last for up to 48 hours. The side effects of oral methionine are similar to those associated with cysteamine; N-acetylcysteine, which is equally effective but less toxic, is now the treatment of choice. This agent should be given in a dose of 150 mg kg^{-1} i.v. over 15 minutes, followed by 50 mg kg^{-1} in 500 ml 5% dextrose over 4 hours and then 100 mg kg^{-1} in 5% dextrose over 16 hours.

When liver damage does occur, the signs of hepatic failure are not usually apparent until 48 hours after the overdose. At this time, the patient may become jaundiced with an enlarged and tender liver. Liver function tests are most abnormal 3–5 days after ingestion. In severe but non-fatal hepatotoxicity a cholestatic picture is usually seen and, in the most serious cases, FHF develops about 3–7 days after ingestion.

Salicylates

The increased use of paracetamol as a mild analgesic has resulted in some reduction in the incidence of salicylate poisoning. Nevertheless, it remains a relatively common cause of poisoning in children.

Aspirin uncouples oxidative phosphorylation, leading to increased metabolism of glucose and fats with a rise in oxygen consumption and carbon dioxide production. The respiratory centre is stimulated both directly and by the increased carbon dioxide production, thereby producing respiratory alkalosis. If salicylate levels are very high, however, respiratory depression may supervene, and respiratory acidosis may occur as a terminal event. Blood levels of pyruvate, lactate and ketone bodies are increased and this, combined with the fact that aspirin is itself an organic acid, produces a metabolic acidosis. In children, although there is also a respiratory alkalosis initially, a metabolic acidosis develops more rapidly and usually becomes the dominant abnormality. Hypoglycaemia may be particularly severe in children. Some patients develop an encephalopathy and hyperthermia.

The majority of patients present within six hours of ingestion and are conscious, alert and orientated, although some are restless and confused. Coma is rare and, in an adult, drowsiness indicates severe poisoning. Confusion and drowsiness are more frequently seen in children. Other clinical features include sweating, tinnitus, deafness, blurred vision and hyperventilation. Less commonly, patients poisoned with aspirin have epigastric pain and vomiting with severe dehydration and oliguria. Occasionally, they may develop acute renal failure. Gastrointestinal bleeding is uncommon but may be related to gastric erosions and a coagulopathy. The latter is usually due to hypoprothrombinaemia, which can be corrected with fresh frozen plasma and vitamin K, but may be due to thrombocytopenia or impaired platelet function. In some cases, pulmonary oedema develops in association with an increase in capillary permeability, proteinuria and hypoproteinaemia. These patients may also be hypotensive and hypovolaemic; cautious administration of colloidal solutions has been recommended (Hormaechea et al, 1979).

The diagnosis should be confirmed, and the severity of poisoning assessed, by measuring plasma salicylate levels. This should be related to the time of ingestion, bearing in mind that absorption of aspirin continues for some time and peak levels may not be attained for up to eight hours. Thus, a level of 300 mg l^{-1} may be significant 12 hours after ingestion, but is almost within the therapeutic range at 4–6 hours. Active treatment should be considered if the level is more than 500 mg l^{-1} within 12 hours of ingestion, and if it is over 300 mg l^{-1} beyond this time. In children, measures to hasten elimination are indicated when the level is more than 300 mg l^{-1} at 12 hours. Respiratory depression is a common mode of death when the plasma salicylate level exceeds 1000 mg l^{-1}.

Gastric aspiration and lavage should be performed regardless of the time elapsed since ingestion. When active treatment is indicated, this should be instituted immediately, since death can occur suddenly and unexpectedly. The excretion of salicylates can be enhanced by forced alkaline diuresis (see Table 17.2), which will also replace water and electrolyte losses and help to maintain blood sugar levels if 5% dextrose is used. If the patient has a marked metabolic acidosis this should be corrected before instituting the alkaline diuresis. In those with renal failure or pulmonary oedema, charcoal haemoperfusion or dialysis has been recommended, but in practice these are rarely necessary.

Opiates

Opiate poisoning is usually encountered in drug abusers who have taken an overdose, either intentionally or accidentally. Occasionally, iatrogenic cases require admission to intensive care. Self-poisoning with distalgesics is now relatively common and this drug contains dextropropoxyphene, which has opiate-like effects, as well as paracetamol (see above). There appears to be a synergism between distalgesic and alcohol, which can cause disproportionate fatal respiratory depression of sudden onset and many victims fail to reach hospital alive (Carson and Carson, 1977).

The triad of coma, respiratory depression (infrequent, deep respirations) and pinpoint pupils (which are equal and reactive) is virtually diagnostic of opiate poisoning. Cardiovascular depression also occurs. Physical examination may reveal evidence of addiction, such as venepuncture scars, or the complications of intravenous drug abuse, such as hepatitis and septicaemia.

Coma and respiratory depression can be reversed by intravenous naloxone 0.1–0.8 mg i.v. or i.m. (in children 0.005–0.01 mg kg^{-1}). Because the half-life of naloxone is short (opiate reversal persists for only 15–30 min), repeated doses or an infusion are usually required. Naloxone can precipitate an acute withdrawal syndrome in addicts and may cause laryngeal spasm. Moreover, a number of adverse reactions to naloxone have been described, including ventricular fibrillation, hypertension and pulmonary oedema. These are presumably related to disinhibition of the sympathetic nervous system. Caution is therefore required in those with known cardiovascular disease.

Benzodiazepines

These agents probably act by occupying specific receptor sites, thereby enhancing the effects of GABA, an inhibitory neurotransmitter. When taken alone, benzodiazepines can produce drowsiness, dizziness, ataxia and slurred speech. More serious manifestations of overdose, such as coma or hypotension, are rarely seen and there are no authenticated deaths due to isolated benzodiazepine poisoning. However, many cases of self-poisoning involve ingestion of a number of drugs and benzodiazepines are included in as many as 40% of overdoses in Britain. Under these circumstances additive effects may aggravate, or precipitate, respiratory failure and hypotension.

Benzodiazepines are absorbed relatively slowly from the gastrointestinal tract and elimination of their active metabolites, as well as the parent compound, may take several days. In general, less than 5% of the ingested dose is recovered unchanged in the urine. Hospital stay may therefore be prolonged and the performance of skilled tasks, e.g. driving a car or operating machinery, can be impaired for weeks after apparent recovery from benzodiazepine poisoning.

In general, management of benzodiazepine poisoning involves supportive care only. However, benzodiazepine agonist–antagonist agents are now available which can effectively reverse coma in such cases (Ashton, 1985) and these may occasionally prove useful. Following isolated benzodiazepine overdose, they may speed recovery, reduce after-effects and shorten hospital stay, while in multiple self-poisoning they may reverse respiratory depression and facilitate diagnosis. Because they have a relatively short half-life (antagonist effects last 3–5 hours), repeated administration is usually required. Moreover, there is a danger of precipitating withdrawal symptoms. Convulsions may be produced in epileptics and in the presence of convulsant agents such as tricyclic antidepressants.

Paraquat (Editorial, 1976)

Paraquat is a herbicide which is available commercially as a 20% solution (Gramoxone) and to the general public in the form of solid granules containing 5% paraquat and diquat (Weedol, Pathclear). Although measures instituted by the manufacturers have reduced the incidence of accidental poisoning with paraquat, this has been largely offset by an increase in the number of cases of deliberate overdose.

Paraquat is a strong corrosive which will burn the skin, tongue, mouth and oesophagus. This may not be apparent until 24–48 hours after ingestion when large white necrotic areas develop; these are often painless. If paraquat contaminates the eyes it will cause extreme irritation with ulceration of the conjunctivae and cornea. Sweating, nausea and repeated vomiting are usual and in some cases the vomitus will contain gastric and oesophageal epithelia. Tremor and convulsions may occur.

Ingestion of large amounts of paraquat may be associated with encephalopathy, myocarditis, liver damage, renal failure and haemorrhagic pulmonary oedema. In such cases death usually occurs within 72 hours. When poisoning is less severe, evidence of myocardial, liver and renal dysfunction may be delayed for several days. However, paraquat can accumulate progressively in the lungs by an energy-dependent process (Rose et al, 1974) even when plasma concentrations are relatively low. Subsequently, the alveolar epithelial lining is destroyed and this is followed by progressive fibrosis culminating in hypoxaemic respiratory failure. Although this lung lesion may take two to three weeks to develop, it is irreversible and death is inevitable.

The diagnosis of paraquat poisoning can be confirmed by examining the urine. Moreover, there is a good correlation between blood levels and the severity of poisoning. An oral dose of approximately 2–3 g is likely to be fatal if untreated and although as many as 90% of those who ingest Weedol survive, the mortality from poisoning with the concentrated solution is approximately 90%.

Gastric aspiration and lavage should be performed, followed by oral administration of Fuller's earth, 250 ml of a 30% suspension with magnesium sulphate 5%. This should be repeated four-hourly. Fuller's earth is unpleasant to take and may have to be given via a nasogastric tube. These measures should be followed by aggressive supportive care since the hepatic lesion, renal failure and pulmonary oedema are all potentially reversible. Unduly high concentrations of oxygen should be avoided since this may accentuate the lung damage.

Cholinesterase inhibitors (organophosphorus compounds and carbamate insecticides)

Most of the organophosphorus compounds are highly lipid-soluble and are therefore well absorbed via all routes, including the skin. They also form very stable links with acetylcholinesterase; recovery of anticholinergic activity is therefore delayed until sufficient quantities of enzyme have been manufactured. This may take days or even months. Carbamates, on the other hand, undergo spontaneous degradation and symptoms of poisoning with these substances last only 6–8 hours.

Poisoning with cholinesterase inhibitors causes an increase in postganglionic parasympathetic nervous activity, muscle fasciculation followed by paralysis and central nervous stimulation followed by depression. There is anorexia, vomiting, abdominal colic and diarrhoea. The patient is restless with constricted pupils; coma and convulsions may occur. Later, respiratory depression supervenes with paralysis of respiratory muscles, laryngobronchospasm, increased tracheobronchial secretions and excessive salivation. Cardiovascular manifestations include bradycardia and hypotension.

Immediate management must include measures to prevent further exposure to the poison, including the removal of contaminated clothing and thorough washing (initially with soap and water and then with ethanol). Those poisoned with an organophosphorus compound should receive pralidoxime (5 ml of a 20% solution) in order to break down the organophosphorus/cholinesterase complex. This is not necessary in the case of carbamate poisoning. Atropine should be administered in large doses for 2–3 days. Otherwise, treatment is supportive and may include mechanical ventilation.

Alcohol

Ethanol poisoning is usually simply related to overindulgence. In large quantities, ethanol can produce a deep, but shortlived, coma which may be complicated by hypothermia and, in a few cases, hypoglycaemia. Children may develop severe hypoglycaemia and a metabolic acidosis. The fatal dose is difficult to determine but it is thought that in adults the equivalent of 600 ml pure ethanol consumed in less than one hour can be lethal.

Treatment consists of gastric aspiration and lavage and, in severe cases, 200 g of fructose 40% infused over 30 minutes to correct hypoglycaemia and increase the rate of fall in blood alcohol levels. Some recommend naloxone administration to lighten coma.

Acute methanol poisoning occurs most frequently in vagrants, although cases of accidental ingestion are occasionally encountered. Methanol is a constituent of antifreeze, paint removers and varnish and is produced in some home-made beverages. Methylated spirit, however, is composed largely of ethanol with only 5% methanol. Methanol is metabolized to formic acid and formaldehyde, both of which are extremely toxic. The central effects of acute methanol intoxication may be delayed for 12–36 hours after ingestion at which time nausea, vomiting, abdominal pain, headache and ataxia can occur and may progress to coma. Often, there is a profound metabolic acidosis with Kussmaul respiration. If poisoning is severe (blood methanol $> 500 \, \text{mg} \, \text{l}^{-1}$, marked acidosis), the patient may develop an acute optic nerve papillitis with blurring of vision which can progress to blindness, dilatation of the pupils and papilloedema.

Gastric aspiration and lavage should be performed if the patient is seen within four hours of ingestion and the metabolic acidosis should be corrected. Because ethanol competes with methanol for the enzyme alcohol dehydrogenase, administration of the former (loading-dose of $0.6 \, \text{mg} \, \text{kg}^{-1}$ followed by an infusion at $66 \, \text{mg} \, \text{kg}^{-1} \, \text{h}^{-1}$) can limit the production of formic acid. Haemodialysis has been recommended if the patient fails to respond to these measures and has visual impairment, a severe metabolic acidosis or a blood methanol level greater than $1 \, \text{g} \, \text{l}^{-1}$. There is no evidence, however, that dialysis is more effective than standard measures.

Cyanide

Cyanides are used industrially in electroplating, and to clean or harden metals, as well as in some chemical laboratories. Most cases of poisoning encountered in clinical practice are caused by ingestion or inhalation of sodium or potassium cyanide; free hydrocyanic acid (prussic acid) is almost instantaneously fatal if taken orally. The effects of inhaled prussic acid depend on the concentration of the vapour. The direct-acting vasodilator sodium nitroprusside is a complex cyanide which releases free hydrogen cyanide in vivo and may produce related toxic effects when a gross overdose has been administered (see Chapter 10).

Cyanide produces its toxic effects by reacting with cytochrome oxidase, thereby inhibiting the final steps in oxidative phosphorylation. If large quantities (1–2 g) are ingested, there is a rapid loss of consciousness, followed by convulsions and death. Lesser amounts produce drowsiness, dizziness, breathlessness, confusion, nausea, vomiting and shock. Coma and death may follow. Severe lactic acidosis and a reduced $P_{a-v}O_2$ are characteristic.

When a patient is known to have ingested or inhaled cyanide, immediate treatment is imperative. A heparinized blood sample should be obtained for blood gas analysis and cyanide assay. General supportive measures, including the administration of oxygen in high concentrations, should be instituted and a specific antidote given. Following massive exposure to cyanide, for example, related to an industrial accident, intravenous dicobalt edetate (CoEDTA) (300–600 mg over 1 min, followed by a further 300 mg if the patient fails to improve) is the ideal antidote since it has a rapid action and, although it is itself toxic, in the presence of HCN it forms a stable non-toxic complex. However, if the patient remains conscious some hours after assumed exposure to cyanide, CoEDTA should not be given since, in the absence of HCN, it is likely to produce an anaphylactic reaction, sometimes with severe laryngeal oedema. It may also precipitate atrial fibrillation, hypocalcaemia and hypomagnesaemia. Because CoEDTA can cause hypoglycaemia, it should be given in dextrose. Thus, when some time has elapsed between ingestion and arrival in hospital, or when there is doubt as to the nature of the poisoning, thiosulphate is the antidote of choice.

Some consider that the administration of a nitrite (e.g. amyl nitrite or sodium nitrite), is a useful adjunct to thiosulphate in acute cyanide poisoning. These agents act by converting haemoglobin to methaemoglobin, the ferric iron of which then combines with HCN. Sodium nitrite (3%) should be given intravenously in divided 10 ml doses in order to convert approximately 25% of the haemoglobin to methaemoglobin and is more effective than amyl nitrite. However, this clearly reduces the amount of haemoglobin available for oxygen transport, and this is a particular hazard in children. Moreover, nitrites can precipitate or exacerbate hypotension.

Iron

Iron tablets are most frequently prescribed to young women and they, or their children, therefore constitute the majority of cases of poisoning.

Initially, most are asymptomatic, although a few develop an acute gastritis with abdominal pain, nausea, vomiting and haematemesis. Some complain of a metallic taste. Those who are seriously poisoned become hypovolaemic and shocked 6–12 hours after ingestion. Convulsions, coma, hepatic necrosis and a metabolic acidosis may supervene approximately 24 hours later.

Iron is slowly absorbed. Gastric aspiration and lavage should be performed and 10 g of desferrioxamine, which chelates iron, instilled into the stomach. The severity of poisoning can be assessed by measuring the serum iron level and, if this is more than twice the upper normal limit, 1–2 g of desferrioxamine should be administered intramuscularly and repeated 12 hours later. If the patient is shocked, this agent should be given intravenously ($15 \, \text{mg} \, \text{kg}^{-1} \, \text{h}^{-1}$ up to a total dose of $80 \, \text{mg} \, \text{kg}^{-1}$ in 24 hours).

β-Blocking drugs

These are extensively prescribed and readily available; poisoning with β-blockers is therefore relatively common.

Manifestations of profound β-blockade include lassitude, drowsiness, bradycardia and hypotension. Peripheral vasospasm and Raynaud's phenomenon may occur. Bronchospasm may be precipitated, particularly in those with asthma or COAD.

Gastric aspiration and lavage should be performed if the patient is seen within four hours of ingestion. Intravenous atropine 1–2 mg and an isoprenaline infusion can be given in an attempt to counteract the bradycardia, although the latter is inefficient and very large doses may be required. Some recommend dopamine or dobutamine as alternatives to isoprenaline. Ideally, cardiac pacing should be instituted in those with extreme bradycardia. Glucagon is of unproven value, although its mechanism of action is thought not to involve the β-adrenoreceptor. Severe bronchospasm should be treated with salbutamol.

Phenothiazines

Although these major tranquillizers are often prescribed for the 'at risk' population of patients with psychotic illnesses, they are a relatively uncommon cause of self-poisoning.

Following an overdose, the patient becomes drowsy or comatose and hypotensive with a tachycardia. Dysrhythmias may occur and the ECG may show prolongation of the Q–T interval and flattening of the T waves. Impaired hypothalamic function, combined with cardiovascular depression, makes the patient susceptible to hypothermia. Extrapyramidal disturbances, such as oculogyric crises, may also occur.

Methods to speed elimination are ineffective and treatment is therefore supportive. Extrapyramidal disturbances can be treated with repeated intravenous administration of benztropine mesylate 2 mg, while dysrhythmias may respond to physostigmine. If hypotension requires specific treatment, an α-stimulant should be used.

Amphetamines

Amphetamines are now prescribed rarely and episodes of poisoning are therefore usually related to illicit use of these drugs.

In overdose, amphetamines produce confusion, anxiety, restlessness, tremor and irritability. The patient may be hyperreflexic with dilated pupils. An initial pallor is followed by flushing, tachycardia and dysrhythmias.

Treatment is supportive and includes sedation with a benzodiazepine or, if this fails, a phenothiazine. Although elimination of amphetamines can be enhanced by using a forced acid diuresis, this is rarely necessary.

Corrosives

Acids and alkalis are used for cleaning, both domestically and industrially, as well as being involved in chemical manufacturing processes.

When swallowed, they can cause extensive burns of the mouth, tongue, pharynx, oesophagus and stomach. These are extremely painful and may cause perforation of the oesophagus or stomach. Oedema of the epiglottis and larynx can produce severe upper airway obstruction necessitating endotracheal intubation. Systemic absorption produces profound acid–base disturbances and shock. Delayed deaths may be associated with necrosis and superimposed infection. Long-term complications in survivors include gastrointestinal scarring and stenosis.

Phenolic compounds are commonly found in antiseptics, disinfectants and preservatives. If swallowed, they cause blanching or erythema around the mouth and chin followed by intense thirst, nausea, vomiting, diarrhoea and sweating. Those who are severely poisoned may develop abdominal pain, convulsions and coma. Acute renal failure is common and hepatic damage may occur.

Gastric lavage should probably be avoided because of the risk of aspiration, although some recommend this procedure as a means of diluting the corrosive. Surgical intervention is required if there are signs of perforation. Otherwise, treatment is supportive and may include total parenteral nutrition.

Carbon monoxide

Since carbon monoxide (CO) is no longer a constituent of domestic gas, the commonest sources of poisoning are motor vehicle exhaust fumes and incomplete combustion of natural gas.

The affinity of CO for haemoglobin is some 300 times greater than that of oxygen, which it therefore displaces. It also shifts the oxyhaemoglobin dissociation curve to the left. The net effect is tissue hypoxaemia, which in many cases is fatal. Manifestations of less severe poisoning include headaches, dizziness, hyperventilation, confusion, disorientation and, in some cases, coma. Nausea, vomiting and faecal incontinence may also occur. Later, pulmonary oedema and respiratory depression may supervene, while extreme hypoxia may produce cerebral oedema, hyperpyrexia and myocardial infarction.

The pink discoloration of the skin caused by the presence of large amounts of COHb is in practice uncommon, except in particularly severe poisoning. Cyanosis and skin pallor is more usual. Skin blisters may occur as a result of tissue hypoxia.

Treatment with high concentrations of oxygen, and IPPV if indicated, should be instituted immediately. The diagnosis may subsequently be confirmed and progress monitored by estimating the percentage of COHb present in the blood. A few recommend hyperbaric oxygen.

Amanita phalloides (death cap) (Editorial, 1972)

Over 90% of those who die as a result of fungal poisoning have eaten *Amanita phalloides*.

This fungus contains two toxins. The phallotoxins (heptapeptides) produce violent nausea, vomiting and diarrhoea within a few hours, while the amatoxins (octapeptides) cause a fatal hepatorenal syndrome.

There is no specific antidote, although it has been suggested that haemodialysis can be effective. Penicillin, chloramphenicol or phenylbutazone may be useful because they displace α-amanitin (the principal amatoxin) from plasma binding sites.

REFERENCES

Ashton CH (1985) Benzodiazepine overdose: are specific antagonists useful? *British Medical Journal* **290:** 805–806.

Carson DJL & Carson ED (1977) Fatal dextropropoxyphene poisoning in Northern Ireland. Review of 30 cases. *Lancet* **i:** 894–897.

Editorial (1972) Death cap poisoning. *Lancet* **i:** 1320–1321.

Editorial (1976) Paraquat poisoning. *Lancet* **i:** 1057.

Hormaechea E, Carlson RW, Rogove H et al (1979) Hypovolemia, pulmonary edema and protein changes in severe salicylate poisoning. *American Journal of Medicine* **66:** 1046–1050.

Lorch JA & Garella S (1979) Hemoperfusion to treat intoxications. *Annals of Internal Medicine* **91:** 301–304.

Masters AB (1967) Delayed death in imipramine poisoning. *British Medical Journal* **iii:** 866–867.

Prescott LF, Park J, Sutherland GR, Smith IJ & Proudfoot AT (1976) Cysteamine, methionine and penicillamine in the treatment of paracetamol poisoning. *Lancet* **ii:** 109–113.

Stern TA, O'Gara PT, Mulley AG, Singer DE & Thibault GE (1985) Complications after overdose with tricyclic antidepressants. *Critical Care Medicine* **13:** 672–674.

Rose MS, Smith LL & Wyatt I (1974) Evidence for energy dependent accumulation of paraquat into rat lung. *Nature* **252:** 314–315.

Sutherland GR, Park J & Proudfoot AT (1977) Ventilation and acid base changes in deep coma due to barbiturate or tricyclic antidepressant poisoning. *Clinical Toxicology* **11:** 403–412.

Wright N (1980) An assessment of the unreliability of the history given by self-poisoned patients. *Clinical Toxicology* **16:** 381–384.

Index